Brian Gray

Fundamentals of Tooth Preparations

for Cast Metal and Porcelain Restorations

Herbert T. Shillingburg, Jr., D.D.S., F.A.C.D.
David Ross Boyd Professor and Chairman

Richard Jacobi, D.D.S.
Associate Professor

Susan E. Brackett, D.D.S.
Assistant Professor

Department of Fixed Prosthodontics
University of Oklahoma College of Dentistry
Oklahoma City, Oklahoma

**Winner, 1988 Book Awards Competition
American Medical Writers Association**

Quintessence Publishing Co
Chicago, London, Berlin, São Paulo, Tokyo, and Hong Kong

Library of Congress Cataloging-in-Publication Data

Shillingburg, Herbert T.
    Fundamentals of tooth preparations for cast metal and
porcelain restorations.

    Includes bibliographies and indexes.
    1. Dental cavity preparations.   2. Dental metallurgy.
3. Dental ceramics.   4. Dental ceramic metals.
I. Jacobi, Richard.   II. Brackett, Susan E.   III. Title.
[DNLM: 1. Dental Cavity Preparation—methods.   2. Dental
Restoration, Permanent—methods.   WU   350   S556f]
RK515.S55   1987   617.6'72   86-18714
ISBN   0-86715-157-9

quinte//ence
book/

Second Printing, 1991

Lithography: Sun Art Printing Co., Osaka
Composition: The Clarinda Co., Clarinda, IA
Printing and binding: Toppan Printing Co. (HK) Ltd.
Printed in China

Contributors

James C. Kessler, D.D.S.
Associate Professor
Department of Fixed Prosthodontics
University of Oklahoma College of
   Dentistry

Robert T. Probst, D.D.S., Ph.D.
Associate Professor
Department of Dental Materials
University of Oklahoma College of
   Dentistry

Frank J. Wiebelt, D.D.S
Associate Professor
Department of Removable
   Prosthodontics
University of Oklahoma School of
   Dentistry

Jack E. Willoughby, D.D.S.
Clinical Assistant Professor
Department of Fixed Prosthodontics
University of Oklahoma School of
   Dentistry

Dedication

This book is dedicated to our parents:

Herbert and Stefi Shillingburg

Herbert and Clara Jacobi

Delbert and Elsie Brackett

We owe them a debt mere words cannot repay.

Contents

Acknowledgments

To Dr. William E. Brown, Dean of the University of Oklahoma College of Dentistry, the authors express their gratitude for creating an atmosphere in which a project of this nature could be done. We also thank the Regents of the University of Oklahoma for granting a sabbatical leave of absence to Dr. Shillingburg. Without that impetus, it is doubtful this book could have been started.

We all tend to view the world in terms of what "I" have done. It is important to remember that we all learn from others and that we all stand on the work of our predecessors. We acknowledge a special debt to Drs. Rex Ingraham, Henry Tanner, Guy Ho, and the late Harold Eissman, all of the University of Southern California, for their unswerving commitment to excellence. We are also indebted to Dr. Donald E. Smith, who is quoted often in this book. His principles and concepts of preparation design form the foundation for much of which appears in the following pages. Thanks to Drs. Robert Dewhirst, Donald Fisher, and Sumiya Hobo. They have been our colleagues and good friends for many years, freely sharing their knowledge and enthusiasm for our profession.

Finally, we express our appreciation to Mr. William Wade of Brasseler, USA, for his repeated assistance in providing information and materials on rotary instruments. Thanks also to Mr. Robert Vaccaro of Syntex Dental Products and Mr. Lonnie Graybill of Union Broach Company for obtaining the information on diamond grits.

Introduction

Cast metal and porcelain restorations are an important part of restorative dentistry. By virtue of their strength and encircling configurations, cast crowns allow the reconstruction of individual teeth and the replacement of lost teeth in a permanent manner not possible by any other treatment mode. Porcelain restorations can be made so that even an expert can have difficulty distinguishing them from their unrestored neighbors. It is quite possible for cast restorations which have been done well and are cared for by well motivated patients to last 30 or even 40 years.[1,2] Unfortunately, we see many that do not.

Successful use of cemented restorations, whether of cast metal, porcelain, or a combination of both, begins with accurate diagnosis and thoughtful treatment planning. Only if the material and preparation design are matched with the patient's needs can the best treatment be rendered. In this age of "fiscodontics" with emphasis placed on daily production quotas, it is worth remembering that the needs of the patient should take precedence over those of the dentist.

The importance of the tooth preparation is often lost in the shuffle of treatment planning, periodontal management, impression materials and techniques, occlusion, cementation, and esthetics. There is a tendency to regard the preparation phase as mundane, *technical,* and unimportant. After all, it will be "covered up." No one will ever see it. One dental curriculum planner went so far as to state that he could train chimpanzees to cut full crown preparations. (Perhaps the same chimpanzees that NASA planned to use in the "manned" space program?)

Tooth preparation is a far more important phase of the treatment than that, although some practitioners never realize this. It must be done with skill and meticulous attention to detail, for everything else that follows—pulpal vitality, periodontal health, a good esthetic result, proper occlusion, protection of remaining tooth structure, and the longevity of the restoration itself—will depend on it. Dr. Lloyd Miller summed it up succinctly when he wrote, "No other clinical procedure in fixed prosthodontics reveals . . . the care, skill, and judgment used by a dentist than the quality of tooth preparation."[3]

Preparations have not always been that important. Their significance grew steadily as technology made possible an increasingly accurate fit of cast restorations. With improvement in the technology of fabricating restorations, there was a concomitant increase in the complexity of restoration designs and in the demands placed on retainers by more sophisticated prostheses.

Although Fauchard employed a pivot crown with a dowel projecting into the root canal for retention as early as 1746,[4] it was Beers' gold shell crown with solder-filled, swaged cusps, developed in 1849 and patented in 1873, that permitted restoration of a tooth by encircling it.[5] This was modified by Matheson to an open-faced crown in 1883, with true partial veneer crowns coming into being with Benneti's vertical half-cap crown in 1885.[4] This concept was developed further as a recognizable three-quarter crown by Carmichael in 1901.[6]

The early three-quarter crown was not a casting. It was made by flowing solder over gold foil that had been adapted to the tooth preparation, with wrought wire staples in the preparation grooves. Inlays were made in a similar fashion by flowing solder into a foil matrix adapted to the cavity preparation. The fit of both intracoronal and extracoronal restorations was improved when Taggart adapted the lost wax technique to dentistry in 1907.[7]

During the same time period that new types of all-metal restorations were evolving, efforts were being made to produce restorations that could restore the patient esthetically as well as functionally. A major step in this direction was the development of the porcelain jacket crown by Land in 1886.[8]

These technological improvements necessitated modifications of existing preparation forms to take full advantage of the restoration design and material. Many dentists in the past 100 years have contributed to the preparation designs and techniques shown on the following pages. Some of the designs and techniques were once tried and abandoned, only to be resurrected years later as a "new development" when instruments or materials became available to make the old concept work.

We have tried whenever we could to identify all of the people associated with an idea, even if they aren't traditionally credited with its development. We undoubtedly have failed at times, and we apologize to those dentists whose work to elevate the quality of restorative dentistry we have not recognized.

From the beginning, restorative dental procedures have been limited far more by the technology available than by a lack of ingenuity on the part of dentists. G. V. Black's concept of extension for prevention was governed in part by the primitive instrumentation available in 1891.[9] The instruments of his time were large and easily dulled. It was nearly a half a century later before diamond and tungsten carbide cutting instruments were developed for use in dentistry, and the effectiveness of those instruments was not fully realized until handpiece speeds were dramatically increased.

These technological improvements have not decreased the need for skilled, knowledgeable restorative dentists. On the contrary, they have made knowledge and skill that much more critical. Technology in the hands of a skilled operator makes it possible to do more work of an even higher quality. But in the hands of one who has not mastered the skills of his or her profession, that technology merely enables one to do tremendous damage.

It is our desire to provide the reader with a better understanding of the rationale for tooth preparation designs. We hope that we have shown actual techniques clearly enough to help the neophyte master the hands-on skills to become a good restorative dentist. For the advanced student of dentistry, this book furnishes detailed information on less frequently used designs as well as serving as a review of basic principles.

References

1. Smith, D. E. Fixed bridgework in the various phases of dental practice. J. South. Calif. Dent. Assoc. 9:13, 1942.
2. Stibbs, G. D. Individual intracoronal cast restorations. Oper. Dent. 10:138, 1985.
3. Miller, L. A clinician's interpretation of tooth preparations and the design of metal substructures for metal-ceramic restorations. pp. 173–206 *In* J. W. McLean (ed.) Dental Ceramics: Proceedings of the 1st International Symposium on Ceramics. Chicago: Quintessence Publishing Co., 1983.
4. Lovel, R. W. The restoration of teeth by crowning. Dent. Pract. 1:336, 1951.
5. Talbot, E. S. Gold crowns. Dent. Cosmos 22:463, 1880.
6. Carmichael, J. P. Attachment for inlay and bridgework. Dent. Rev. 15:82, 1901.
7. Taggart, W. H. A new and accurate method of making gold inlays. Dent. Cosmos 49:1117, 1907.
8. Land, C. H. A new system of restoring badly decayed teeth by means of an enamelled coating. Independent Pract. 7:407, 1886.
9. Sigurjons, H. Extension for prevention: Historical development and current status of G. V. Black's concept. Oper. Dent. 8:57, 1983.

Chapter 1

Biomechanical Principles of Preparations

The design and preparation of a tooth for a cast metal or porcelain restoration are governed by five principles:

1. Preservation of tooth structure
2. Retention and resistance form
3. Structural durability of the restoration
4. Marginal integrity
5. Preservation of the periodontium

At times it may be necessary to compromise one or more for the sake of another. For example, sound tooth structure may have to be sacrificed in order to produce a more retentive form, to create space for the bulk of restorative material necessary for structural durability or an esthetic veneer, and to allow the restoration to seat with close-fitting margins. Sound judgment must be exercised in making these compromises, with the requirements of the individual situation taken into careful consideration.

Preservation of tooth structure

Excessive removal of tooth structure can have many ill effects. If a tooth is overtapered or shortened too much, there will be an unnecessary sacrifice of retention and resistance. Thermal hypersensitivity, pulpal inflammation, and necrosis can result from approaching the pulp too closely. As a guide to how much tooth structure can be safely removed, or how deeply a preparation may extend, the average thicknesses of enamel and dentin for permanent maxillary teeth are given in Table 1-1. Those for mandibular teeth are shown in Table 1-2.

One of the most common violations of this principle is seen in the indiscriminate use of full-coverage porcelain veneered crowns in situations where partial veneer coverage with an all-metal restoration could be used. It is true that full-coverage restorations have long been recognized by clinicians as offering superior retention and resistance.[1] This has been borne out in recent years by several studies.[2-4] However, the shift in emphasis from partial veneer to full veneer restorations is more probably related to the ease and convenience associated with the design.[5-7] The decision to use full coverage should be reached only after a partial veneer crown has been considered and found wanting because of inadequate retention or esthetics.[8-11]

Preservation of tooth structure entails more than simply avoiding excessive destruction. It also requires designing the restoration so that it will reinforce and protect the remaining enamel and dentin even when this means sacrificing a small amount of additional tooth structure on the occlusal surface to protect underlying cusps.

Table 1-1 Enamel and dentin thicknesses in maxillary teeth (mm)*

Material		Incisal	Occlusal					Midcrown				CEJ			
			MF/F	DF	Cent	ML/L	DL	M	F	D	L	M	F	D	L
Central incisor	Enamel	0.9						0.7	1.0	0.7	0.7				
	Dentin	3.4						1.6	1.4	1.6	1.0	2.2	2.5	2.3	3.1
Lateral incisor	Enamel	0.9						0.8	1.0	0.6	0.7				
	Dentin	3.3						1.2	1.1	1.2	0.9	1.8	2.2	1.7	2.4
Canine	Enamel	1.1						0.7	0.8	0.8	0.7				
	Dentin	4.4						1.8	2.0	2.2	2.0	2.0	2.7	2.2	2.9
First premolar	Enamel		Cusp 1.5		Groove 1.3	Cusp 1.8		1.2	1.3	1.3	1.4				
	Dentin		3.0		3.1	3.3						2.2	2.6	2.2	2.7
Second premolar	Enamel		Cusp 1.7		Groove 1.3	Cusp 1.7		1.1	1.3	1.1	1.4				
	Dentin		3.3		3.2	3.4						2.0	2.2	1.9	2.3
			MF	DF	Cent	ML	DL								
First molar	Enamel		Cusp 1.8	Cusp 1.9	Fossa 0.6	Cusp 1.9	Cusp 1.9	1.3	1.5	1.4	1.6				
	Dentin		3.9			4.0						2.5	2.8	2.6	2.8
Second molar	Enamel		Cusp 2.0	Cusp 1.9	Fossa 0.5	Cusp 2.1	Cusp 1.9	1.3	1.4	1.3	1.6				
	Dentin		3.8			4.4						2.6	2.9	2.6	3.0

*Modified from H. T. Shillingburg and C. S. Grace, Thickness of enamel and dentin, J. South. Calif. Dent. Assoc., 41:33, 1973.

Table 1-2 Enamel and dentin thicknesses in mandibular teeth (mm)*

Material	Incisal	Occlusal MF/F	DF	D	CENT/Cent	ML/L	DL	Midcrown M	F	D	L	CEJ M	F	D	L
Incisor															
Enamel	0.9							0.6	0.9	0.7	0.6				
Dentin	3.7							1.1	1.1	1.2	0.9	1.5	2.3	1.5	2.4
Canine															
Enamel	1.0							0.6	0.8	0.8	0.6				
Dentin	3.6							2.0	2.0	2.1	1.7	2.1	2.8	2.2	2.9
First premolar		F			Cent	L									
Enamel		Cusp 1.3			Groove 1.2	Cusp 1.1		1.0	1.2	1.0	1.1				
Dentin		3.2			2.0	3.0						2.1	2.5	2.1	2.8
Second premolar		F			Cent	L									
Enamel		Cusp 1.6			Groove 1.3	Cusp 1.6		1.1	1.3	1.1	1.2				
Dentin		3.4			2.7	3.8						2.2	2.6	2.2	2.5
		MF	DF	D	CENT	ML	DL								
First molar															
Enamel		Cusp 2.0	Cusp 1.8	Cusp 1.9	Fossa 0.5	Cusp 1.9	Cusp 1.8	1.2	1.5	1.3	1.3				
Dentin		3.8	3.3			3.7	3.3					2.5	2.8	2.7	2.6
Second molar															
Enamel		Cusp 2.0	Cusp 1.9	Cusp 1.9	Fossa 0.5	Cusp 1.8	Cusp 1.8	1.4	1.6	1.5	1.5				
Dentin		3.6	3.6			3.3	3.6					2.5	3.0	2.8	2.6

*Modified from H. T. Shillingburg and C. S. Grace, Thickness of enamel and dentin, J. South. Calif. Dent. Assoc., 41:33, 1973.

Retention and resistance

If it does not remain firmly attached to the tooth, a restoration cannot meet its functional, biological, and esthetic requirements. Its capability for retention and resistance must be great enough to withstand the dislodging forces it will encounter in function. Some estimate of the prevailing occlusal forces in an individual patient can be made by noting the degree of wear on the other teeth, the firmness of the opposing teeth, the thickness of the supporting bone, and the bulk of the masticatory muscles. Contrary to the expectations of students, a retainer for a prosthesis requires greater, not less, retention and resistance than does a single tooth restoration.

The geometric form of the preparation is perhaps the most important of the factors under the operator's control which determine whether or not a restoration will remain cemented to its preparation. It is the geometric form that determines the orientation of the tooth-restoration interfaces to the direction of forces encountered. This in turn determines whether the cement in a given area will be subjected to tension, shear, or compression.

All cements exhibit their greatest strength under compression. They are weakest under tension, with the value for shear strength lying in between. Zinc phosphate cement, for example, has compressive, shear, and tensile strengths, which have been measured at 14,000 psi, 7,900 psi, and 1,300 psi, respectively.[12] Where a part of the restoration is pulled directly from the tooth, separation is prevented only by the relatively weak tensile strength and adhesive properties of the cement (Fig. 1-1, A).

Dental cements hold mainly through the mechanical interlocking of projections of cement into small irregularities of the surfaces being joined. Zinc phosphate cement exhibits no specific adhesion, so even its modest tensile strength is not fully utilized before it separates from one of the bonded surfaces. Polycarboxylate and glass ionomer cements claim some true adhesion under proper conditions, but their tensile strengths are still very weak when compared with their respective compressive strengths. The newer technique of bonding etched metal to etched enamel with resins can achieve tensile bonds of 2,270 psi[13] to 2,500 psi[14] under optimum conditions, but these values are still too low to permit us to ignore geometric retention and resistance form.

If the applied force is parallel with the cement film (Fig. 1-1, B), movement at the cement-tooth and cement-metal interfaces is more effectively impeded by the minute projections of cement into the surface irregularities than when the force is tensile in nature. Movement within the cement film itself is resisted by its relatively greater shear strength. A force directed at an angle toward the restoration has one component parallel with and one component perpendicular to the joined surfaces (Fig. 1-1, C). Thus the cement is subjected to a combination of shear and compression, and movement is resisted more effectively than if the forces were purely tensile or shear in nature. A compressive force perpendicular to the cement film can produce no movement of the restoration relative to the tooth unless it is great enough to crush the cement or deform the structures (Fig. 1-1, D). Such forces are seldom encountered in function.

Retention and resistance can be maximized by shaping the preparation so that as much of its surface as possible will experience compression and

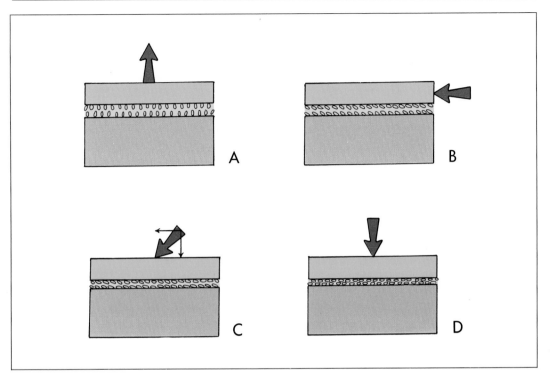

Fig. 1-1 The direction of the force acting upon a segment of a restoration determines the type of stress to which the cement film is subjected. A resultant force directed away from the tooth produces tensile stress *(A)*, while a force parallel with the interface produces shear *(B)*. A force directed at an angle toward the tooth will produce a combination of shear and compression *(C)*. When the force is perpendicular to the tooth, compression results *(D)*.

shear when the restoration is subjected to an unseating force.

In practice, *retention* and *resistance* are closely related, and they are not always clearly distinguishable. *Retention* is the ability of the preparation to impede removal of the restoration along its path of insertion. Under this condition, the cement bond is subjected to tension and shear. *Resistance,* on the other hand, is the ability of the preparation to prevent dislodgment of the restoration by forces directed in an apical, oblique, or horizontal direction. Where there is effective resistance, much of the cement film will be placed under

compression, although some parts will still be subjected to tension and shear.

Retention

A restoration can experience withdrawing forces along its path of insertion during mastication of sticky foods. If the restoration is a retainer for a bridge, an apically directed force elsewhere on the prosthesis can produce occlusally directed tensile force on the retainer through leverage. There are four factors under the control of the operator during tooth preparation which influence reten-

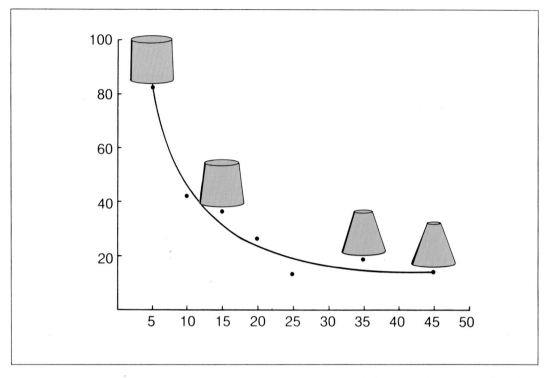

Fig. 1-2 As the degree of taper of a preparation increases, its ability to retain a restoration decreases (after Jørgensen[15]).

tion: (1) degree of taper,[15] (2) total surface area of the cement film,[16] (3) area of cement under shear, and (4) roughness of the tooth surface.[17]

Taper and retention

The ability of a cement bond to withstand a force depends largely on the direction of the force in relation to the cemented surfaces. From this we would expect that the more nearly parallel the opposing walls of a preparation, the greater will be the retention. This has been verified experimentally by Jorgensen,[15] who found that retention decreases as taper increases (Fig. 1-2).

Theoretically, the most retentive preparation would be one with parallel walls. However, in order to avoid undercuts and to allow complete seating of the restoration during cementation, the walls must have some taper. One which lies within the range of 2 to 6.5 degrees has been considered to be optimal.[18-23] This is based on an inclination of approximately 3 degrees being produced on each surface, external or internal, by the sides of a tapered instrument. The result would be an overall taper or angle of convergence of 6 degrees (Fig. 1-3).

Studies of actual crown preparations made by students have shown aver-

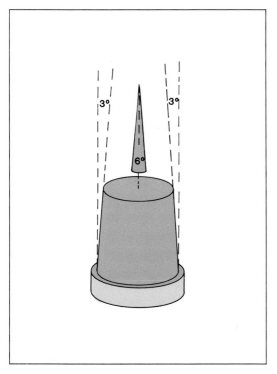

Fig. 1-3 To produce an optimal 6-degree taper, or convergence angle, each opposing axial wall should have an inclination of 3 degrees to the path of insertion.

age tapers between 13 and 29 degrees.[24–26] Dies taken at random from commercial laboratories by Eames et al. were found to have an average overall taper of 20 degrees.[27] Kent and associates found the tapers of preparations done by an experienced operator to average from 8.6 to 26.6 degrees, depending upon location in the mouth and visual accessibility. Grooves and boxes were observed to be markedly less tapered. The overall mean in that study was reported as 14.7 degrees.[28]

A taper or total convergence of 16 degrees has been proposed as being clinically achievable, while also affording adequate retention.[29,30] The tenden-

cy for operators to overtaper preparations needlessly must be guarded against in order to produce preparations with minimum taper and maximum retention for any given situation.

Surface area

Obviously, the greater the area of the cement film bound to the preparation and to the internal detail of the casting, the greater the retention of the casting will be. Therefore, the greater the surface area of the preparation, the greater the retention of its restoration.[16,31–33] The total surface area of the preparation is influenced by the size of the tooth, the extent of coverage by the restoration, and features such as grooves and boxes that are placed in the preparation.

Area under shear

More important for retention than the total surface area is the area of cement that will experience shearing rather than tensile stress when the restoration is subjected to forces along the path of insertion. To decrease the failure potential, it is essential to minimize tensile stress.[34] For the shear strength of the cement to be utilized, the preparation must have opposing walls, i.e., two surfaces of the preparation in separate planes must be nearly parallel with each other and the line of draw. The opposing surfaces may be internal, as the facial and lingual walls of the proximal box of an inlay preparation (Fig. 1-4), or external, such as the axial walls of a full veneer crown preparation (Fig. 1-5). There may also be a combination of internal and external walls in opposition. With the walls in this configuration, the restoration cannot be removed in any direction without overcoming the shear

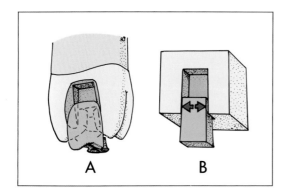

Fig. 1-4 An inlay *(A)* depends on internal retention to hold it within its preparation. Internal retention is created by the close adaptation of a restoration to two or more opposing, slightly divergent internal walls *(arrows, B)*.

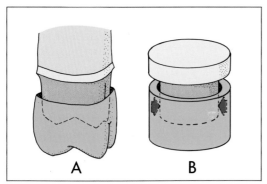

Fig. 1-5 A crown *(A)* depends primarily on external retention to resist removal. External retention is provided by approximation of the restoration to the opposing external axial walls of the preparation *(arrows, B)*.

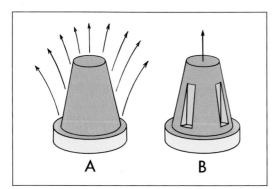

Fig. 1-6 Retention is enhanced by restricting the possible paths of withdrawal or paths of insertion. The excessively tapered truncated cone has an infinite number of paths along which a crown could be withdrawn *(A)*. The addition of parallel-sided grooves *(B)* limits the path of withdrawal to one direction, thereby reducing the possibility of dislodgment.

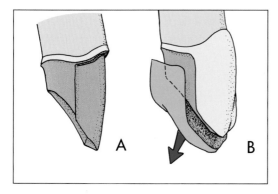

Fig. 1-7 A preparation for a porcelain-fused-to-metal crown has a limited path of insertion and excellent retention *(A)*. However, if one of the four axial walls is missing or left uncovered *(B)*, the potential paths of withdrawal are greatly increased and retention is compromised.

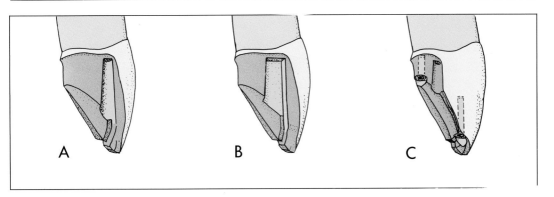

Fig. 1-8 When an axial wall is left unveneered, retention is achieved by substituting grooves *(A)*, boxes *(B)*, or pinholes *(C)* for the missing wall.

strength of the cement contacting the opposing walls.

To obtain the greatest area of cement under shear, the directions in which a restoration can be removed must be limited to essentially one path.[35] As much of the preparation surface as possible must be made nearly parallel with that line of draw. A severely overtapered preparation has many paths along which a tensile force could remove a crown (Fig. 1-6, *A*); a restoration on such a preparation would encounter many such forces during function. If features are added to the preparation so that only a force in *one* direction can move a restoration without compressing the cement film against one or more surfaces, retention is enhanced (Fig. 1-6, *B*). Even against a force along the line of draw, such features enhance retention, not only because they increase the total surface area of the cement film, but because most of the added area is subjected to pure shear with no component of tension.

A full veneer crown preparation has excellent retention because the mesial, distal, lingual, and facial walls limit the possible paths of insertion to a narrow range (Fig. 1-7, *A*). However, if the fa-

cial surface is left unveneered, the crown placed on this preparation could be removed toward the lingual, the incisal, or any direction in between (Fig. 1-7, *B*). To create a more retentive form, grooves, boxes, or pinholes are substituted for the missing axial wall (Fig. 1-8).[36] These features are also useful for augmenting retention on severely damaged teeth.

In order for a groove to effectively substitute for the uncovered facial wall, the lingual wall of the groove must be distinct and perpendicular to the adjoining axial surface (Fig. 1-9, *A*). Otherwise a lingually directed displacing force could cause the ribs of metal in the crown to slide along the inclined planes of the lingual walls of grooves, spreading the axial walls and opening the margins (Fig. 1-9, *B*).

The length of the preparation is an important factor in retention: a long preparation has greater retention than does a short preparation.[31,32,37] This is due, at least in part, to its greater surface area (Fig. 1-10), and to the fact that most of the additional area is under shear rather than tension.

Because of its greater surface area, a preparation with a larger diameter (and

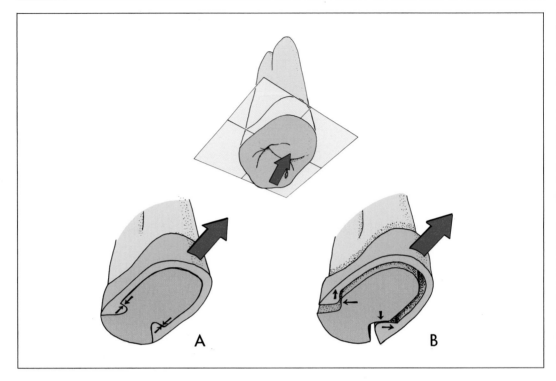

Fig. 1-9 A lingually directed force acting on a three-quarter crown is effectively resisted if the lingual walls of the groove are perpendicular to the path of displacement *(A)*. However, the walls of V-shaped grooves will act as inclined planes which will eventually cause the walls of the restoration to spread *(B)*.

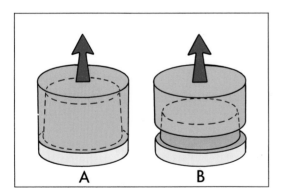

Fig. 1-10 All other factors remaining constant, the greater the surface area of cement film, the greater the retention. Therefore, a restoration on a long preparation *(A)* can withstand a force that could remove a restoration from a shorter preparation of equal diameter *(B)*. Doubling the height of a preparation would nearly double the area of its axial walls.

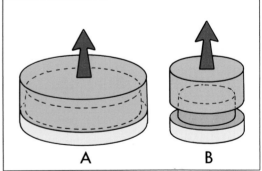

Fig. 1-11 Of two preparations of equal height and taper, the wider *(A)* will have greater retention than the narrower *(B)*. Doubling the diameter of a preparation doubles the area of its axial walls under shear, and quadruples the area of the occlusal surface, where the cement is under tension.

circumference) will have greater retention than will a narrow preparation of the same length (Fig. 1-11).[31,38]

Surface roughness

Because the adhesion of dental cements depends primarily on projections of the cement into microscopic irregularities and recesses on the surfaces being joined, the prepared tooth surface should not be highly polished. Øilo and Jorgensen found retention of castings cemented with zinc phosphate cement on test dies with a 10-degree taper to be twice as great on preparations with 40 μm scratches as on those with 10 μm scratches,[17] while Smith found no significant difference in castings cemented on 14-degree taper preparations whose roughness varied by a factor of 24 from smoothest to roughest.[39]

Resistance

Resistance prevents dislodgment of a restoration by forces directed in an apical, oblique, or horizontal direction. If the cement film is disrupted by the restoration's sliding or tipping on its preparation the smallest fraction of a millimeter, the restoration is doomed through percolation of fluids, dissolution of the cement, and recurrent caries. Resistance to sliding and tipping must be designed into a preparation by forming walls to block the anticipated movements. The more nearly perpendicular it lies to the force, the greater is the resistance provided by the supporting surface, because the cement will be compressed,[40] and failures are less likely to occur from compression than shear.[41]

Leverage and resistance

The strongest forces encountered in function are apically directed and can produce tension and shear in the cement film only through leverage. Leverage, probably the predominant factor in the dislodgment of cemented restorations, occurs when the line of action of a force passes outside the supporting tooth structure, or when the structures flex. For the sake of simplicity, all structures in the following situations will be considered to be rigid.

If the force passes within the margin of a crown, there will be no tipping of the restoration (Fig. 1-12, A). The margin on all sides of the restoration is supported by the preparation. The torque produced merely tends to seat the crown further. If the occlusal table of the restoration is wide, even a vertical force can pass outside the supported margin and produce destructive torque (Fig. 1-12, B). This can also occur in crowns on tipped teeth and retainers for cantilever bridges.

A force applied to a cemented crown at an oblique angle can also produce a line of action which will pass outside the supporting tooth structure (Fig. 1-13). The point on the margin that lies closest to the line of action is the fulcrum point, or center of rotation. The magnitude of the torque produced is equal to the applied force multiplied by its lever arm, which is the closest distance between the line of action and the fulcrum. In equilibrium, this torque is balanced by the sum of all the resisting tensile, shear, and compressive stresses generated in the cement film. The farther these resisting forces lie from the fulcrum, the greater their mechanical advantage is.

If a line is drawn from the center of rotation perpendicular to the cement film

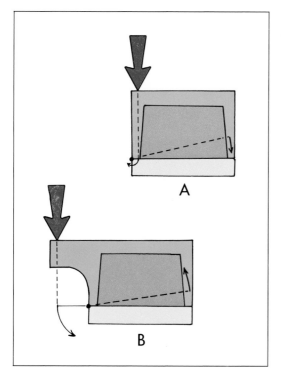

Fig. 1-12 When the line of action of an applied force passes within the margins of the restoration, no secondary lifting forces are produced *(A)*. When the line of action passes outside the margins of the restoration, a torque is produced that will tend to tip or rotate the crown around a point on the margin *(B)*.

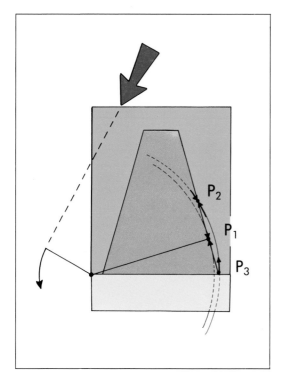

Fig. 1-13 At P_1 the arc of rotation is tangent to the surface of the preparation, and the cement film is subject only to shear. There is a component of compression at P_2 and at all points occlusal to P_1, which becomes greater the higher the point is located. At P_3 and all points apical to the tangent point, stresses have a component of tension. Mechanical resistance is provided only by points occlusal to the tangent point.

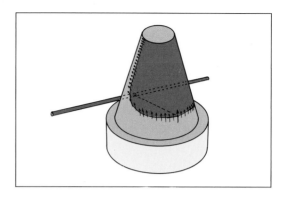

Fig. 1-14 If the tangent points of all the arcs of rotation around a given axis are connected, they form the *tangent line*. The area above the tangent line *(red)* is the *resisting area*, which prevents tipping of a restoration around the axis (after Hegdahl and Silness[42]). For a preparation to have effective resistance, the tangent line should extend at least halfway down the preparation.

on the opposite wall of the preparation, the point where this line intercepts the cement film can be referred to as the *tangent point*. At this point, the arc of rotation around the fulcrum is tangent to the surface of the preparation, and the cement film is subject to shear only. All points occlusal to the tangent point are subject to shear *and* compression. The compression component becomes greater the farther a point lies above the tangent point. A point near the occlusal end of the preparation would contribute more to resistance than would a site near the tangent point, not only because of the mechanical advantage of its longer lever arm, but also because the force is directed at a steeper angle toward the surface of the preparation.

If a line is drawn connecting the tangent points of all the arcs around the axis of rotation, the cement film along that line would be subjected to pure shear by any force applied perpendicularly to the axis of rotation (Fig. 1-14). The area encompassed by this tangent line has been referred to as the "resisting area" by Hegdahl and Silness.[42] Within this area, the luting material is subjected to varying degrees of compression as well as shear, while all other points on the surface of the preparation will experience some degree of tension and will contribute little to the resistance of the preparation.

Preparation length and resistance

The length of a preparation has a strong influence on its resistance. Shortening a preparation will produce a proportionally greater diminution of the resisting area (Fig. 1-15). The ability of a restoration to resist tipping depends not only on the preparation, but also on the magnitude of the torque. If two crowns of unequal length on two preparations of equal length are subjected to identical forces, the longer crown is more likely to fail because the force on it acts through a longer lever arm (Figs. 1-16 and 1-17).

When a relatively long crown must be made on a short preparation, additional resistance form, usually in the form of a pin-retained core, must be created before the cast restoration can be made. Techniques for this are discussed in greater detail in chapter 16.

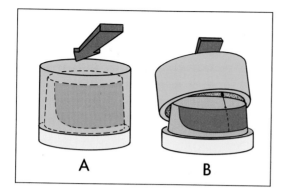

Fig. 1-15 Decreasing the length of a tapered preparation causes a disproportionate decrease in the resisting area. A crown with relatively long axial walls can resist a strong tipping force *(A)*. Although preparation *B* still has more than half the length of preparation *A*, it has less than half the resisting area. Its crown will fail under a force that would be easily resisted by the longer preparation *(B)*.

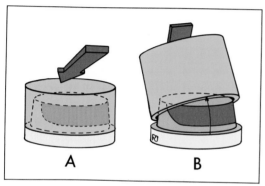

Fig. 1-16 A short restoration on a short preparation is less likely to fail through tipping than is a long restoration on the same preparation. The resistance of this preparation is adequate to prevent the crown from tipping under the applied force *(A)*. Although the preparation and the applied force in *(B)* are identical to those in *(A)*, the crown fails because of the greater height of the restoration.

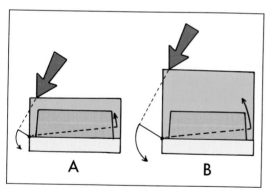

Fig. 1-17 The length of the primary lever arm is the shortest distance from the line of action of the force to the nearest margin. On the short crown the lifting force is small because the primary lever arm is short *(A)*. With a long crown *(B)*, the same force produces a greater torque because its line of action passes farther from the point of rotation.

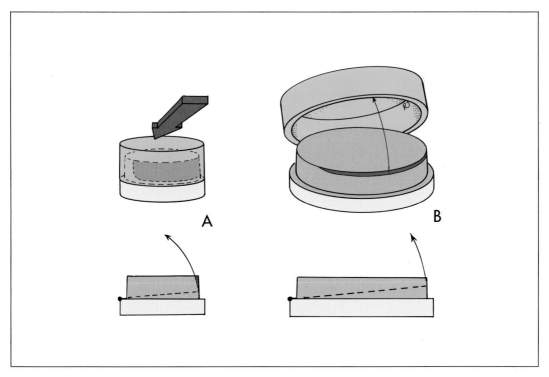

Fig. 1-18 Because of the small diameter, the tangent line of this narrow preparation falls low on the wall opposite the axis of rotation, resulting in a large resisting area *(A)*. Preparation A is wider than preparation B, but its height and taper are the same. Because of the much greater radius of the arc of rotation, its resisting area is smaller than that of the narrower preparation.

Resistance and tooth width

As explained earlier, a wide preparation has greater retention than a narrower one of equal height. Under some circumstances a crown on the narrow tooth can have greater resistance to tipping than one on the wider tooth. This occurs because the crown on the narrower tooth has a shorter radius of rotation resulting in a lower tangent line and a larger resisting area (Fig. 1-18). This advantage is offset, in part, by the shorter lever arm of the narrow tooth and by its diminished axial surface area.

The resistance of a preparation on a wide, short tooth can be greatly enhanced by the addition of grooves (Fig. 1-19). The shorter radius of rotation between the fulcrum point and the groove causes the arc of rotation to be tangent to the resisting surface on the groove wall at a lower point than does the longer radius on the more distant axial wall. A large area of the groove wall lies at a relatively steep angle to the arc of rotation, affording increased resistance.

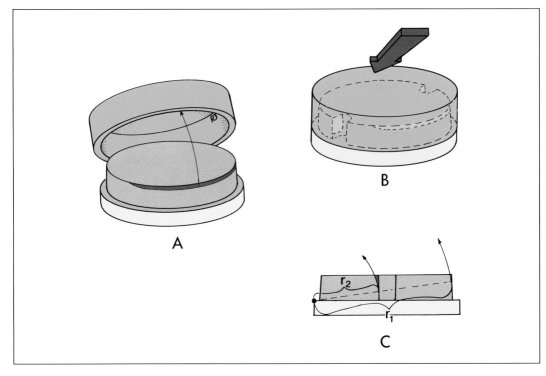

Fig. 1-19 The weak resistance of a short, wide preparation *(A)* can be enhanced by the addition of vertical grooves *(B)*. From the side *(C)*, it can be seen that the arc of radius r_2 is effectively blocked by the resisting area of the groove walls, while the arc of radius r_1 encounters little or no resistance on the far axial wall.

Fig. 1-20 The resisting area decreases as the preparation taper increases. For a cylinder with no taper, the resisting area would cover half the axial walls *(A)*. For an ideally-tapered tooth preparation the resisting area covers somewhat less than half the axial walls *(B)*. An over-tapered (20 degrees) preparation has only a small resisting area near the occlusal surface *(C)*.

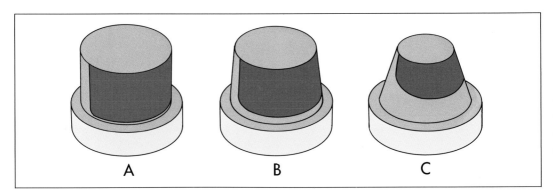

Table 1-3 Preparation dimensions and maximum preparation tapers*

Preparation height (mm)	Preparation diameter (mm)											
	3	4	5	6	7	8	9	10	11	12	13	14
	degrees											
2	16	12	10	8	7	6	6	5	5	4	4	4
3	24	18	14	12	10	9	8	7	7	6	6	5
4	33	24	19	16	14	12	11	10	9	8	8	7
5	33[†]	31	24	20	17	15	13	12	11	10	9	9
6	28[†]	37	29	24	21	18	16	14	13	12	11	10
7	24[†]	32[†]	35	28	24	21	19	17	15	14	13	12
8	21[†]	28[†]	35[†]	33	28	24	21	19	17	16	15	14
9	19[†]	25[†]	31[†]	37[†]	31	27	24	22	20	18	17	15
10	17[†]	23[†]	28[†]	33[†]	35	31	27	24	22	20	18	17

*Calculations are based on an assumption of a symmetrical tooth preparation, with straight axial walls and an area of maximum resistance that is 80% of the preparation height.
†This is the maximum possible preparation taper for the given preparation height and diameter.

Taper and resistance

The resisting area of a cylindrical preparation would include half of its axial surface (Fig. 1-20, A). As the degree of taper increases, the tangent line approaches the occlusal surface, and the resisting area decreases (Fig. 1-20, B and C). The more tapered a preparation, the less its resistance. A short tooth can be easily overtapered to the extent that it has no resistance form at all.

A long, narrow preparation can have a greater taper than a short and wide one without jeopardizing resistance. Conversely, the walls of a short, wide preparation must be kept nearly parallel to achieve adequate resistance form. The permissible taper of a preparation is directly proportional to the height/width ratio. The preparation taper that will still permit an effective resisting area, for a preparation in which the height equals the width, is double that permissible in a preparation in which the height is only one-half of the width (Fig. 1-21). The maximum allowable preparation tapers for various preparation height and width combinations are shown in Table 1-3.

The formulas used in calculating allowable preparation tapers (convergence angles) and for determining the height of the tangency point and preparation height are:

$$T = \text{arc sin } (2r/w),$$
$$r = (w \sin T) / 2, \text{ and}$$
$$h = [w \tan (90° - T/2)] / 2.$$

T = preparation taper in degrees
r = height of tangency point in mm
w = preparation width in mm
h = preparation height in mm

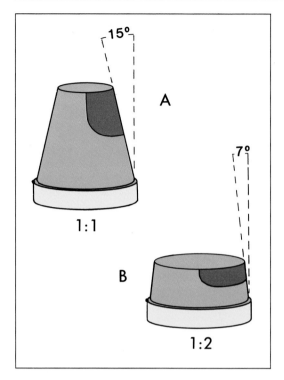

Fig. 1-21 The inclination of the walls of a preparation that will still provide effective resistance is dependent on the height/width ratio. A preparation with a height/width ratio of 1:1 *(A)* can have a wall inclination of 15 degrees and still have effective resistance. A preparation with a ratio of 1:2 *(B)* can have an individual wall inclination no greater than 7 degrees without seriously compromising resistance. Resistance is arbitrarily considered effective if the resisting area extends at least halfway down the axial wall.

Rotation around a vertical axis

Although the previous examples have dealt exclusively with tipping or rotation of the restoration around a horizontal axis, rotation about a vertical axis is also possible. When a crown is subjected to an eccentric horizontal force, moments of torque occur around a vertical as well as a horizontal axis (Fig. 1-22). A three-quarter crown without grooves has little resistance to rotational dis-

placement (Fig. 1-23, *A*). The addition of grooves places a resisting surface at right angles to the arc of rotation, effectively blocking it (Fig. 1-23, *B*).

It is possible for a full crown on a cylindrical preparation to rotate enough to break the cement bond before any compressive resistance is encountered (Fig. 1-24, *A*). Geometric forms such as grooves or "wings" (Fig. 1-24, *B*) increase resistance by blocking rotation around a vertical axis.

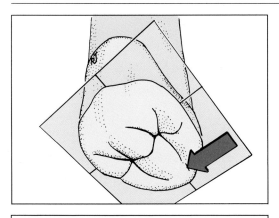

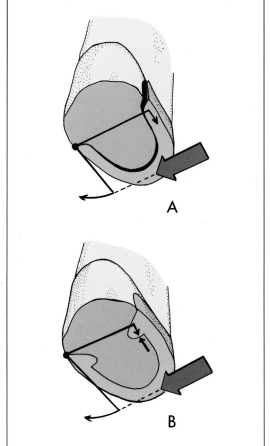

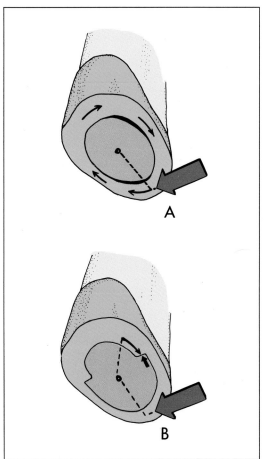

Fig. 1-22 The horizontal component of occlusal force can have a rotating influence on a crown in a horizontal plane.

Fig. 1-23 A partial veneer crown which has no grooves *(A)* has little resistance to rotation around a vertical axis. When grooves are present, their lingual walls provide resistance by blocking the arc of rotation *(B)*.

Fig. 1-24 The axial symmetry of a full veneer crown preparation may allow rotation of the restoration around the preparation *(A)*. Resistance can be gained by forming vertical planes (wings) which are perpendicular to the arc of rotation *(B)*.

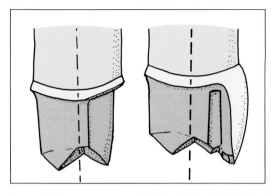

Fig. 1-25 The ideal path of insertion for a posterior full or partial veneer crown is parallel with the long axis of the tooth.

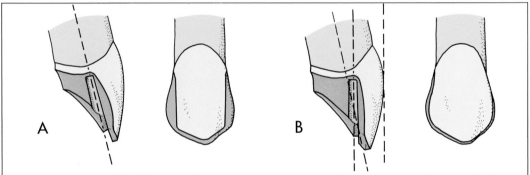

Fig. 1-26 Making the path of insertion of an anterior three-quarter crown parallel with the long axis of the tooth would result in an unnecessary display of metal *(A)*. The preferred path of insertion for an anterior preparation parallels the incisal two-thirds of the labial surface *(B)*. This not only will minimize the display of metal, but allow the grooves to be longer and more retentive.

Path of insertion

Before any tooth structure is cut, the path of insertion should be decided upon, keeping in mind the principles discussed previously. This is especially important when preparing bridge abutments, because multiple paths of insertion must be parallel. A path must be selected that will allow the margins of the retainers to fit against their respective preparation finish lines with the removal of minimum sound tooth structure. This path should not encroach upon the pulp or adjacent teeth.

The path of insertion for posterior full and partial veneer crowns is usually parallel with the long axis of the tooth (Fig. 1-25). However, paralleling the path of insertion of an anterior three-quarter crown with the long axis of the tooth will produce an unesthetic display of metal on the facial surface (Fig. 1-26, *A*). The remaining incisal tooth structure will also be undermined, making it susceptible to fracture. Instead, the path of insertion for an anterior three-quarter crown should be inclined to parallel the incisal two-thirds of the facial surface (Fig. 1-26, *B*), enabling the restoration to have almost no metal visible on the facial surface. This inclination also permits longer grooves with better retention and resistance.

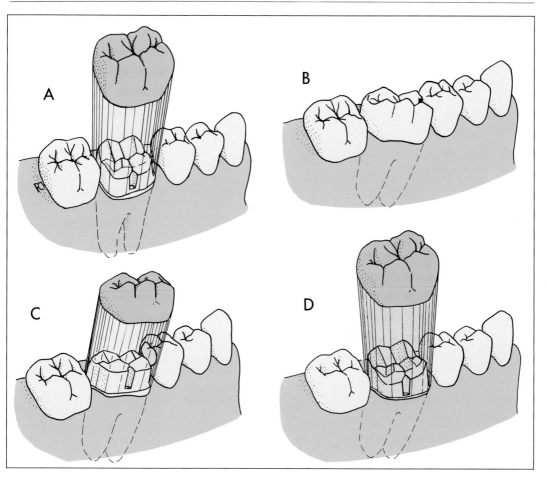

Fig. 1-27 The path of insertion for a full veneer crown on a posterior tooth in normal alignment parallels the long axis of the tooth *(A)*. A tipped tooth must be handled differently *(B)*. If the path of insertion on a tipped tooth parallels the long axis, the crown will be prevented from seating by those parts of the adjacent teeth which protrude into the path of insertion *(C)*. The correct path of insertion for such a tooth is perpendicular to the occlusal plane *(D)*.

Normally, for a full crown to have structural durability with proper contours, its path of insertion would parallel the long axis of the tooth (Fig. 1-27, *A*). However, if the tooth is tilted (Fig. 1-27, *B*), a path of insertion paralleling the long axis of the tooth may be blocked by the proximal contours of the adjacent tooth (Fig. 1-27, *C*). In this case, the path of insertion is made perpendicular to the occlusal plane (Fig. 1-27, *D*).

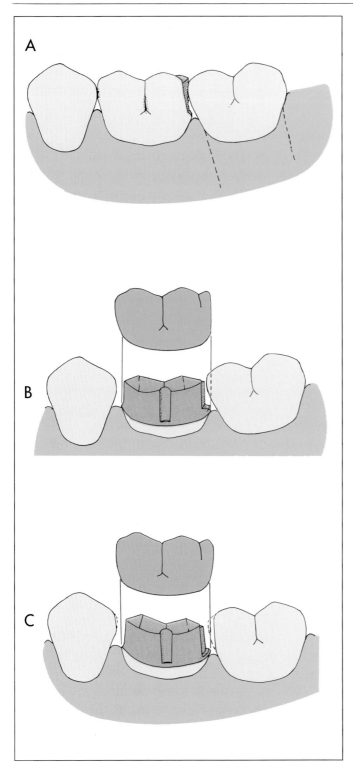

Fig. 1-28 A tooth has migrated into the space formed by a long-standing carious lesion *(A)*. A vertical path of insertion will not permit seating without removal of excessive amounts of tooth structure from the proximal surface of the adjacent tooth *(B)*. The problem can be solved less destructively by inclining the path of insertion slightly to the mesial, and removing small amounts of enamel from *both* adjacent teeth *(C)*. More severe collapse may require orthodontic uprighting to regain needed space.

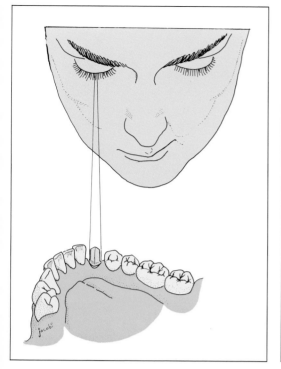

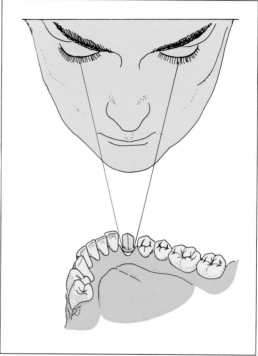

Fig. 1-29 When viewed with one eye from a distance of 30 cm, all the axial surfaces of a preparation with an ideal taper or angle of convergence of 6 degrees can be seen.

Fig. 1-30 Binocular vision should never be employed to evaluate a preparation for correct taper. With both eyes open, a preparation that is undercut can appear to have an acceptable degree of taper.

Long-standing loss of proximal contact is usually accompanied by tipping of the adjacent tooth into the space (Fig. 1-28, *A*). When this occurs, a path of insertion parallel with the long axis of the tooth might not allow a crown to seat even if its distal wall were grossly undercontoured (Fig. 1-28, *B*). The space between the adjacent teeth must be made greater than the mesiodistal diameter of the prepared tooth at the gingival finish line. An acceptable compromise can be reached by inclining the path of insertion so that removal of equal amounts of enamel from each of the adjacent teeth will allow a crown

to seat on the prepared tooth (Fig. 1-28c). If the loss of space is so great that more than 50% of the thickness of enamel would have to be removed from either adjacent tooth, or if there isn't space for adequate gingival embrasures, the teeth should be separated and uprighted orthodontically.

All negative taper, or undercut, must be eliminated or it will prevent the restoration from seating. To evaluate preparation taper, view it with one eye from a distance of approximately 30 cm or 12 in. (Fig. 1-29). In this way it is possible to simultaneously see all the axial walls of a preparation with an adequate

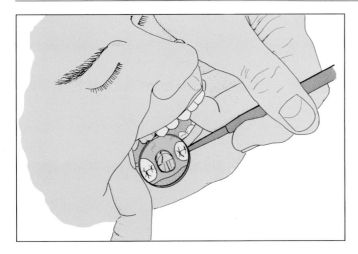

Fig. 1-31 A mirror is used to evaluate a preparation where direct vision is not possible. An unobstructed view of the entire finish line barely outside the circumference of the occlusal surface indicates correct taper.

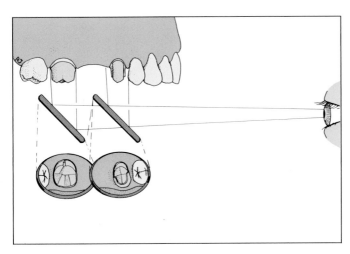

Fig. 1-32 Matching bridge abutment paths of insertion can be evaluated by centering the image of one preparation in the mirror and then moving the mirror bodily, *without tilting,* until the second preparation is centered. The entire finish line of the second preparation should be visible. If the angulation of the mirror must be changed to see the finish line of the second preparation, the paths of insertions of the two preparations do not match, and corrections must be made.

taper. An undercut as great as 8 degrees can be overlooked if both eyes are used (Fig. 1-30).

Where it is difficult to survey the preparation with direct vision, use a mouth mirror (Fig. 1-31). The entire finish line should be visible to one eye from one fixed position with no obstruction by any part of the prepared tooth or any adjacent tooth. To verify parallel paths of insertion of bridge abutments, the image of one preparation is centered in the mirror. Then, using firm finger rests, the mirror is moved bodily without changing its angulation, until the image of the second preparation is also centered (Fig. 1-32). If the angulation of the mirror must be changed in order to see all of the finish lines, there is a discrepancy between the paths of insertion of the preparations.

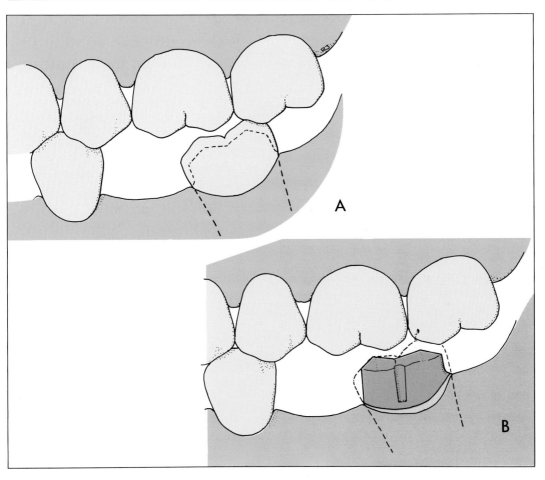

Fig. 1-33 The interocclusal space over the mesial cusps of a tipped tooth may be sufficient for a crown preparation without any reduction. Uniform occlusal reduction in such a case would produce excessive occlusal clearance and an unnecessarily shortened mesial axial wall (A). Only enough tooth structure to provide necessary space for the restoration should be removed (B). Some of the original occlusal surface may not need to be cut at all.

Structural durability of the restoration

The casting must be rigid enough not to flex and break the cement film.[43] Sufficient tooth structure must be removed to create space for an adequate bulk of restorative material to accomplish this without departing from the normal contours of the tooth. There are three preparation features that contrib-ute to the durability of the restoration: (1) occlusal reduction, (2) axial reduction, and (3) provision for reinforcing struts.

Occlusal reduction

Enough tooth structure must be removed from the occlusal surface of the preparation so that when the restora-

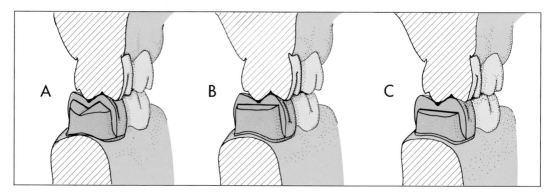

Fig. 1-34 Correct occlusal reduction parallels the major planes of the tooth *(A)*. Flat, single-plane occlusal reduction may result in insufficient thickness of the restoration over the grooves and fossae *(B)*. Single plane reduction deep enough to provide adequate thickness of metal in the central groove area will result in unnecessary loss of dentin over the pulp horns and excessive shortening of the axial walls with loss of retention *(C)*.

tion is built back to ideal occlusion it will be thick enough to prevent wearing through or distorting. The occlusal thickness will vary with the restorative material used. A gold crown requires approximately 1.5 mm clearance over the functional cusps and 1.0 mm over the nonfunctional cusps. Harder metals require slightly less. If a porcelain veneer is extended onto the occlusal surface, an additional 0.5 mm of space is needed.

The amount of occlusal reduction is not always the same as the clearance needed. Often part of a tipped tooth is already short of the ideal occlusal plane and will require less reduction than would a tooth in ideal occlusion (Fig. 1-33).

Occlusal reduction should reflect the geometric inclined planes underlying the morphology of the finished crown[44] and follow the major planes of the opposing facial and lingual cusps as well (Fig. 1-34, *A*). Avoid creating steep planes with sharp angles, since these can increase stress and hinder complete seating of the casting. To diminish stress, round the angles and avoid deep grooves in the center of the occlusal surface,[45] keeping the angulation of the occlusal planes shallow.[46]

Any necessary equilibration of the opposing teeth should be done before the restorative procedure is begun. Opposing cusps that are missing or otherwise short of their ideal position should be replaced in a diagnostic wax-up on a cast so that the required amount of occlusal reduction can be determined.

A flat occlusal surface is undesirable.[21] If the occlusal surface is made flat and reduction is conservative, metal in the area of the developmental grooves will be too thin, with a risk of perforation (Fig. 1-34, *B*). An attempt to avoid this problem by lowering the entire occlusal table will cause excessive destruction of tooth structure, and the axial walls will be overshortened with a resultant loss of retention and resistance (Fig. 1-34, *C*).

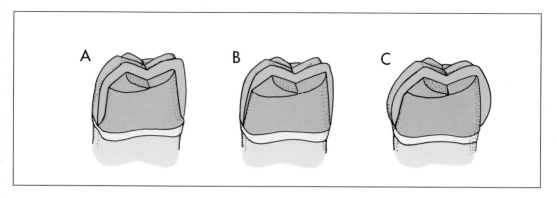

Fig. 1-37 Adequate axial reduction creates space for a strong bulk of metal within the normal contours of the tooth *(A)*. Inadequate axial reduction can result in a crown with thin, weak walls *(B)*. More probably, a restoration with bulky, plaque-promoting contours will result *(C)*.

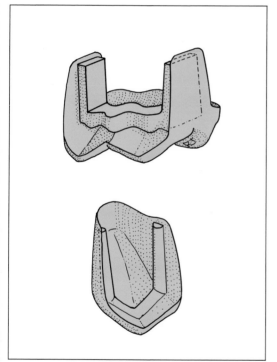

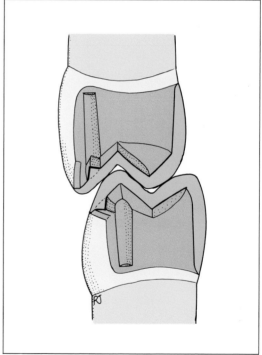

Fig. 1-38 Partial veneer castings are reinforced by a bar of thickened metal across their occlusal portions. This joins the metal occupying the proximal boxes or grooves to form rigid trusses.

Fig. 1-39 Spaces for the reinforcing ribs of metal across the occlusal surfaces of standard posterior three-quarter crowns are created by cutting occlusal offsets into the nonfunctional buccal cusps of maxillary teeth, and shoulders into the functional buccal cusps of mandibular teeth.

(Fig. 1-38). In a three-quarter crown it is a connecting rib of metal that joins the grooves to provide a "trussing effect."[56,57] This reinforcing rib takes the form of an offset on a maxillary preparation and an occlusal shoulder on a mandibular one (Fig. 1-39). The occlusal offset is used on nonfunctional cusps because it displays less metal. The shoulder is indicated on functional cusps to protect the margins from distortion by nearby occlusal impacts.

References

1. Knapp, K. W. A modern conception of proper bridge attachments for vital teeth. J. Am. Dent. Assoc. 14:1027, 1927.
2. Lorey, R. E., and Myers, G. E. The retentive qualities of bridge retainers. J. Am. Dent. Assoc. 76:568, 1968.
3. Reisbick, M. H., and Shillingburg, H. T. Effect of preparation geometry on retention and resistance of cast gold restorations. J. Calif. Dent. Assoc. 3:51, 1975.
4. Potts, R. G., Shillingburg, H. T., and Duncanson, M. G. Retention and resistance of preparations for cast restorations. J. Prosthet. Dent. 43:303, 1980.
5. Ingraham, R., Sochat, P., and Hausing, F. J. Rotary gingival curettage—A new technique for tooth preparation and management of the gingival sulcus for impression taking. Int. J. Periodont. Rest. Dent. 1(4):9, 1981.
6. Maxwell, E. L., and Wasser, V. E. Debate: Full vs. partial coverage as the abutment of choice in fixed bridgework. J. D. C. Dent. Soc. 36:9, 1961.
7. Grosso, F. P., and Carreno, J. A. Partial or full coverage restorations: A survey of prevailing criteria. J. Prosthet. Dent. 40:628, 1978.
8. Hollenback, G. M. A plea for a more conservative approach to certain dental procedures. J. Ala. Dent. Assoc. 46:16, 1962.
9. Kahn, A. E. Partial vs. full coverage. J. Prosthet. Dent. 10:167, 1960.
10. Yock, D. H. The anterior three-quarter crown abutment preparation and retainer. Dent. Clin. North Am. 9:43, 1965.
11. Perel, M. L. Crown and bridge and partial coverage castings. R.I. Dent. J. 14:19, 1981.
12. Civjan, S., and Brauer, G. M. Physical properties of cements, based on zinc oxide, hydrogenated rosin, o-ethoxybenzoic acid and eugenol. J. Dent. Res. 43:281, 1964.
13. Dhillon, M., Fenton, A. H., and Watson, P. A. Bond strengths of composite to perforated and etched surfaces. Abstract no. 1219. J. Dent. Res. 62:304, 1983.
14. Sloan, K. M., Lorey, R. E., and Meyers, G. E. Evaluation of laboratory etching of cast metal resin-bonded retainers. Abstract no. 1220. J. Dent. Res. 62:305, 1983.
15. Jorgensen, K. D. The relationship between retention and convergence angle in cemented veneer crowns. Acta Odontol. Scand. 13:35, 1955.
16. Lorey, R. E., and Myers, G. E. The retentive qualities of bridge retainers. J. Am. Dent. Assoc. 76:568, 1968.
17. Øilo, G., and Jorgensen, K. D. The influence of surface roughness on the retentive ability of two dental luting cements. J. Oral Rehabil. 5:377, 1978.
18. Minker, J. S. Simplified full coverage preparations. Dent. Clin. North Am. 9:355, 1965.
19. Sanell, C. Vertical parallel pins in occlusal rehabilitation. Dent. Clin. North Am. 7:755, 1963.
20. El-Ebrashi, M. K., Craig, R. G., and Peyton, F. A. Experimental stress analysis of dental restorations: IV. The concept of parallelism of axial walls. J. Prosthet. Dent. 22:346, 1969.
21. Guyer, S. E. Multiple preparations for fixed prosthodontics. J. Prosthet. Dent. 23:529, 1970.
22. Lum, L. B. Management of virgin teeth in fixed prosthodontics. Gen. Dent. 23:38, 1975.
23. Turner, C. H.: Bevels and slots in full crown preparations. Dent. Update. 4:161, 1977.
24. Ohm, E., and Silness, J. The convergence angle in teeth prepared for artificial crowns. J. Oral Rehabil. 5:371, 1978.
25. Mack, P. J. A theoretical and clinical investigation into the taper achieved on crown and inlay preparations. J. Oral Rehabil. 7:255, 1980.
26. Weed, R. M., Suddick, R. P., and Kleffner, J. H. Taper of clinical and typodont crowns prepared by dental students. Abstract no. 1036. J. Dent. Res. 63:286, 1984.
27. Eames, W. B., O'Neal, S. J., Monteiro, J., Roan, J. D., and Cohen, K. S. Techniques to improve the seating of castings. J. Am. Dent. Assoc. 96:432, 1978.
28. Kent, W. A., Shillingburg, H. T., and Duncanson, M. G. A clinical study of preparations for cast restorations. I. Taper. Quint. Int. (in press).
29. Weed, R. M. Determining adequate crown convergence. Dent. J., 98:14, 1980.
30. Dodge, W. W., Weed, R. M., Baez, R. J. and Buchanan, R. N. The effect of convergence angle on retention and resistance form. Quint. Int. 16:191, 1985.
31. Kaufman, E. G., Coelho, D. H., and Colin, L. Factors influencing the retention of cemented gold castings. J. Prosthet. Dent. 11:487, 1961.

32. Gilboe, D. B., and Teteruck, W. R. Fundamentals of extracoronal tooth preparation. I. Retention and resistance form. J. Prosthet. Dent. 32:651, 1974.

33. Douglass, G. D. Principles of preparation design in fixed prosthodontics. Gen. Dent. 21:25, 1973.

34. Mahler, D. B., and Terkla, L. G. Analysis of stress in dental structures. Dent. Clin. North Am. 2:789, 1958.

35. Rosenstiel, E. The retention of inlays and crowns as a function of geometrical form. Br. Dent. J. 103:388, 1957.

36. Shillingburg, H. T., and Fisher, D. W. The partial veneer restoration. Aust. Dent. J. 17:411, 1972.

37. Danielson, G. L. Stress analysis related to tooth preparation and fixed partial denture design. J. South. Calif. Dent. Assoc. 40:928, 1972.

38. Collett, H. A. Cast shell veneer crowns. J. Prosthet. Dent. 25:177, 1971.

39. Smith, B. G. N. The effect of the surface roughness of prepared dentin on the retention of castings. J. Prosthet. Dent. 23:187, 1970.

40. Bodecker, H. W. C. The Metallic Inlay. New York: William R. Jenkins Co., 1911.

41. Smyd, E. S. Dental engineering applied to inlay and fixed bridge fabrication. J. Prosthet. Dent. 2:536, 1952.

42. Hegdahl, T., and Silness, J. Preparation areas resisting displacement of artificial crowns. J. Oral Rehabil. 4:201, 1977.

43. Smyd, E. S. The role of torque, torsion, and bending in prosthetic failures. J. Prosthet. Dent. 11:95, 1961.

44. Shillingburg, H. T. Conservative preparations for cast restorations. Dent. Clin. North Am. 20:259, 1976.

45. Craig, R. C., El-Ebrashi, M. K., and Peyton, F. A. Experimental stress analysis of dental restorations. II. Two-dimensional photoelastic stress analysis of crowns. J. Prosthet. Dent. 17:292, 1967.

46. El-Ebrashi, M. K., Craig, R. C., and Peyton, F. A. Experimental stress analysis of dental restorations. V. The concept of occlusal reduction and pins. J. Prosthet. Dent. 22:565, 1969.

47. Nicholls, J. I. Crown retention. I. Stress analysis of symmetric restorations. J. Prosthet. Dent. 31:179, 1974.

48. Tjan, A. H., and Miller, G. D. Common errors in tooth preparation. Gen. Dent. 28:20, 1980.

49. Morris, M. L. Artificial crown contours and gingival health. J. Prosthet. Dent. 12:1146, 1962.

50. Stein, R. S., and Kuwata, M. A dentist and a dental technologist analyze current ceramo-metal procedures. Dent. Clin. North Am. 21:729, 1977.

51. Higdon, S. J. Tooth preparation for optimum contour of full coverage restorations. Gen. Dent. 26:47, 1978.

52. Lustig, L. P. A rational concept of crown preparation revised and expanded. Quint. Int. 7:41, 1976.

53. Perel, M. L. Axial crown contours. J. Prosthet. Dent. 25:642, 1971.

54. Carmichael, J. P. Attachment for inlay and bridgework. Dent. Rev. 15:82, 1901.

55. Rhoads, J. E. Preparation of the teeth for cast restorations. pp. 34–67 In G. M. Hollenback, Science and Technic of the Cast Restoration. St. Louis: The C. V. Mosby Co., 1964.

56. Willey, R. E. The preparation of abutments for veneer preparations. J. Am. Dent. Assoc. 53:141, 1956.

57. Ingraham, R., Bassett, R. W., and Koser, J. R. An Atlas of Cast Gold Procedures. 2nd ed. Buena Park, CA: Unitro College Press, 1969, 161–165.

Chapter 2

Finish Lines and the Periodontium

There are three requirements for successful restoration margins: *(1)* they must fit as closely as possible against the finish line of the preparation to minimize the width of exposed cement; *(2)* they must have sufficient strength to withstand the forces of mastication; and *(3)* whenever possible, they should be located in areas where the dentist can finish and inspect them, and the patient can clean them.

A properly tapered preparation is essential for close-fitting margins. There can be no undercuts or irregularities on the axial walls that will prevent complete seating or cause the margins to spread as the restoration is being inserted. Roughness of the tooth surface under margins can prevent close adaptation,[1,2] therefore all bevels and flares should be given a smooth finish line with as fine an instrument as will fit into the area being finished. Fine discs and carbide burs are preferred.[3]

Historically, the bevel was used as a device for compensating for the solidification shrinking of alloys used in fabricating cast restorations.[4]

Metal margins should be acute in cross-section rather than right-angled to facilitate a closer fit. [2,3,5–12] To accomplish this, preparation finish lines should take forms that permit acute edges in the restoration margins.

Even the best crowns fail to seat completely by several microns (Fig. 2-1). If the prepared surface that is adjacent to a finish line is perpendicular to the path of insertion, as a shoulder is, the marginal gap, *d*, will be as great as the distance by which the crown fails to seat, *D*. However, if the inner surface of the metal margin forms an angle, *m*, of less than 90 degrees with the path of insertion, as does a bevel or a chamfer, *d* will be smaller than *D*.

The shortest distance from the casting margin to tooth structure, *d*, can be stated as a function of *D* and the sine of the angle *m* or the cosine of angle *p*, which is the angle between the surface of the bevel and the path of insertion $(180 - m)$:

$$d = D \sin m, \text{ or}$$
$$d = D \cos p.$$

As the angle *m* is reduced, its sine becomes smaller (Table 2-1), and so does *d*.[8] The more obtuse the angle of tooth structure at a horizontal finish line, and therefore, the more acute the restoration margin, the shorter the distance between the restoration margin and the tooth. Obviously the margin angle must become quite acute before the actual distance is diminished to a great extent (Fig. 2-2). An angle of 30 to 45 degrees is considered optimal.[2,13] If it is made much more acute it becomes weak. An acute edge of some kinds of alloys can

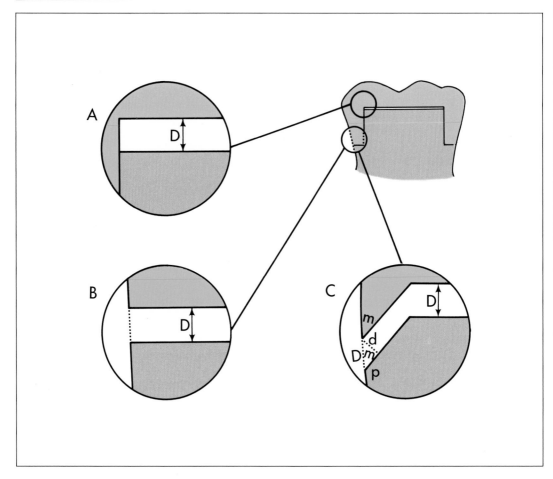

Fig. 2-1 A bevel allows closer approximation of a crown margin to the tooth. The distance, *D*, by which a crown fails to seat *(A)*, is reflected in the marginal opening, *d*, in a butt joint *(B)*. However, in the presence of a bevel, the shortest distance from the margin to tooth structure is less than *D* and is a function of the sine of the acute angle of the margin, *m*, or of the cosine of the obtuse angle of the finish line, *p (C)*.

Table 2-1 Sines and cosines for various angles

Function	Angle (degrees)						
	0	15	30	45	60	75	90
Sine	0	0.259	0.500	0.707	0.866	0.966	1.000
Cosine	1.000	0.966	0.866	0.707	0.500	0.259	0

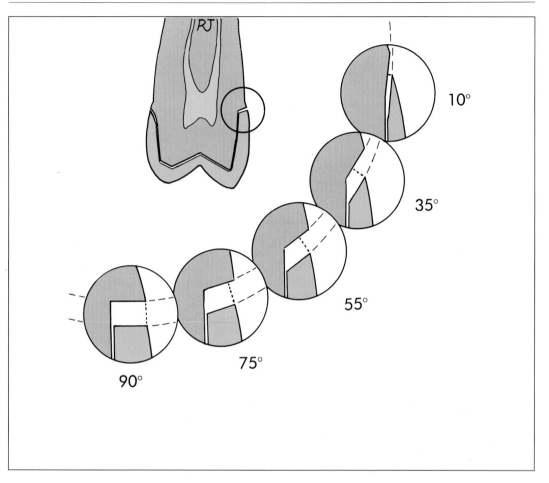

Fig. 2-2   The smaller the angle between the prepared tooth surface at the finish line and the path of insertion, the less the marginal opening for the same amount of incomplete seating. The width of the marginal opening for selected angles is given as a percentage of the distance by which the restoration fails to seat. For angles greater than 50 degrees the reduction is not significant. Angles of less than 25 degrees may produce a margin that is too thin and weak.

also be burnished against the tooth to further improve marginal fit.[10,14]

McLean and Wilson refute the superiority of bevels where a ceramic veneer is employed. They state that the margin must reach an angle of 10 to 20 degrees before it can fulfill its intended role.[15] While the bevel's use can enhance the fit of a metal margin, how-

ever minimally, the deep subgingival extensions required for its use with a ceramic veneer are unacceptable. Pascoe found oversize castings with bevels had greater marginal discrepancies than those with shoulders.[16] Pardo, on the other hand, advocated differentially oversized castings (created with die relief short of the finish lines) with

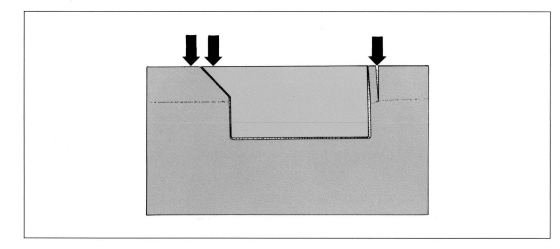

Fig. 2-3 Impacts striking enamel next to a bevel can be withstood without damage *(left)*. Where there is no bevel, however, the unprotected enamel rods near the restoration can be more easily fractured *(right)*.

Fig. 2-4 Without a bevel, the preparation would have an acute edge of unsupported enamel *(A)*. Occlusal forces can deform the thin overlying gold sufficiently to fracture the brittle enamel *(B)*. The margin can be strengthened by placing a simple finishing bevel *(C)* or, if the esthetic situation allows, a contrabevel *(D)*. If the inclination of the occlusal surface is relatively flat, the cavosurface angle may be so obtuse that a bevel for strength is unnecessary *(E)* (After Ingraham [53]).

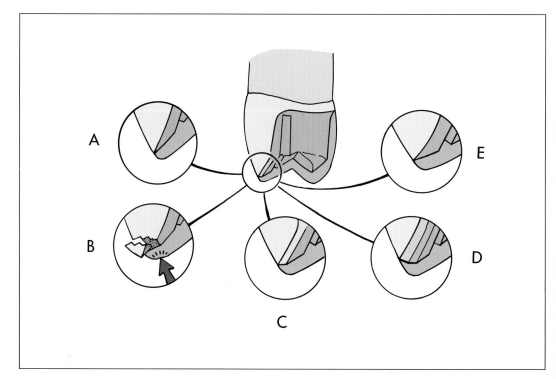

bevels.[17] Gavelis et al. found that knife-edge margins produced the best seal, while shoulders allowed the most complete seating of any of the margin configurations they tested.[18]

To impart strength and rigidity to a margin, there should be a nearby bulk of metal. This can be provided by an occlusal offset or shoulder, an isthmus, a vertical groove, a box, or a gingival shoulder. Bulk is an integral part of the chamfer margin.

Occlusal bevels

Margins must always be placed at least 1.0 mm away from centric occlusal contacts to avoid distortion of the margin or fracture of the adjoining enamel.[19] The cavosurface line angles of the preparation in the occlusal portion of the tooth should be finished with a bevel to avoid a right angle "butt joint" which would leave a brittle, easily fractured edge of tooth structure. The acute edge of metal and obtuse angle of enamel created by a bevel can withstand impacts much better than can a square edge of enamel (Fig. 2-3).

The bevel used as the occlusal finish line of maxillary MOD onlays and partial veneer crowns provides a combination of tooth protection, casting reinforcement, and margin finishibility (Fig. 2-4). It meets the requirement of having an acute edge with a nearby bulk of metal. A thin extension of metal over a cusp is made more rigid with only a small addition of bulk by placing a bevel at an angle to the inclined plane of the cusp. This effect can be demonstrated by placing creases near the edges of a sheet of paper. The creased paper can be held horizontally by one edge, whereas an uncreased paper will bend under its own weight.

Flares

The vertical finish line of the inlay, onlay, or partial veneer crown preparation is finished with a flare, which forms an acute edge of metal in the casting and extends it into an accessible area. A flare differs from a bevel in that a flare is a geometric plane inclined slightly to the path of insertion (Fig. 2-5, A), and cutting through the contour of the tooth. A bevel, on the other hand, follows the contour of the tooth and should be used only on finish lines that are more or less perpendicular to the path of insertion. A bevel placed on a vertical finish line would inevitably produce undercuts because of the convexity of the tooth (Fig. 2-5, B).

On mesial surfaces that are easily visible, the flare should extend just far enough toward the facial surface to be reached by the tip of an explorer. In less visible areas, it can extend farther onto the facial or lingual surfaces.

The planes of two facial flares on the same tooth should lean toward each other and converge toward a point somewhat facial to the tooth. The planes of lingual flares should likewise converge lingual to the tooth (Fig. 2-6). A flare with the proper inclination will be narrow near the gingival finish line, becoming wider toward the occlusal surface. It should be cut equally at the expense of the external axial tooth sur-

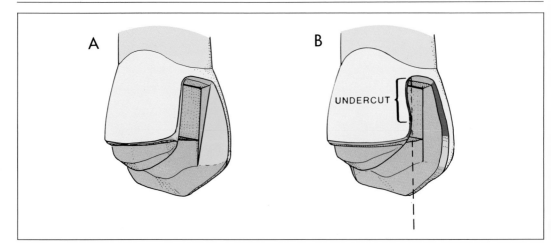

Fig. 2-5 A properly formed flare is a flat plane that cuts through the tooth at an acute angle *(A)*. Incorrect use of a bevel in place of a flare on vertical finish lines will produce undesirable undercuts because of the natural contours of the tooth *(B)*.

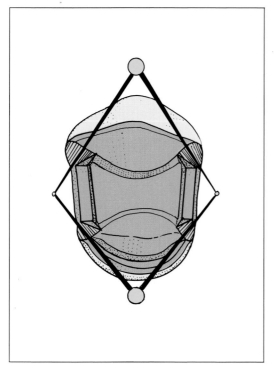

Fig. 2-6 The planes of two facial flares should intersect slightly facial to the path of insertion and well above the occlusal surface. The planes of the lingual flares should intersect lingual to the path of insertion. In this occlusal view, the heavy lines are projections of lines drawn along the lengths of properly placed flares.

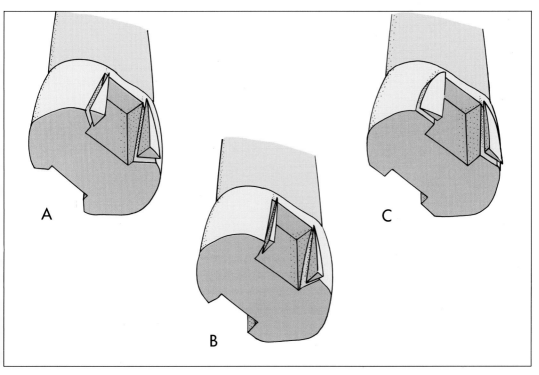

Fig. 2-7 Flares are properly formed by removing equal amounts of tooth structure from the walls of a box or groove and from the outer surface of the tooth *(A)*. Flares cut more at the expense of internal tooth structure will be too nearly parallel with the walls of the box *(B)*, resulting in margins that are not sufficiently acute, and probably underextended as well. Flares cut too much at the expense of the outer tooth surface are too flat *(C)*. The resulting margins will be thin, weak, and possibly overextended, and undercut gingivally as well.

face and the wall of the adjoining box or groove (Fig. 2-7, *A*). If the flare is cut too much from the wall of the box or the groove, the margin of the restoration will meet the finish line of the preparation in a butt joint and will not extend far enough buccally or lingually for access (Fig. 2-7, *B*). If, on the other hand, it is cut too much at the expense of the outer axial surface of the tooth, the margin of the restoration will be thin and weak (Fig. 2-7, *C*).

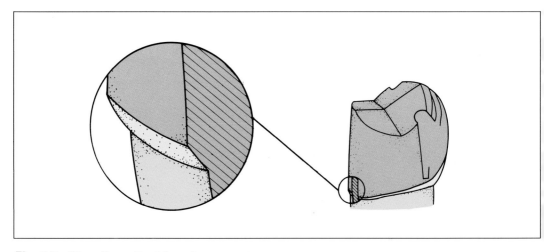

Fig. 2-8 When the path of insertion must deviate markedly from the long axis of a tooth, a knife-edge finish line is indicated on the axial wall toward which the tooth is tipped. Formation of a shoulder or a chamfer here would necessitate removal of too much tooth structure, and the enamel at the finish line would be very fragile.

Gingival finish lines

The more commonly used forms of gingival finish lines are the knife-edge, the shoulder, the beveled shoulder, and the chamfer. The knife-edge finish line was popular before the development of high-speed cutting instruments and accurate impression materials. It is still used on tipped teeth where the axial surface of the tooth meets the path of insertion at an angle greater than 15 degrees (Fig. 2-8). Not only will it produce a distinct finish line in this situation with less destruction of tooth structure than is necessary for a shoulder or a chamfer, but it does not leave a fragile lip of unsupported enamel such as that which can result from using one of those finish lines on an inclined surface.

Because the cut surface is more nearly parallel with the path of insertion, the knife-edge finish line produces the best marginal seal.[18] For most situations, however, the knife-edge finish line is not recommended because it is difficult to follow on both tooth and die. Although it produces a good fit, the margin is weak.[20] The most likely result of this type of finish line is overcontouring.[21,22]

In contrast, the shoulder is a distinct finish line and provides an adequate bulk of material at the margin (Fig. 2-9). However, it does not have the recommended acute edge of metal and can leave a fragile, unprotected edge of tooth structure. This finish line is recommended for porcelain restorations only.

The beveled shoulder is recommended for extremely short walls, since it permits that critical portion of the axial walls just coronal to the finish line to be formed nearly parallel with the path of insertion (Fig. 2-10). These nearly parallel walls enhance retention, while providing adequate reduction to prevent overcontouring.[23] A 0.3 to 0.5 mm bevel

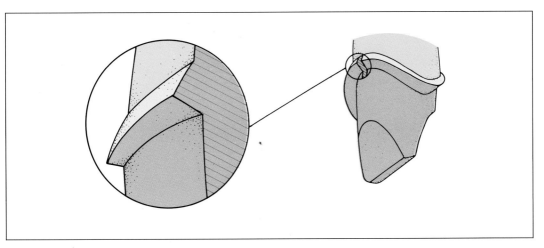

Fig. 2-9 An ordinary shoulder is indicated where the margin of the restoration will be formed of porcelain. Porcelain fractures too easily when it terminates in an acute edge.

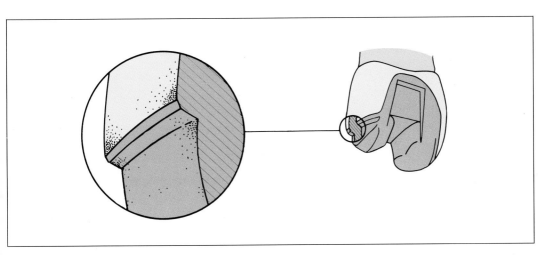

Fig. 2-10 A shoulder with a bevel can be used on short axial walls to create maximum retention and resistance form. A chamfer here would leave the greater part of the wall overtapered. The bevel allows an acute edge of metal in the margin.

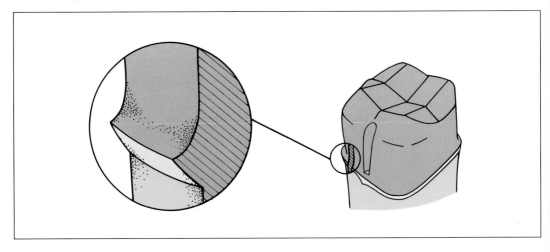

Fig. 2-11 In the majority of instances the chamfer best fulfills the requirements of a finish line for metal restorations. It allows an acute edge of metal with a nearby bulk, and it minimizes stress in the cement film.

is placed to form the recommended obtuse finish line, which, in turn, will accommodate an acute restoration margin. The beveled shoulder can also be used for porcelain-fused-to-metal restorations in areas of the mouth where a small metal collar will not be cosmetically offensive, or where a shoulder results from removal of caries or an existing restoration.

The chamfer is widely regarded as the gingival finish line of choice for most veneer cast metal restorations (Fig. 2-11).[20,21,24–29] It makes possible the desired acute margin of metal with sufficient thickness for strength. The rounded concavity produces lower stress concentrations within the cement film than does the sharp internal angle of a shoulder.[30,31] It can be formed easily using a sharp-nosed, torpedo diamond and carbide bur.[22,32] These instruments produce lines that are easily discernible on both tooth and die.

Preservation of the periodontium

While the location of preparation finish lines is governed by all of the principles of preparations previously discussed, the single most important factor is the preservation of the periodontium. Traditionally, gingival margins have been placed subgingivally. This concept originally grew from a mistaken belief that the gingival sulcus represented a caries-free zone. In 1891 G. V. Black stated, "Decay does not occur at . . . margins as long as they are covered by reasonably healthy gum tissue."[33] As a result, the recommended position has ranged from just below the gingival crest[26,34] to halfway into the sulcus,[35] and, in some cases, almost to the epithelial attachment.[36]

However, numerous clinicians and investigators have observed a correlation between subgingival margins and gingival inflammation or periodontitis.[37–44] Larato found gingival inflammation around 83% of 219 crowns with subgingival margins, but adjacent to only 21% or 327 crowns whose margins were flush with or above the gingiva.[45] In a subsequent study he found pockets in proximity to subgingival margins that had a mean depth 0.7 mm greater than those around unrestored teeth.[46] The mechanism by which subgingival margins cause periodontal damage appears to be direct irritation and plaque retention.[47] Lang found an increase in Gram-negative bacteria in the sulcus in association with subgingival margins, representing a disturbance in the ecological balance within this microcosm.[48]

Not too surprisingly, several studies have determined that the deeper the restoration margin extends into the gingival sulcus, the more severe the inflammatory response.[49–52] Silness, comparing the lingual surfaces of 385 abutment teeth with contralateral unrestored teeth, found the greatest inflammation surrounding subgingival margins, with less around crowns with margins even with the tissue. There were no significant differences in gingival health between teeth with supragingival margins and unrestored control teeth.[53] These findings are somewhat at variance with an experimental study by Marcum, which indicated that margins even with the gingival crest produced less inflammation than either subgingival or supragingival margins.[54]

Richter and Ueno found no difference in gingival response to subgingival or supragingival margins and concluded that fit and finish of margins are more important than their location. Nonetheless, they recommended that margins be placed supragingivally.[55] Koth reported no relationship between margin location and gingival health in a careful-ly selected population of patients on a strict oral hygiene and recall regimen.[56] These studies do not refute the abundant evidence linking margin placement with gingival inflammation. They do show that location is not as critical when a skillful operator places well-fitting margins in the mouth of a motivated, cooperative patient.

It is important to remember that subgingival margins can be difficult to evaluate. Christensen demonstrated that experienced restorative dentists could miss marginal defects as great as 120 μm when the margins were subgingival.[57] In a study of 225 full-mouth sets of radiographs, Bjorn et al. found that 83% of the proximal margins on gold crowns and 74% of the proximal margins on porcelain crowns were defective! Of the defects on gold crowns, 68% were greater than 0.2 mm, while 57% of the porcelain defects exceeded 0.3 mm.[58]

The weight of evidence makes the practice of routinely placing margins subgingivally no longer acceptable. Margins of cast restorations should be placed supragingivally whenever possible.[59–67] There will often be occasions when subgingival margins are unavoidable. Schöler has estimated, that in spite of the desirability of supragingival margins, subgingival margins are necessary in over 50% of the crowns placed.[5] Among the legitimate reasons for extending margins subgingivally are existing caries,[27,32,44,65,67–69] extensions of previous restorations,[27,32,44,65,67,69] retention,[27,32,44,65,67–70] esthetics,[27,44,59,65,67–69,71] subgingival tooth fracture,[45,65] and root sensitivity.[32,67]

A crown margin should not be placed any closer than 2.0 mm away from the alveolar crest, or bone resorption will occur.[72] The combined width of the epithelial and connective tissue attach-

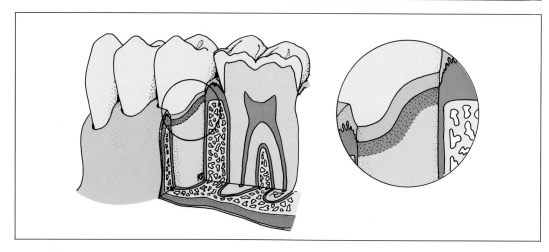

Fig. 2-12 The distance from the epithelial attachment to the crest of the alveolar bone has been described as the "biologic width." It is normally about 2.0 mm wide, including the epithelial attachment and the connective tissue attachment.

ments is normally about 2.0 mm (Fig. 2-12).[73] If the margin intrudes into this "biological width," inflammation will result (Fig. 2-13), and the bone will recede until it is once again at least 2.0 mm from the crown margin (Fig. 2-14). This can result in an interproximal cul de sac or an infrabony pocket that would be impossible to maintain in a healthy state.

When conditions dictate that a margin be placed at or near the level of the alveolar crest, periodontal surgery may be required to maintain correct con-tours. Care must be taken that the surgery itself does not cause other problems through the excessive loss of attached gingiva or bone support for the adjacent teeth. Another approach is the forcible eruption of the tooth before restoration.[72] Either solution will result in a less favorable crown/root ratio. If restoring a tooth with extensive subgingival damage would jeopardize the health of adjacent teeth, it might be preferable to extract the tooth and replace it with a fixed bridge.

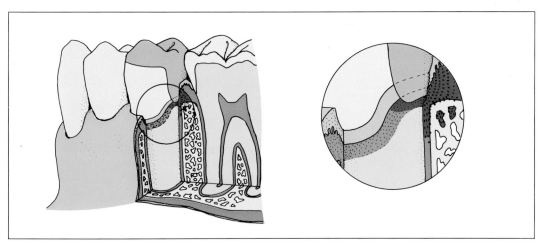

Fig. 2-13 When the margin of a restoration intrudes into the biologic width, inflammation and osteo clastic activity are stimulated.

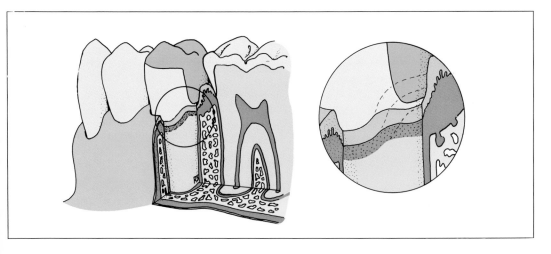

Fig. 2-14 Bone resorption will continue until the alveolar crest is at least 2.0 mm from the restoration margin. The best outcome that can be expected is that the epithelial and connective tissue attachments will reestablish themselves at a more apical level. Continued inflammation with pocket formation is likely.

References

1. Charbeneau, G. T., and Peyton, F. A. Some effects of cavity instrumentation on the adaptation of gold castings and amalgam. J. Prosthet. Dent. 8:514, 1958.
2. Kashani, H. G., Khera, S. C., and Gulker, I. A. The effects of bevel angulation on marginal integrity. J. Am. Dent. Assoc. 103:882, 1981.
3. Barkmeier, W. W., Kelsey, W. P., Blankenau, R. J., and Peterson, D. S. Enamel cavosurface bevels finished with ultraspeed instruments. J. Prosthet. Dent. 49:481, 1983.
4. Rosenstiel, E. To bevel or not to bevel. Br. Dent. J. 138:389,1975.
5. Schöler, A. Ueberlegungen, Analysen and Praktische Erkenthisse zur Kronenstumpfpräparation (II). Die Quint. 31:47–53, 1980.
6. Gillett, H. W., and Irving, A. J. Gold Inlays by the Indirect System. Brooklyn: Dental Items of Interest Publ. Co., 1932, 22–37.
7. Bassett, R. W. How we can improve our operative dentistry. J. Prosthet. Dent. 3:542, 1953.
8. Rosner, D. Function, placement and reproduction of bevels for gold castings. J. Prosthet. Dent. 13:1160, 1963.
9. Mahler, D. B., and Terkla, L. G. Relationship of cavity design to restorative materials. Dent. Clin. North Am. 9:149, 1965.
10. Eames, W. B., and Little, R. M. Movement of gold at cavosurface margins with finishing instruments. J. Am. Dent. Assoc. 75:147, 1967.
11. Barnes, I. E. The production of inlay cavity bevels. Br. Dent. J. 137:379, 1974.
12. Metzler, J. C., and Chandler, H. H. An evaluation of techniques for finishing margins of gold inlays. J. Prosthet. Dent. 36:523, 1976.
13. Rosenstiel, E. The marginal fit of inlays and crowns. Br. Dent. J. 117:432, 1964.
14. Kishimoto, M., Hobo, S., Shillingburg, H. T., and Duncanson, M. G. Effectiveness of margin finishing techniques on cast gold restorations. Int. J. Periodont. Rest. Dent. 1(5):21, 1981.
15. McLean, J. W. and Wilson, A. D. Butt joint versus bevelled gold margin in metal ceramic crowns. J. Biomed. Mater. Res. 14:239, 1980.
16. Pascoe, D. F. Analysis of the geometry of finishing lines for full crown restorations. J. Prosthet. Dent. 40:151, 1978.
17. Pardo, G. I. A full cast restoration design offering superior marginal characteristics. J. Prosthet. Dent. 48:539, 1982.
18. Gavelis, J. R., Morency, J. D., Riley, E. D., and Sozio, R. B. The effect of various finish line preparations on the marginal seal and occlusal seat of full crown preparations. J. Prosthet. Dent. 45:138, 1981.
19. Willey, R. E. The preparation of abutments for veneer preparations. J. Am. Dent. Assoc. 53:141, 1956.
20. Guyer, S. E. Multiple preparations for fixed prosthodontics. J. Prosthet. Dent. 23:529, 1970.
21. Higdon, S. J. Tooth preparation for optimum contour of full coverage restorations. Gen. Dent. 26:47, 1978.
22. Lustig, L. P. A rational concept of crown preparation revised and expanded. Quint. Int. 7:41, 1976.
23. Gage, J. P. Rationale for bevelled shoulder veneer crown preparations. Aust. Dent. J. 22:432, 1977.
24. Douglass, G. D. Principles of preparation design in fixed prosthodontics. Gen. Dent. 21:25, 1973.
25. Danielson, G. L. Stress analysis related to tooth preparation and fixed partial denture design. J. South. Calif. Dent. Assoc. 40:928, 1972.
26. Herlands, R. E., Lucca, J. J., and Morris, M. L. Forms, contours and extensions of full coverage restorations in occlusal reconstruction. Dent. Clin. North Am. 6:147, 1962.
27. Mount, G. J. Crowns and the gingival tissue. Aust. Dent. J. 15:253, 1970.
28. Rogers, E. T. The partial veneer crown: Preparation, construction and application. Dent. Items Interest 50:397, 1928.
29. Thom, L. W. Principles of cavity preparation in crown and bridge prostheses. I. The full crown. J. Am. Dent. Assoc. 41:284, 1950.
30. El-Ebrashi, M. K., Craig, R. G., and Peyton, F. A. Experimental stress analysis of dental restorations. III. The concept of the geometry of proximal margins. J. Prosthet. Dent. 22:333, 1969.
31. Farah, J. W., and Craig, R. G. Stress analysis of three margin configurations of full posterior crowns by three-dimensional photoelasticity. J. Dent. Res. 53:1219, 1974.

32. Ingraham, R., Sochat, P., and Hausing, F. J. Rotary gingival curettage—A new technique for tooth preparation and management of the gingival sulcus for impression taking. Int. J. Periodont. Rest. Dent. 1(4):9, 1981.
33. Black, G. V. The management of enamel margins. Dent. Cosmos 33:85, 1891.
34. Smith, G. P. Full crown preparation. N. Y. J. Dent. 26:307, 1956.
35. Minker, J. S. Simplified full coverage preparations. Dent. Clin. North Am. 9:355, 1965.
36. Abrahams, E. J. Combination shoulder-feather edge veneer crown preparation. J. Prosthet. Dent. 13:901, 1963.
37 Waerhaug, J. Tissue reactions around artificial crowns. J. Periodontol. 24:172, 1953.
38. Weinberg, L. A. Esthetics and the gingivae in full coverage. J. Prosthet. Dent. 10:737, 1960.
39. Alexander, A. G. Periodontal aspects of conservative dentistry. Br. Dent. J. 125:111, 1963.
40. Silness, J. Periodontal conditions in patients treated with dental bridges. J. Periodont. Res. 5:60, 1970.
41. Mormann, W., Regolati, B., and Renggli, H. H. Gingival reaction to well-fitted subgingival proximal gold inlays. J. Clin. Periodontol. 1:120, 1974.
42. Janenko, C., and Smales, R. J. Anterior crowns and gingival health. Aust. Dent. J. 24:225, 1979.
43. Romanelli, J. H. Periodontal considerations in tooth preparation for crowns and bridges. Dent. Clin. North Am. 24:271, 1980.
44. Wilson, R. D. Intracrevicular restorative dentistry. Int. J. Periodont. Rest. Dent. 1(4):35, 1981.
45. Larato, D. C. Effect of cervical margins on gingiva. J. Calif. Dent. Assoc. 45:19, 1969.
46. Larato, D. C. Effects of artificial crown margin extension and tooth brushing frequency on gingival pocket depth. J. Prosthet. Dent. 34:640, 1975.
47. Loe, H. Reactions of marginal periodontal tissues to restorative procedures. Int. Dent. J. 18:759, 1968.
48. Lang, N. P., Kiel, R. A., and Anderhalden, K. Clinical and microbiological effects of subgingival restorations with overhanging or clinically perfect margins. J. Clin. Periodontol. 10:563, 1983.
49. Silness, J. Fixed prosthodontics and periodontal health. Dent. Clin. North Am. 24:317, 1980.
50. Karlsen, K. Gingival reactions to dental restorations. Acta Odontol. Scand. 28:895, 1970.
51. Newcomb, G. M. The relationship between the location of subgingival crown margins and gingival inflammation. J. Periodontol. 45:151, 1974.
52. Jameson, L. M., and Malone, W. F. P. Crown contours and gingival response. J. Prosthet. Dent. 47:620, 1982.
53. Silness, J. Periodontal conditions in patients treated with dental bridges. III. The relationship between the location of the crown margin and the periodontal condition. J. Periodont. Res. 5:225, 1970.
54. Marcum, J. J. The effect of crown marginal depth upon gingival tissue. J. Prosthet. Dent. 17:479, 1967.
55. Richter, W. A., and Ueno, H. Relationship of crown margin placement to gingival inflammation. J. Prosthet. Dent. 30:156, 1973.
56. Koth, D. L. Full crown restorations and gingival inflammation in a controlled population. J. Prosthet. Dent. 48:681, 1982.
57. Christensen, G. J. Marginal fit of gold inlay castings. J. Prosthet. Dent. 16:297, 1966.
58. Bjorn, A. L., Bjorn, H., and Grkovic, B. Marginal fit of restorations and its relation to periodontal bone level. II. Crowns. Odontol. Rev. 21:337, 1970.
59. Tjan, A. H., and Miller, G. D. Common errors in tooth preparation. Gen. Dent. 28:20, 1980.
60. Selberg, A. Cast gold crowns. J. Tenn. State Dent. Assoc. 29:21, 1949.
61. Karlstrom, G. Parallel pins and fixed partial dentures. J. Prosthet. Dent. 19:613, 1968.
62. Silness, J. Periodontal conditions in patients treated with dental bridges. II. The influence of full and partial crowns on plaque accumulation, development of gingivitis and pocket formation. J. Periodont. Res. 5:219, 1970.
63. Eissmann, H. F., Radke, R. A., and Noble, W. H. Physiologic design criteria for fixed dental restorations. Dent. Clin. North Am. 15:543, 1971.
64. Grosso, F. P., and Carreno, J. A. Partial or full coverage restorations: A survey of prevailing criteria. J. Prosthet. Dent. 40:628, 1978.
65. Becker, C. M., and Kaldahl, W. B. Current theories of crown contour, margin placement, and pontic design. J. Prosthet. Dent. 45:268, 1981.
66. Behrand, D. A. Ceramometal restorations with supragingival margins. J. Prosthet. Dent. 47:625, 1982.
67. Nevins, M., and Skurow, H. M. The intracrevicular restorative margin, the biologic width, and the maintenance of the gingival margin. Int. J. Periodont. Rest. Dent. 4(3):31, 1984.
68. Berman, M. H. The complete coverage restoration and the gingival sulcus. J. Prosthet. Dent. 29:301, 1973.
69. Gardner, F. M. Margins of complete crowns—Literature review. J. Prosthet. Dent. 48:396, 1982.
70. Stein, R. S., and Kuwata, M. A dentist and a dental technologist analyze current ceramo-metal procedures. Dent. Clin. North Am. 21:729, 1977.
71. Goldstein, R. E. Esthetics in Dentistry. Philadelphia: J. B. Lippincott Co., 1976, 804.
72. Ingber, J. S., Rose, L. F., and Coslet, J. G. The "biologic width"—A concept in periodontics and restorative dentistry. Alpha Omegan 10:62, 1977.
73. Garguilo, A. W., Wentz, F. M., and Orban, B. Dimensions of the dentogingival junction in humans. J. Periodontol. 32:261, 1961.

Chapter 3

Instrumentation

Tooth preparations for cast restorations have been influenced, at least in part, by the technology of instrumentation. This is seen in the development of handpieces and power sources as well as in the evolution of abrasives and cutting instruments. Singer and Howe's sewing machine is credited with stimulating Morrison to develop the first dental foot engine.[1] The adaptation of electric motors for powering dental instruments was the only major advance made in equipment for preparing teeth during the first four decades of the 20th century.

Significant changes began to occur at about the time of World War II. Among these were the development of diamond cutting instruments in Germany in the late 1930s and the introduction of carbide burs in 1947.[1] A milestone in the history of restorative dentistry was the increase of handpiece speeds in the late 1950s, as first the belt-driven handpieces were improved, and then the air turbine handpieces were introduced.

Prior to that time, instruments that rotated at speeds of less than 12,000 rpm were in general use. Tooth preparation was laborious for the dentist and uncomfortable for the patient. To achieve sufficient surface speed for effective cutting, large diameter diamond stones, wheels, and disks were used for bulk removal of enamel and dentin. These instruments influenced the design of preparations; slice preparations with knife-edge finish lines and overextended flares were popular. Inlay and onlay preparations confined largely to existing cavities were frequently used as abutment preparations for bridge retainers.

The advent of handpieces capable of speeds in excess of 100,000 rpm made possible efficient cutting with smaller instruments, which in turn made more sophisticated preparation designs practical. It also made removal of sound enamel much easier than ever before. Unfortunately, some dentists greeted the new technology more as a way to increase their productivity than as a means of producing higher quality conservative preparations, and more destructive preparation designs gained in popularity.

Water-air cooling

With high-speed instrumentation, the problem of overheating the tooth during preparation is critical. Cutting dry at high speeds will produce nearly three times as much dentinal burning as cutting with a water spray,[2] and thermal changes can result in pulpal inflammation[3] or necrosis.[4]

Brown et al. calculated the temperature of dentin at a distance of 0.5 mm from a high-speed bur cutting dry to be 245°F (118°C).[5] In light of this, Zach's contention that a temperature rise of only 20°F will lead to pulpal death in 60% of teeth is most serious indeed.[6] Even in nonvital teeth, dry cutting at high speeds should be avoided, since the thermal stresses will cause microfractures in the enamel. This could contribute to marginal failure of the restoration at some future time.[5]

The use of air alone as a coolant is harmful to the pulp,[7] and is therefore not an acceptable substitute for a water-air spray. Prolonged dehydration of freshly cut dentin will increase pulpal damage,[8] producing odontoblastic displacement.[4] To minimize pulpal trauma, a water spray should always be used when cutting a tooth preparation at high speeds.[9–18]

The use of a water spray does not in itself guarantee that the pulp will be protected from damage. A low quantity of water, poorly directed, will result in a weak spray that can permit localized dentinal scorching.[4] A small orifice that produces a higher water velocity is more likely to allow penetration of the air vortex around the instrument tip.[18]

A water spray also increases the efficiency of high-speed rotary instruments by keeping the cutting edges washed clean of debris. Eames et al. found that a greater flow of water coolant is required to prevent clogging when diamonds are used under increased pressure.[19] Diamond stones used under heavy pressure (150 g) became more effective as the water flow rate increased from 3 to 21 ml/min. If light pressure (50 g) was used, there was still an increase in effectiveness, but it leveled off after the flow rate reached 7 ml/min.

Novices often dislike using water spray because they feel it interferes with their vision—probably a holdover from dental school exercises on dry tooth models. Actually, the spray enhances visibility in many instances by flushing away blood and debris. Even indirect vision can be utilized while cutting wet, if the mirror is first coated with a film of detergent. This allows the water to form a smooth transparent film on the surface of the mirror with only a moderate decrease in visibility.

Most patients will not object to the flow of water if proper suction and patient position are utilized. From the patient's point of view, a little water in the mouth is undoubtedly less objectionable than the "burnt chicken feathers" odor of scorched dentin anyway.

Armamentarium

Based on their mode of operation, the rotary instruments commonly used for tooth preparation can be classified in one of three categories: stones, burs, and drills (Fig. 3-1). Stones remove tooth structure by abrading, or wearing away, the surface. The most efficient abrasive for removing tooth structure is the diamond chip.[20] Burs are miniature milling cutters with blades that shear tooth structure from the tooth surface, cutting primarily on the sides of the instrument. Twist drills, with cutting edges on their tips, are used for boring small-diameter holes in tooth structure. They are the least frequently used of the rotary instruments.

The preparation of teeth for cast metal and porcelain restorations does not demand an extensive armamentarium. In fact, it is important that the novice learn to perform the task with the smallest number of instruments possible. Otherwise, considerable time can be

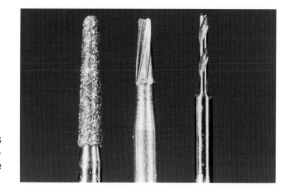

Fig. 3-1 The three types of rotary instruments used in tooth preparation are, left to right: the diamond stone, the tungsten carbide bur, and the twist drill.

lost in trying many instruments that are either unsuited for the job or very similar to ones already tried. The inexperienced operator may switch instruments needlessly to find the "right one," when what is really needed is mastering the skills to use the instrument already in the handpiece.

Diamond stones

Numerous small, irregularly shaped, sharp-edged diamond chips are electroplated with a nickel or chromium bonding medium to steel instrument blanks whose heads have been machined to the desired shapes of the final instruments.[21] Each chip cuts away a minute quantity of tooth structure. Rotary diamond instruments are made in an ever growing array of sizes, shapes, and grits. They are most effective for removing enamel and for cutting through porcelain. Eames et al. found that they cut tooth structure two to three times as quickly as burs.[19] They are deposited in one to three layers on the surface of the instrument. The best diamond stones have abrasive particles evenly spaced over the surface of the instrument.[22]

There also should be intimate contact between the chips and the binding material.

In addition to being described by the configuration and size of the blank on which the diamond abrasive particles are deposited, diamond rotary instruments are also classified by the size or coarseness of the grains with which they are coated. The actual size of the chips used for any given class, such as "regular," will vary somewhat from manufacturer to manufacturer. The particle size used by four major U. S. dental firms are compared by both U. S. Mesh-Standard and equivalent metric size (Table 3-1).

While there are many sizes and shapes of diamonds to be used for special applications and to suit the taste of every operator, there are a few diamond stones which should be included in a basic set of instruments: the round-end tapered, flat-end tapered, long-needle, short-needle, and small round-edge wheel diamonds (Fig. 3-2). Two other diamonds also commonly used, the torpedo and flame, are frequently paired with carbide burs of matching shapes (Fig. 3-3). Dimensions for these instruments are shown in Table 3-2.

Table 3-1 Comparison of diamond rotary instrument grits by particle size

	Brasseler*		Denscot		Star‡		Union Broach§	
				Range of particle size				
Grit	U.S. std. mesh	μm	U.S. std. mesh	μm	U.S. std. mesh	μm	U.S. std. mesh	μm
Extra fine	—	15–30	320–400	38–45	325–400	38–45	X	X
Fine	—	24–40	230–270	53–63	200–230	63–75	270	53
Regular	120–200	75–125	100–170	90–150	140–170	90–106	140	106
Coarse	100–140	100–150	100–120	125–150	100–120	125–150	120–130	115–125
Extra coarse	80–120	125–180	60–80	180–250	X	X	X	X

*Brasseler USA Inc., Savannah, Ga.
†Teledyne Densco, Denver, Colo.
‡Syntex Dental Products, Valley Forge, Pa.
§Union Broach Corp. New York

Table 3-3 Dimensions of nondentate tapered fissure burs

Bur	Tip diameter (mm)	Base diameter (mm)	Cutting length (mm)	Inclination per side (degrees)
169	0.54	0.9	4.2	2.5
169L	0.50	0.9	5.2	2.0
170	0.56	1.0	4.2	3.0
170L	0.58	1.0	6.0	2.0
171	0.76	1.2	4.2	3.0
171L	0.78	1.2	6.0	2.0
172	1.14	1.6	4.4	3.0
172L	1.18	1.6	6.0	2.0
H375-012†	0.8	1.2	7.0	3.0
H375-014†	0.8	1.4	8.0	2.0
7702-010*	0.7	1.0	5.2	2.0
7713-012*	0.8	1.2	5.2	2.0
7204-014*	0.6	1.4	9.0	2.5
7205-016*	0.7	1.6	9.0	3.0

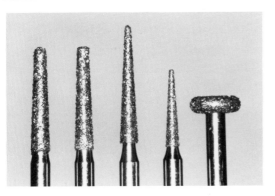

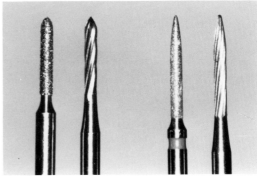

Fig. 3-2 These five diamonds are part of the standard general instrument set used for preparing teeth for cast metal and ceramic restorations. They are (*left to right*): the round-end tapered diamond (856–016),* the flat-end tapered diamond (847–016),* the long-needle diamond (30006–012),* the short-needle diamond (852–012),* and the small round-edge wheel diamond (909–040).*

Fig. 3-3 The concept of diamond/bur dual instrumentation, first developed by Lustig in his RCB series,[36] is based on diamonds and carbide burs of matching sizes and shapes. The torpedo diamond (877–010)* and bur (282–010)* on the left are part of the original RCB kit. A fine-grit flame diamond (862–010)* and bur (H48L–010) are seen on the right.

Some instruments of a particular size and shape are made by many manufacturers, while others are made only by one manufacturer. Instruments used for cutting specific preparation features should be substituted only after a careful examination under some form of magnification to insure that they are similar enough to be used interchangeably.

All small-diameter diamonds, or those with small-diameter tips, must be used cautiously. To preserve instrument configuration and to prevent excessive loss of diamond particles from the binding material, some manufacturers use a finer particle size on those portions of the instruments with small diameters. These areas of a diamond stone also will have lower peripheral speeds than parts of the instrument with larger diameters, making the thinner segments less

effective. The normal response—which should be avoided—is to use heavier pressure. This will result in failure of the bonding medium and loss of the abrasive.[23]

Tungsten carbide burs

Tungsten carbide burs are best for making precise preparation features and smooth surfaces in enamel or dentin. A logical application of their planing capability is the production of smooth finish lines. Carbide burs can also be used to cut through metal, while both carbide burs and diamonds can be used to cut sound dentin.

The metal in the head of a tungsten carbide bur is formed by *sintering,* or pressure molding, tungsten carbide

*Brasseler USA Inc., Savannah, Ga.

*Brasseler USA Inc., Savannah, Ga.

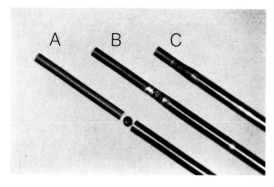

Fig. 3-4 A tungsten carbide dowel *(A, left)* is attached to a steel rod *(A, right)* with a small piece of solder interposed. The soldered carbide tip is machined *(B)* and shortened *(C)* to form the blank from which the bur will be cut.*

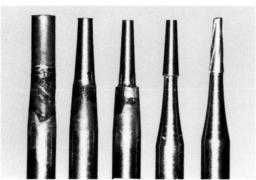

Fig. 3-5 The carbide-tipped blank goes through several machining processes *(left to right)*: shortening, head prefinishing, head finishing, neck prefinishing, and head and blade finishing (grinding).*

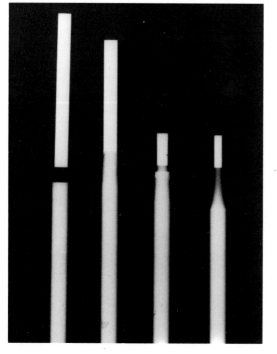

Fig. 3-6 This radiograph shows the carbide blank and steel shaft before *(left)* and after soldering *(second from left)*, after initial head finishing *(second from right)*, and after blade grinding *(right)*. The tungsten carbide segments appear as dense white areas in the radiographs. At this magnification, there are no voids in the attachment areas between the steel shaft and the carbide blank.* (Radiograph courtesy of Ms. Beverly Dye of Oklahoma City.)

*Specimens shown are courtesy of Brasseler USA Inc., Savannah, Ga.

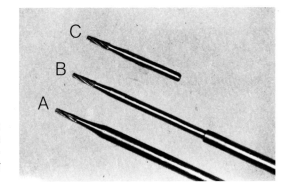

Fig. 3-7 After the head of the bur has been completely formed *(A)*, the shank is cut down *(B)*, and then shortened to form the final instrument, which in this case is a friction grip bur *(C)*.*

powder and cobalt powder under heat and vacuum.[20] The tungsten carbide is cut into small cylinders and then attached to steel rods by soldering or welding to form blanks (Fig. 3-4). The tungsten carbide head is machined with large diamond disks to create the specific head for the type of bur being formed (Fig. 3-5). The attachment of the carbide head is quite secure (Fig. 3-6), and loss of the carbide portion of a bur is rare. Only when the process has been completed is the shank of the instrument shortened, notched, or diminished in diameter to make a straight handpiece, latch, or friction grip bur (Fig. 3-7).

Most burs intended primarily for cutting are made with six and occasionally eight blades. Those burs made for finishing usually have 12 blades, but they can have 20, or even as many as 40. The cutting edge of each blade is formed by the junction of two surfaces, the *face* and the *land* (Fig. 3-8).

The *clearance angle,* which is the angle formed between the back of the

blade and the surface being cut by the bur, is one factor which affects the bulk of metal found near the cutting edge of a bur blade. There is an optimum clearance angle for each diameter of bur, and the larger the diameter, the smaller the clearance angle that is required.[24] The smaller the clearance angle, the stronger the cutting blade. However, if the angle becomes too small, the back of the blade may rub against the cut surface, generating heat and decreasing efficiency.

The angle at which the face of the blade meets a line extending from the cutting edge to the bur axis is known as the *rake angle.*[25] The more positive the rake angle (Fig. 3-9), the more acute the edge of the blade, and the more effective the cutting action. A positive rake angle, unfortunately, also has a weaker edge. Therefore, the blades are usually made with either negative or neutral (radial) rake angles, and wider bases. These are slightly less efficient for cutting, but because of their greater bulk they are less likely to chip.

The blades usually spiral around the bur, separated from each other by *flutes,* which are the grooves between the blades. The amount of spiral, or *he-*

*Specimens shown are courtesy of Brasseler USA Inc., Savannah, Ga.

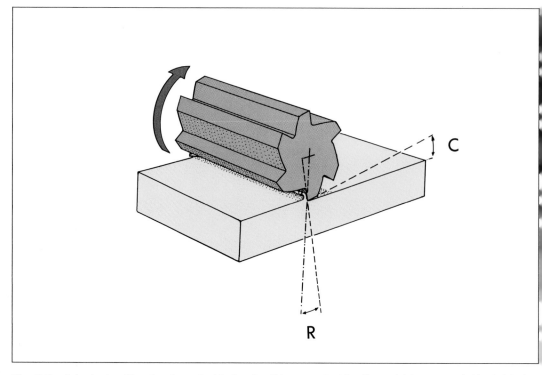

Fig. 3-8 A typical cutting bur has six *blades* (teeth) separated by *flutes* (chip spaces). Each blade has three surfaces: a *face*, a *land*, and a *back*, although the land and back may blend together into a single curved surface. The angle between the face and the radial line is called the *rake angle (R)*. The angle between the land and the surface being cut is the *clearance angle (C)*. These two angles determine the sharpness of the blade edge.

lical angle, of the blades affects the cutting characteristics of the bur. A greater helical angle produces a smoother surface on the preparation, and reduces the "chatter," or vibration of the bur on the tooth surface.[24] This also reduces chipping of the tungsten carbide during use on a tooth, and it prevents debris from clogging the flutes between the blades.[26]

In some burs, the blades are interrupted by cuts across the edge. Burs made in this configuration are described as *dentate,* or *cross-cut* burs. Dentate burs have been shown to be somewhat more effective than nondentate burs.[27] Notwithstanding this finding, nondentate burs are still preferred over the crosscut fissure bur for preparations for cast restorations. The crosscut bur will leave deep, severe striations at right angles to the path of insertion of the preparation.[28,29]

Several carbide burs of specific shapes are included in the standard armamentarium. These include at least two tapered fissure burs, long and standard length, an end-cutting bur, and a friction grip no. 4 round bur (Fig. 3-10). For removal of deep caries, a low-

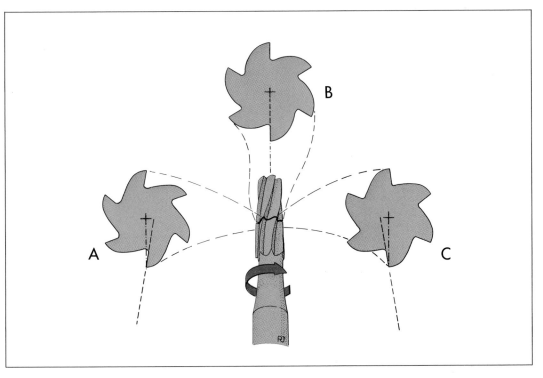

Fig. 3-9   The three types of rake angle are: *(A)* Positive rake angle: The plane of the face lies behind the radial line. Although this forms the most effective cutting blade initially, the sharp edge chips and dulls quickly against enamel. *(B)* Radial or neutral rake angle: The plane of the face coincides with the radial line. *(C)* Negative rake angle: the plane of the face lies in front of the radial line. This allows a greater bulk of metal just behind the cutting edge for longer bur life. Most dental burs have either a neutral or a negative rake angle.

speed handpiece no. 6 round bur is used so that sound dentin can be distinguished from softer carious dentin by its greater resistance to cutting.

Tapered fissure burs have a number of uses in preparing teeth for cast metal and porcelain restorations. In addition to the placement of grooves, box forms, and isthmuses, they are especially useful for planing vertical axial surfaces. The burs in the conventional nondentate, six-bladed 170 series are not always long enough to accomplish this, and the relatively small tips may create a rough shoulder at the base of the wall.

There are a number of tapered finishing burs whose greater length and diameter make them better suited for this task. Some of the more commonly used sizes are shown in Fig. 3-11. Dimensions are given in Table 3-3.

Other rotary instruments used frequently enough to be included in the standard armamentarium are a no. 34 inverted cone bur, a no. 1/2 round bur, and a 0.6-mm (.024-in.) twist drill (Fig. 3-12).

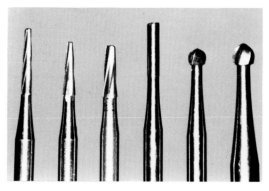

Fig. 3-10 These tungsten carbide burs are needed in the basic set of instruments for tooth preparations for cast metal and porcelain restorations. *Left to right:* nos. 169L, 170, 171, 957, 4, and 6.

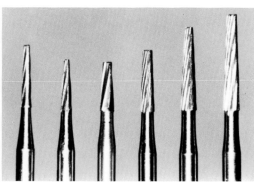

Fig. 3-11 Several tapered fissure burs can be used more or less interchangeably: nos. 169L, 170, 171, 713–012, 375–012, and 375–014. The smaller-diameter instruments are best used for starting grooves and accentuating boxes, while the larger ones will do a better job of planing axial walls.

Table 3-2 Dimensions of diamond stones and diamond/bur combinations

	Tip diameter (mm)	Base diameter (mm)	Cutting length (mm)	Inclination per side (degrees)	Convergence angle of tip (degrees)
Round-end tapered diamond	1.0	1.6	8.0	2.0	–
Flat-end tapered diamond	1.0	1.6	8.0	2.0	–
Long-needle diamond	0.5	1.2	9.0	3.0	–
Short-needle diamond	0.5	1.2	6.0	3.5	–
Small-wheel diamond	–	4.0	1.4	0	–
Torpedo diamond	–	1.0	6.0	0	60
Torpedo bur	–	1.0	6.0	0	60
Flame diamond	–	1.0	8.0	0	12
Flame bur	–	1.0	8.0	0	12

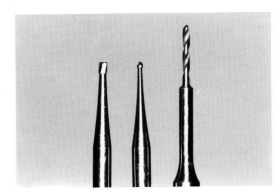

Fig. 3-12 These three rotary instruments also may be used for preparing teeth: no. 34, no. 1/2, and a 0.6-mm (.024-inch) drill.

Twist drills

The twist drill, which is made of steel, cuts only at its tip as it is pushed into the tooth in the direction of the long axis of the instrument. It has deep twin helical flutes that wind around the shaft in a tight spiral (Fig. 3-13), helping to remove chips from the hole. The drill can be used to produce small, uniform-diameter, parallel-sided holes in dentin to receive retentive pins for restorations. Because the holes are untapered, precise alignment is imperative.

The drill diameter is slightly larger than the pins that are incorporated into cast restorations to allow for a small cement space. The working portion of this type of drill should be 3.0 to 5.0 mm long. The drill for the threaded pins used to retain composite resin and amalgam cores is slightly smaller than the ultimate pin diameter. It has a self-limiting collar to keep the pinhole an optimum 2.0 mm deep (Fig. 3-14).

Twist drills must be used differently than regular burs. They do not cut through enamel, and they tend to "crawl" when a hole is attempted on a sloping surface. Therefore, a shallow pilot hole is made with a no. 1/2 round bur on a narrow horizontal ledge to insure that the hole will be drilled precisely in its intended position.

The pilot hole is deepened with the drill in a low-speed latch-type handpiece, using a pumping motion to aid chip removal and to prevent excessive heat. Spiral drills are never used in a high-speed handpiece. They cannot be adequately cooled, and the danger of drill breakage within the hole is too great.

The drill must not stop rotating while it is in the hole. If it does, it may bind and shear off, and a broken drill is virtually impossible to remove from the tooth. If a drill does bind in a hole, the safest way to remove it is to disengage the latch and remove the handpiece from the drill. Then back the drill out of the hole with finger and thumb. This produces less stress on the drill than the handpiece would.

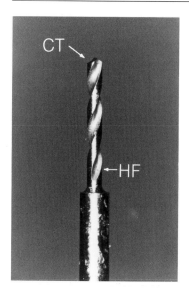

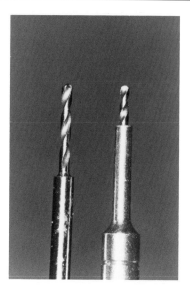

Fig. 3-13 A closeup view of a 0.6-mm-diameter twist drill shows the cutting tip *(CT)* and helical flutes *(HF)*.

Fig. 3-14 The 0.6-mm-diameter twist drill on the left, used in drilling pinholes for parallel pins, which are an integral part of a cast restoration, has a cutting portion 5.0 mm long.* The 0.5-mm Kodex drill† on the right, used for creating pinholes for Minim threaded pins,† which retain amalgam and composite resin cores, has a collar 2.0 mm from the end to prevent overcutting the depth of the pinhole.

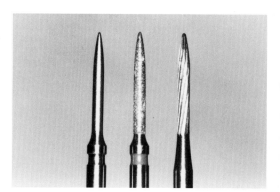

Fig. 3-15 To produce the most consistent results, the diamond used to prepare the tooth and the carbide bur used to finish it should be made from blanks machined to the same configuration. The configuration of the blank on the left is used for the flame diamond (862–010)* in the middle and the carbide bur (H48L–010)* on the right.

*Brasseler USA Inc., Savannah, Ga.
†Whaledent International, New York.

Diamond/bur dual instrumentation

Diamonds remove tooth structure more efficently than do burs, but they leave undesirably rough surfaces and irregular cavosurface finish lines.[30-34] Tungsten carbide burs produce smooth finish lines and precise internal features, but they cut more slowly. Therefore, to take advantage of the best features of both types of instrument, diamonds should be used for the bulk reduction and carbide burs for finishing the preparation and placing internal features such as grooves, box forms, isthmuses, etc.

The technique of choice in this situation utilizes diamonds and carbide burs of matching size and configuration as described by Lustig.[35,36] These instruments are manufactured by making both the diamond and the bur from a common blank configuration (Fig. 3-15). This assures that the shape of the instrument and the resultant contour of the tooth will match exactly when the diamond and carbide finishing bur are used for each step of the preparation.

The potential role of surface roughness in the retention of cast restorations was discussed in chapter 1. While scratches and irregularities on the preparation surface may aid the retention of the casting, this advantage must be weighed against the disadvantages. A smooth surface will allow a more accurate impression.[37] If the surface is too rough, it may be difficult to withdraw the impression without distorting it and losing fine detail in the die. Perhaps more importantly, excessive roughness at the finish line may prevent close adaptation of the restoration margin.[38] The microscopic scratches left by carbide burs (2 μm) and fine diamond stones (10 μm) are deep enough to enhance retention without compromising accuracy.[39]

No matter how carefully the axial reduction of a veneer restoration is done with a torpedo diamond, the surface will exhibit some roughness. Close examination of the finish line discloses chips that will be difficult to duplicate in the casting margin (Figs. 3-16a and b). If a 12-blade torpedo carbide bur is used to finish the axial surface after reduction has been completed with a diamond, the surface will be much smoother, and the finish line itself will have minimal defects (Figs. 3-17a and b). Schärer has demonstrated in SEM studies that a smooth, distinct finish line is essential if a technician is to be able to produce a well-adapted restoration margin.[40]

Barkmeier et al. found a straight fissure bur produced the smoothest and most distinct bevel of the instruments they tested, which included a 12-blade and 40-blade bur as well as a superfine diamond.[30] Examination of an occlusal bevel prepared with a nondentate tapered fissure bur (Figs. 13-18a and b), reveals a markedly smoother bevel and more distinct finish line than a bevel made with a fine flame diamond (Figs. 3-19a and b).

A gingival bevel, however, must be created by the tip of the instrument, rather than its side. In this location on the tooth, it is not practical to use a tapered fissure bur for placing a bevel, since the squared tip will gouge either the bevel or adjacent teeth, or lacerate the tissue. A fine flame diamond will produce a bevel that exhibits some horizontal striations (Fig. 3-20). If the bevel formed by the flame diamond is then retraced and finished with the tip of a long-flame carbide bur,* the result will

*No. H48L-010, Brasseler USA Inc., Savannah, Ga.

73

Figs. 3-16a and b SEMs of a preparation axial wall and finish line instrumented with a torpedo diamond show the surface roughness near the chamfer.

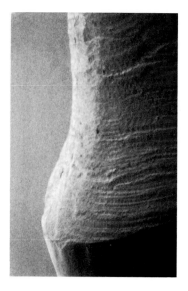

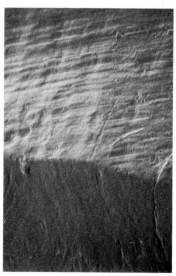

Fig. 3-16b 700×.

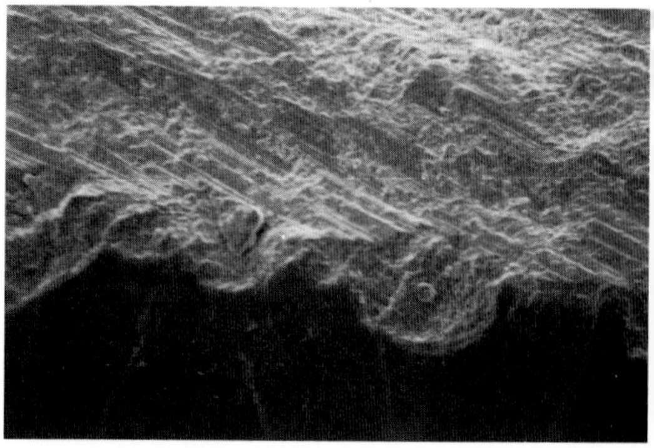

Fig. 3-16a 35×.

Figs. 3-17a and b These SEMs demonstrate full-crown axial reductions and chamfer finish lines that were done with a torpedo diamond and then smoothed with a torpedo carbide bur.

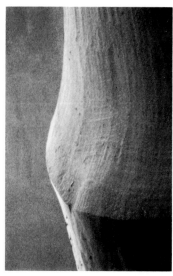

Fig. 3-17a 35×.

Fig. 3-17b 700×.

Figs. 3-18a and b An occlusal bevel prepared with a diamond is rough.

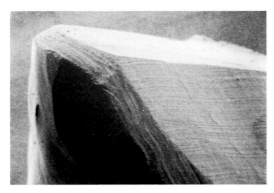

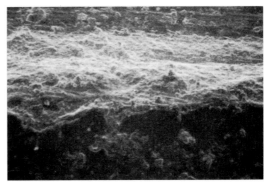

Fig. 3-18a 35×.

Fig. 3-18b 700×.

Figs. 3-19a and b An occlusal bevel cut with a no. 170 carbide bur is much smoother than one made with a diamond.

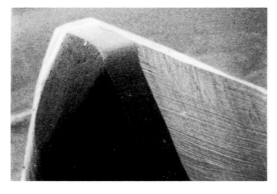

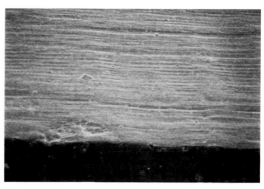

Fig. 3-19a 35×.

Fig. 3-19b 700×.

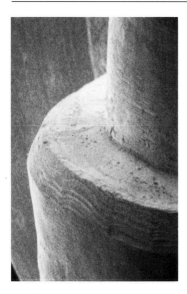

Fig. 3-20 This gingival bevel was made with a flame diamond (35×).

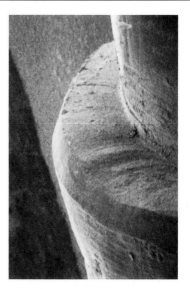

Fig. 3-21 If a gingival bevel prepared with a flame diamond is retraced and retouched with a flame carbide bur, the bevel will be much smoother (35×).

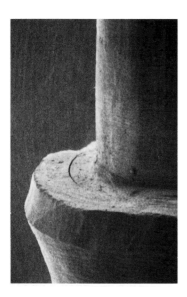

Fig. 3-22 Gingival bevels made with torpedo burs are smoother than those made with diamonds, but the surface is scalloped (35×).

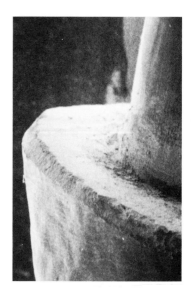

Fig. 3-23 The bevel created by a 40-blade finishing bur is not as smooth and well instrumented as one created by a 6- or 12-blade bur (35×).

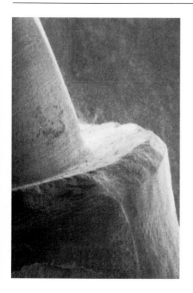

Fig. 3-24 The bevel created by a gingival margin trimmer is unacceptably rough (35×).

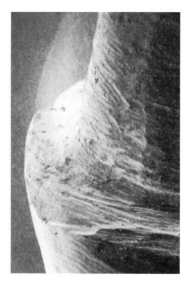

Fig. 3-25 A shoulder created with nothing more than a flat-end diamond will be a very rough finish line (35×).

be a much smoother gingival bevel (Fig. 3-21).

Gingival bevels made with the tips of other rotary instruments can produce good results in the hands of experienced operators, but they are more technique-sensitive and difficult to use. The torpedo bur tends to produce scalloping in the bevel and the finish line, since the bur cannot be guided by contact with a longer axial wall (Fig. 3-22). The 40-blade bur produces an irregular, choppy bevel when the tip of the instrument must be used (Fig. 3-23). Gingival margin trimmers, widely used on the gingival floors of amalgam preparations, are not suitable instruments for the gingival bevels of preparations for cast restorations. They produce a rough, irregular bevel (Fig. 3-24).

A shoulder cut with a regular-grit flat-end tapered diamond is much too rough to allow fabrication of an ade-

quately fitting restoration margin (Fig. 3-25). Shoulders should be finished with an end-cutting bur and an enamel hoe to insure the smoothest possible finish line (Fig. 3-26).

Distinct, well-finished proximal flares can be made with abrasive paper disks.[41–43] However, they require a light touch to avoid overheating, and they must be changed frequently to insure that they will cut tooth structure effectively. They are limited to those areas of the mouth with good access, and extreme caution must be exercised when using them to avoid injury to the patient. Although they can produce a very smooth flare with a distinct finish line, too coarse a disk will cut grooves in the flare, and worn-out disks will round over the finish line (Fig. 3-27).

A flame diamond with parallel sides rather than slightly convex ones can be used to produce a flare. The ability of

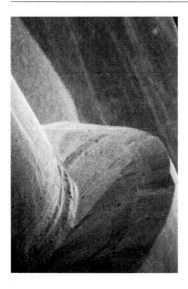

Fig. 3-26 The shoulder can be improved by instrumenting it further with an endcutting bur and sharp hand instruments (40×).

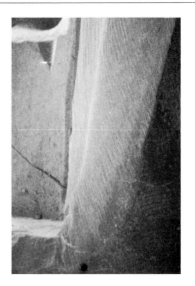

Fig. 3-27 This proximal flare was made with a medium emery disk, followed by a coarse cuttle disk. Notice the rounding over of the finish line in the gingival segment (35×).

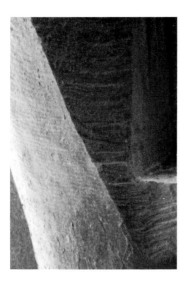

Fig. 3-28 A flame diamond was used to prepare this flare. It blends well with the gingival bevel, but there are horizontal striations on the surface (25×).

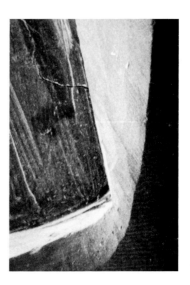

Fig. 3-29 A 12-blade flame finishing bur was used to smooth this flare after it was made with a flame diamond (25×).

this instrument to smoothly blend vertical flares into the horizontal gingival bevel helps to produce a finish line that flows from one tooth surface to another. Nonetheless, it cannot compensate completely for the fact that the cut surface of the flare or bevel and the finish line itself are less than perfectly smooth (Fig. 3-28).

A long 12-blade flame-shaped carbide finishing bur* is used to create a distinct finish line with a smooth surface on horizontal bevels and vertical flares (Fig. 3-29). This 1.0 mm diameter instrument is cut from a blank stock of

the same configuration as the flame-shaped bur. To achieve maximum effectiveness, it should be used only to finish the bevel or flare *after* it has been cut with the flame diamond. Use of the bur as the primary cutting instrument will quickly dull it and will produce a less-than-optimal finish line in the process.

Use of large diamond disks has not been described for these preparations because it is the opinion of the authors that there is no place in modern restorative dentistry for such instruments for either proximal reduction or flare placement. They are dangerous for the patient, and it is easy to overextend a preparation using one.

*No. H48L-010, Brasseler USA Inc., Savannah, Ga.

References

1. McKay, R. C. Evolution of tooth cutting techniques and its influence on restorative dentistry. J. Prosthet. Dent. 8:843, 1958.
2. Kramer, I. R. H. Changes in dentine during cavity preparation using turbine handpieces. Br. Dent. J. 109:59, 1960.
3. Arnim, S. S. Conservation of the dental pulp: Cavity preparation. J. Prosthet. Dent. 9:1017, 1959.
4. Langeland, K. Pulp reactions to cavity preparation and to burns in the dentin. Odont. Tidskr. 68:463, 1960.
5. Brown, W. S., Christensen, D. O., and Lloyd, B. A. Numerical and experimental evaluation of energy inputs, temperature gradients and thermal stresses during restorative procedures. J. Am. Dent. Assoc. 96:451, 1978.
6. Zach, L., and Cohen, G. Pulp response to externally applied heat. Oral Surg. 19:515, 1965.
7. Brannstrom, M. Dentinal and pulpal response. II. Application of an airstream to exposed dentine. Short period observation. Acta Odont. Scand. 18:19, 1960.
8. Hamilton, A. I., and Kramer, I. R. H. Cavity preparation with and without waterspray: Effects on the human dental pulp and additional effects of further dehydration of the dentine. Br. Dent. J. 123:281, 1967.
9. Smith, G. P. Full crown preparation. N. Y. J. Dent. 26:307, 1956.
10. Ingraham, R., and Tanner, H. M. The adaptation of modern instruments and increased operating speeds to restorative procedures. J. Am. Dent. Assoc. 47:311, 1953.
11. Lieban, E. A. Pulpal irritation and devitalization as a result of preparation of teeth for complete crowns. J. Am. Dent. Assoc. 51:679, 1955.
12. Nuttal, E. B. Abutment preparations using high speed instruments. J. Ky. Dent. Assoc. 13:161, 1961.
13. Langeland, K., and Langeland, L. K. Pulp reactions to crown preparation, impression, temporary crown fixation, and permanent cementation. J. Prosthet. Dent. 15:129, 1965.
14. Tucker, R. V. Variation of inlay cavity design. J. Am. Dent. Assoc. 84:616, 1972.
15. Miller, L. A clinician's interpretation of tooth preparations and the design of metal substructures for metal-ceramic restorations. p. 156 In J. W. McLean (ed.) Dental Ceramics: Proceedings of the 1st International Symposium on Ceramics. Chicago: Quintessence Publishing Co., 1983.
16. Stanley, H. R. Traumatic capacity of high-speed and ultra-sonic dental instrumentation. J. Am. Dent. Assoc. 63:749, 1961.
17. Diamond, R. D., Stanley, H. R., and Swerdlow, H. Reparative dentin formation resulting from cavity preparation. J. Prosthet. Dent. 16:1127, 1966.
18. Lloyd, B. A., Rich, J. A., and Brown, W. S. Effect of cooling techniques on temperature control and cutting rate for high-speed dental drills. J. Dent. Res. 57:675, 1978.
19. Eames, W. B., Reder, B. S., and Smith, G. A. Cutting efficiency of diamond stones: Effect of technique variables. Oper. Dent. 2:156, 1977.
20. Phillips, R. W. Skinner's Science of Dental Materials. 8th ed. Philadelphia: W. B. Saunders Co., 1982, 563, 581.
21. Dentists' Desk Reference. 2nd ed. Chicago: American Dental Association, 1983, 286.
22. Janota, M. Use of scanning electron microscopy for evaluating diamond points. J. Prosthet. Dent. 29:88, 1973.
23. Hartley, J. L., Hudson, D. C., Sweeney, W. T., and Dickson, G. Methods for evaluation of rotating diamond abrasive dental instruments. J. Am. Dent. Assoc. 54:637, 1957.
24. Lou, R. Personal communication, Apr. 1986.
25. Henry, E. E., and Peyton, F. A. The relationship between design and cutting efficiency of dental burs. J. Dent. Res. 33:281, 1954.
26. Osborne, J., Anderson, J. N., and Lammie, G. A. Tungsten carbide and its application to the dental bur. Br. Dent. J. 110:230, 1951.
27. Eames, W. B., and Nale, J. L. A comparison of cutting efficiency of air-driven fissure burs. J. Am. Dent. Assoc. 86:412, 1973.
28. Schuchard, A., and Watkins, E. C. Cutting effectiveness of tungsten-burs and diamond points at ultra-high rotational speeds. J. Prosthet. Dent. 18:58, 1967.
29. Allan, D. N. Cavity finishing. Br. Dent. J. 125:540, 1968.
30. Barkmeier, W. W., Kelsey, W. P., Blankenau, R. J., and Peterson, D. S. Enamel cavosurface bevels finished with ultraspeed instruments. J. Prosthet. Dent. 49:481, 1983.

31. Barnes, I. E. The production of inlay cavity bevels. Br. Dent. J. 137:379, 1974.
32. Leidal, T. I., and Tronstad, L. Scanning electron microscopy of cavity margins finished with ultraspeed instruments. J. Dent. Res. 54:152, 1975.
33. Kinzer, R. L., and Morris, C. Instruments and instrumentation to promote conservative operative dentistry. Dent. Clin. North Am. 20:241, 1976.
34. Rodda, J. C., and Gavin, J. B. A scanning electron microscope study of cavity margins finished by different methods. N. Z. Dent. J. 73:64, 1977.
35. Lustig, L. P., Perlitsh, M. J., Przetak, C., and Mucko, K. A rational concept of crown preparation. Quint. Int. 3:35, 1972.
36. Lustig, L. P. A rational concept of crown preparation revised and expanded. Quint. Int. 7:41, 1976.
37. Clayman, L. H. Modern techniques for the full crown and plastic faced gold veneer crown preparations using diamond instruments. J. Prosthet. Dent. 2:260, 1952.
38. Charbeneau, G. T., and Peyton, F. A. Some effects of cavity instrumentation on the adaptation of gold castings and amalgam. J. Prosthet. Dent. 8:514, 1958.
39. Schöler, A. Ueberlegungen, analysen und praktische erkentnisse zur Kronenstumpfpräparation (II). Die Quint. 31:47, 1980.
40. Schärer, P. A closer look at the crown margin. Presented at the 33rd Annual Meeting of the American Academy of Crown and Bridge Prosthodontics, Chicago, Feb. 18, 1984.
41. Street, E. V. Effect of various instruments on enamel walls. J. Am. Dent. Assoc. 46:274, 1953.
42. Boyde, A. Finishing techniques for the exit margin of the approximal portion of class II cavities. Br. Dent. J. 134:319, 1973.
43. Tronstad, L., and Leidal, T. I. Scanning electron microscopy of cavity margins finished with chisels or rotating instruments at low speed. J. Dent. Res. 53:1167, 1974.

Chapter 4

Full Veneer Crowns

The full veneer crown, for many years the workhorse of cast restorations, is a restoration for which there are many indications. It can be used where breakdown of tooth structure is severe,[1-3] to the extent that it has been described in operative dentistry as "the final attempt to preserve a tooth."[4] It is also extremely useful in those situations where the tooth to be restored needs to be recontoured,[1,2,4,5] since those changes can be blended into the normal contours of the tooth when all of the axial surfaces are involved.

Although the full veneer crown is a valuable, irreplaceable part of the restorative dentist's armamentarium, the design is probably overused. Dental insurance statistics indicate that as many as 93% of the cast restorations done are full-coverage restorations in some form.[6] The popularity of the full veneer crown is probably due, at least in part, to its ease of use.[7]

Clinicians have known empirically that full crowns are superior to other designs in retention[2-4,8-13] and resistance.[14] This has been confirmed in laboratory studies by Lorey and Meyers,[15] Reisbick and Shillingburg,[16] and Potts et al.[17] When maximum retention is needed, a full-coverage restoration is indicated, and if the cosmetic result is not a concern, an all-metal crown can be used.

The terms "full crown," "full cast crown," and "complete crown" can be used interchangeably with "full veneer crown" to describe a restoration made entirely of cast metal. The declining use of gold and its replacement by other noble or base metals, make "full gold crown," once a common term, unacceptable as a generic description.

Removing the entire anatomical form of the clinical crown is a radical procedure,[18] and is sometimes performed with the mistaken belief that it will protect the tooth from caries. While any decalcified axial surfaces of a tooth should be veneered when a restoration is done, it is erroneous to think that all surfaces should be covered on the chance that they might become cariously involved at some future time. Full coverage should not be used to prolong the longevity of a crown in a mouth in which the biological environment has not been brought under control. In such cases, no cast restoration is indicated until the carious process has been controlled.

Figures 4-1 through 4-33 illustrate the steps in cutting a classic full veneer crown preparation on a mandibular molar. The basic steps are the same for any posterior tooth except that the functional cusp bevel would be placed on the lingual cusp of maxillary teeth.

Figures 4-34 to 4-37 are clinical examples of full veneer crowns and full veneer crown preparations used to restore mandibular and maxillary molars.

Mandibular full veneer crown preparation (Figs. 4-1 through 4-33)

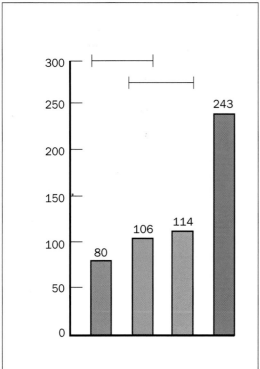

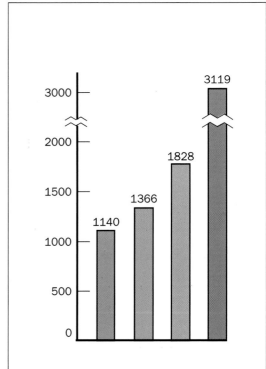

Fig. 4-1 Retention values are compared for five commonly used preparation designs.[17,19,20] The retention of the full crown is significantly greater than that of the various partial veneer crown designs.

Fig. 4-2 Resistance values are shown for the same five preparations shown in Fig. 4-1.[17,19,20] The resistance afforded by the full crown is clearly superior to that of the other preparation designs.

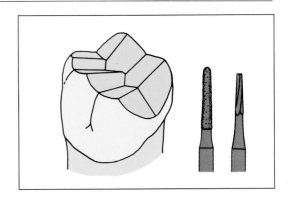

Fig. 4-3 Planar occlusal reduction: round-end tapered diamond and no. 171 bur.

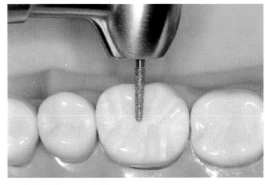

Fig. 4-4 Use a round-end tapered diamond to make depth orientation grooves on the triangular ridges and in the primary developmental grooves.

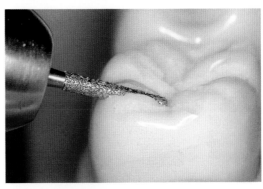

Fig. 4-5 To achieve a desired occlusal reduction of 1.0 to 1.5 mm,[21] the depth-orientation grooves should be 1.5 mm deep on the functional cusps (maxillary lingual and mandibular facial cusps) and 1.0 mm deep on the nonfunctional cusps (maxillary facial and mandibular lingual cusps). Depth can be gauged from the diameter of the diamond used for the reduction.

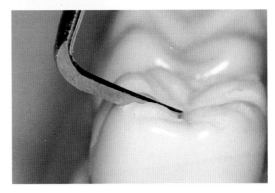

Fig. 4-6 A 1.0- or 1.5-mm enamel chisel (depending on the depth of reduction desired) can also be used in the depth-orientation groove to more precisely judge the depth of the groove.

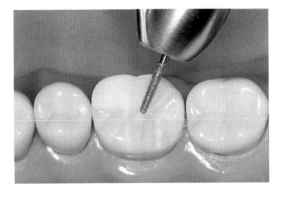

Fig. 4-7 Occlusal reduction consists of removing the tooth structure remaining between the orientation grooves. It is done in an inclined-plane pattern,[22] which can also be described as following cuspal contours,[3] or preserving general occlusal morphology.[23] By using this form, adequate occlusal reduction is insured without overreducing the tooth.

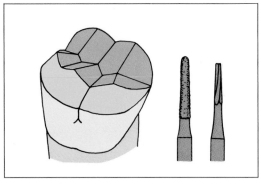

Fig. 4-8 Functional cusp bevel: round-end tapered diamond and no. 171 bur.

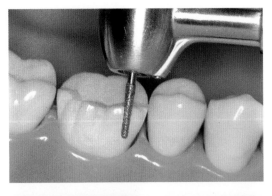

Fig. 4-9 Place depth-orientation grooves for a functional cusp bevel across the facial occlusal line angle of a mandibular premolar or molar, and across the lingual occlusal of a maxillary tooth.

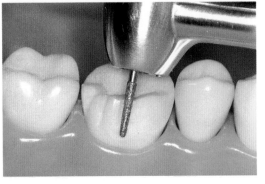

Fig. 4-10 The functional cusp bevel should be made with the same round-end tapered diamond used in the preceding steps. It should parallel the inward facing inclines of the cusps of the opposing tooth, at a depth of 1.5 mm, usually forming a 45-degree angle with the axial wall.[24]

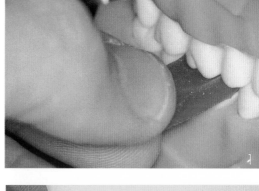

Fig. 4-11 Check the occlusal clearance by having the patient close completely on a strip of red utility wax of approximately the same width as the mesiodistal dimension of the prepared tooth.

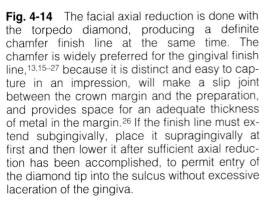

Fig. 4-12 Examine the imprint of the occlusal surface in the wax. Compare the translucency of the wax over portions of the preparation that have known adequate clearance with the translucency of those cusps and areas of the preparation that are too far lingual to be seen in the mouth. If the imprints of unseen segments are more translucent than those known to have adequate clearance, more reduction is needed in the unseen regions. Although the thickness of the wax can be measured with a thickness gauge, it is very difficult to do because of the softness of the wax.

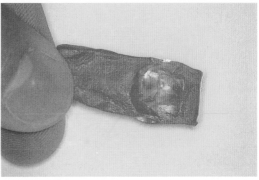

Fig. 4-13 Facial and lingual axial reduction: torpedo diamond.

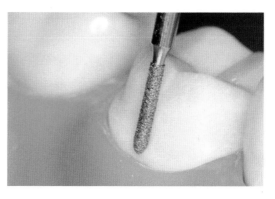

Fig. 4-14 The facial axial reduction is done with the torpedo diamond, producing a definite chamfer finish line at the same time. The chamfer is widely preferred for the gingival finish line,[13,15–27] because it is distinct and easy to capture in an impression, will make a slip joint between the crown margin and the preparation, and provides space for an adequate thickness of metal in the margin.[26] If the finish line must extend subgingivally, place it supragingivally at first and then lower it after sufficient axial reduction has been accomplished, to permit entry of the diamond tip into the sulcus without excessive laceration of the gingiva.

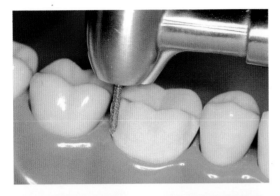

Fig. 4-15 The facial axial reduction is carried as far as possible into interproximal embrasures without nicking the adjacent teeth.

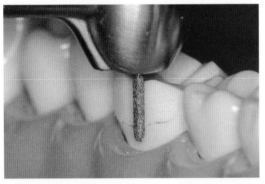

Fig. 4-16 Lingual axial reduction is done with the same diamond. Because of the lingual inclination of many mandibular molars, the chamfer in this area might be less pronounced. Every effort should be made to produce a chamfer rather than a knife edge to insure sufficient space for the restoration. Inadequate reduction will usually result in overcontouring of the restoration.[26] A minimum inclination of the prepared surface in relation to the uncut facial surface of 2.5 to 6.5 degrees is preferred.[24,28–30]

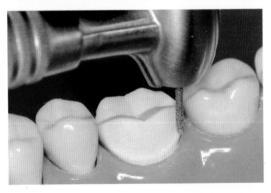

Fig. 4-17 The lingual axial reduction also extends as far interproximally as can be easily accomplished.

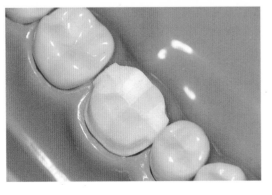

Fig. 4-18 An occlusal view of the tooth preparation at this stage reveals isolated areas of intact tooth structure surrounding each proximal contact.

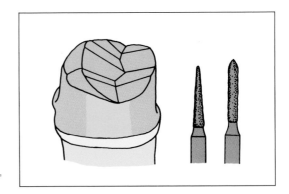

Fig. 4-19 Complete axial reduction: short, thin, tapered diamond and torpedo diamond.

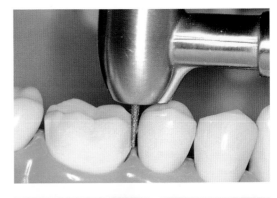

Fig. 4-20 The short, thin, tapered diamond is placed against the facial surface of the remaining interproximal tooth structure. It is held upright and moved up and down, directing it lingually with light pressure.

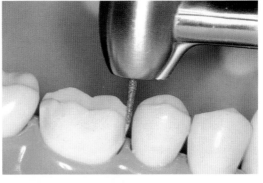

Fig. 4-21 It may be necessary to use the tip in especially tight areas, or to lay the diamond horizontally along the marginal ridge. Don't use the tip exclusively for any extended periods of time, because the diamond chips may be stripped from the end of the instrument.

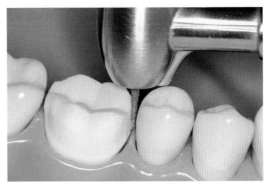

Fig. 4-22 Once sufficient space has been produced, sweep the short thin diamond back and forth, planing the mesial surface to smoothness. Be careful not to incline the diamond toward the center of the tooth being prepared, or the preparation will be overtapered.

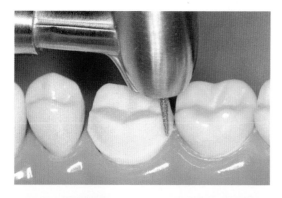

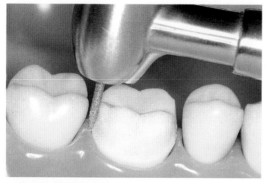

Fig. 4-23 Repeat the process on the distal surface with the short, thin, tapered diamond, working it through in short movements first. When you have gained sufficient space, make longer, sweeping strokes to smoothen the surface.

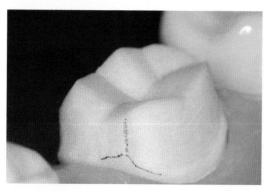

Fig. 4-24 Now go back over both proximal surfaces with the torpedo diamond. This will produce a chamfer finish line and increase the axial depth of reduction. It will also avoid the common problem of an underprepared proximal surface, which leads to overcontouring of the restoration.[31]

Fig. 4-25 A common error may occur at the line angles of the preparation, where the proximal reduction and the facial or lingual axial reduction meet. These surfaces are cut with long sweeps of the handpiece in one plane, tending to produce a "scallop" at each line angle. The result is likely to be inadequate reduction adjacent to the finish line. This is an especially critical area for inadequate reduction and resultant overcontouring of the crown.[23,26]

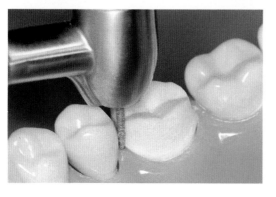

Fig. 4-26 Make a special effort to do more axial reduction in each transition area around a line angle, paying particular attention to creating a smooth, continuous finish line. Be careful not to incline the torpedo diamond while doing this, or the angles of the preparation will be overtapered.

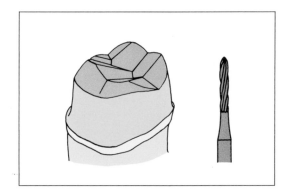

Fig. 4-27 Chamfer finishing: torpedo bur.

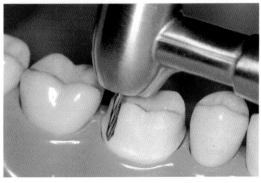

Fig. 4-28 Go over the axial walls with the torpedo bur, making sure that you also retouch the chamfer to produce a crisp, distinct finish line.

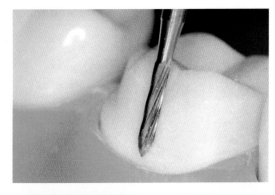

Fig. 4-29 Take special care to round off the angles of the preparation and produce a smooth, continuous chamfer in this area of the preparation, too.

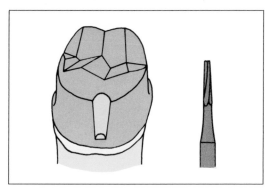

Fig. 4-30 Seating groove: no. 171 bur.

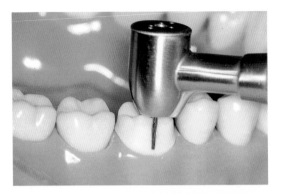

Fig. 4-31 A seating groove is placed on the axial surface with a large nondentate tapered fissure bur. The groove should be cut to the full diameter of the bur, and it should extend gingivally to a point just 0.5 mm above the chamfer. This groove primarily helps to guide the crown into place during cementation. A second groove can be added elsewhere on the preparation, which, if not reproduced in the final restoration, will be an excellent cement escape vent that will permit more complete seating of the crown.[32,33]

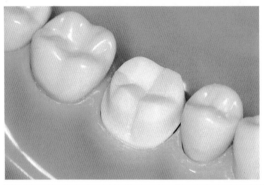

Fig. 4-32 The completed full veneer crown preparation.

Fig. 4-33 The features of a full veneer crown preparation and the function served by each.

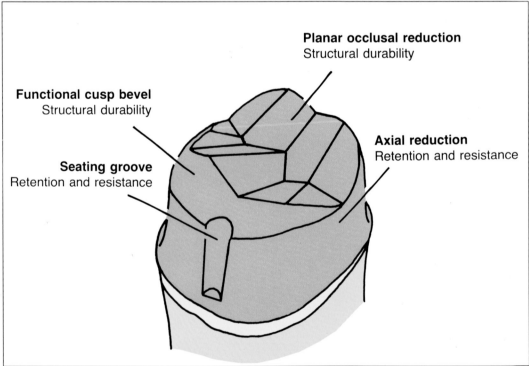

Planar occlusal reduction
Structural durability

Functional cusp bevel
Structural durability

Axial reduction
Retention and resistance

Seating groove
Retention and resistance

Clinical examples: Mandibular and maxillary (Figs. 4-34 through 4-37)

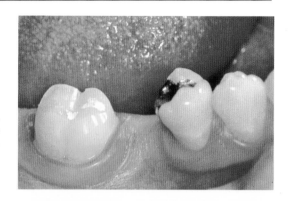

Fig. 4-34 A full veneer crown preparation is shown on a mandibular molar, which will serve as a bridge abutment. Because of the nonconservative nature of this preparation, it is seldom seen in an unmodified classic form cut in natural tooth structure.

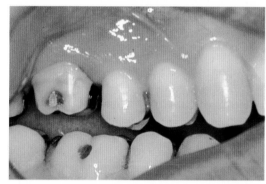

Fig. 4-35 A full veneer crown preparation on a maxillary molar is seen from the facial view.

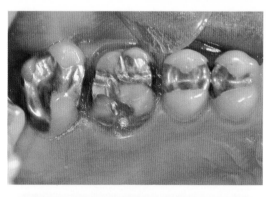

Fig. 4-36 The occlusal aspect of the same preparation displays a more common classic full veneer crown preparation in which the tooth has been built up with an amalgam core.

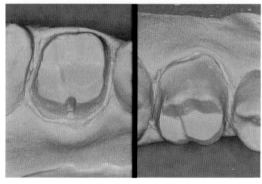

Fig. 4-37 Occlusal *(left)* and facial *(right)* views of a stone cast of the maxillary molar full veneer crown preparation exhibit all of the features discussed previously. If damage to the tooth is less extensive, a modified tooth preparation will be used (see chapter 16).

References

1. Dressel, R. P. The three-quarter crown as a bridge abutment for posterior teeth. Dent. Cosmos 72:730, 1930.
2. Pruden, W. H., II. Full coverage, partial coverage, and the role of pins. J. Prosthet. Dent. 26:302, 1971.
3. Shooshan, E. D. The full veneer cast crown. J. South. Calif. Dent. Assoc. 23:27, 1955.
4. Selberg, A. A full cast crown technique. J. Prosthet. Dent. 7:102, 1957.
5. Smith, G. P. What is the place of the full crown in restorative dentistry? Am. J. Orthod. Oral Surg. 33:471, 1947.
6. Howard, W. W. Full coverage restorations: Panacea or epidemic? Gen. Dent. 27:6, 1979.
7. Kahn, A. E. Partial vs. full coverage. J. Prosthet. Dent. 10:167, 1960.
8. Klaffenbach, A. O. Retention factors in fixed bridge prosthesis. Iowa Dent. Bull. 34:224, 1948.
9. Leander, C. T. Preparation of abutments for fixed partial dentures. Dent. Clin. North Am. 3:59, 1959.
10. Maxwell, E. L., and Wasser, V. E. Debate: Full vs. partial coverage as the abutment of choice in fixed bridgework. J. D. C. Dent. Soc. 36:9, 1961.
11. Nelson, E. A., and Hinds, F. W. Abutments as applied to fixed as well as removable partial denture prostheses. J. Am. Dent. Assoc. 29:534, 1942.
12. Smith, D. E. Abutment preparations. J. Am. Dent. Assoc. 18:2063, 1931.
13. Thom, L. W. Principles of cavity preparation in crown and bridge prostheses. I. The full crown. J. Am. Dent. Assoc. 41:284, 1950.
14. Knapp, K. W. A modern conception of proper bridge attachments for vital teeth. J. Am. Dent. Assoc. 14:1027, 1927.
15. Lorey, R. E., and Myers, G. E. The retentive qualities of bridge retainers. J. Am. Dent. Assoc. 76:568, 1968.
16. Reisbick, M. H., and Shillingburg, H. T. Effect of preparation geometry on retention and resistance of cast gold restorations. Calif. Dent. Assoc. J. 3:51, 1975.
17. Potts, R. G., Shillingburg, H. T., and Duncanson, M. G. Retention and resistance of preparations for cast restorations. J. Prosthet. Dent. 43:303, 1980.
18. Wheeler, R. C. Complete crown form and the periodontium. J. Prosthet. Dent. 11:722, 1961.
19. Kishimoto, M., Shillingburg, H. T., and Duncanson, M. G. Influence of preparation features on retention and resistance. I. MOD onlays. J. Prosthet. Dent. 49:35, 1983.
20. Kishimoto, M., Shillingburg, H. T., and Duncanson, M. G. Influence of preparation features on retention and resistance. II. Three-quarter crowns. J. Prosthet. Dent. 49:188, 1983.
21. Clayman, L. H. Modern techniques for the full crown and plastic-faced gold veneer crown preparations using diamond instruments. J. Prosthet. Dent. 2:260, 1952.
22. Shillingburg, H. T. Conservative preparations for cast restorations. Dent. Clin. North Am. 20:259, 1976.
23. Tjan, A. H., and Miller, G. D. Common errors in tooth preparation. Gen. Dent. 28:20, 1980.
24. Turner, C. H. Bevels and slots in full crown preparations. Dent. Update 4:161, 1977.
25. Herlands, R. E., Lucca, J. J., and Morris, M. L. Forms, contours, and extensions of full coverage restorations in occlusal reconstruction. Dent. Clin. North Am. 6:147, 1962.
26. Higdon, S. J. Tooth preparation for optimum contour of full-coverage restorations. Gen. Dent. 26:47, 1978.
27. Grundy, J. R. Color Atlas of Conservative Dentistry. Chicago: Year Book Medical Publ., Inc., 1980, 68.
28. Minker, J. S. Simplified full coverage preparations. Dent. Clin. North Am. 9:355, 1965.
29. El-Ebrashi, M. K., Craig, R. G., and Peyton, F. A. Experimental stress analysis of dental restorations. IV. The concept of parallelism of axial walls. J. Prosthet. Dent. 22:346, 1969.
30. Guyer, S. E. Multiple preparations for fixed prosthodontics. J. Prosthet. Dent. 23:529, 1970.
31. Weisgold, A. S., and Feder, M. Tooth preparation in fixed prosthesis. (Part I). Comp. Cont. Educ. Dent. 1:375, 1980.
32. Webb, E. L., Murray, H. V., Holland, G. A., and Taylor, D. F. Effects of preparation relief and flow channels on seating full coverage castings during cementation. J. Prosthet. Dent. 49:777, 1983.
33. Tjan, A. H. L., and Sarkissian, R. Internal escape channel: An alternative to venting complete crowns. J. Prosthet. Dent. 52:50, 1984.

Chapter 5

Maxillary Posterior Three-Quarter Crowns

The partial veneer crown represents a philosophy of practice as much as it does a form of treatment. It is generally a more conservative restoration requiring less destruction of tooth structure than most. Its use is based on the simple tenet that sound tooth structure should not be needlessly removed.[1] The partial veneer crown should be employed judiciously, so it will not be subjected to demands it is unable to meet.

In addition to preserving sound tooth structure, the partial veneer crown permits the accuracy of fit to be evaluated at exposed margins. Cement can escape more easily, allowing more complete seating. Finally, the uncut wall serves as a guide in reproducing natural contours in the restoration, and makes pulp testing possible.[2]

That large segments of the partial veneer crown's margins are supragingival is a distinct plus for the health of the gingiva surrounding it.[2-5] Some clinicians eschew the use of a three-quarter crown on the grounds that it will have a greater length of margin than would a full crown. That is true, although it is not necessarily relevant. There is additonal margin in a three-quarter crown, but it is entirely vertical and will fit better than the horizontal segment of the margin will.[6]

The consideration of a three-quarter crown is a matter of mental discipline. This conservative design should be considered first whenever a cast restoration is to be done, or it is not likely to be used at all.[7] The three-quarter crown is inadequate where there is extensive tooth destruction, a need for maximum retention, or a demand for maximum esthetics.

Partial veneer crowns are indicated in those situations where there is an intact facial surface,[8,9] minimal caries,[8-10] average or greater tooth length, and good hygiene.[10] They have been demonstrated to have less retention and resistance than full veneer restorations,[11-13] and therefore should be restricted to use in those situations where less than maximum retention will suffice. This type of crown can be used very sucessfully as a retainer for short-span bridges.

In a recent survey of dental educators, Grosso and Carreno found some controversy surrounding the use of partial veneer crowns in situations where esthetics were considered important. Educators in several regions of the United States felt that these crowns should be reserved for those situations in which esthetics were of no concern.[10] This judgment was by no means unanimous, nor should it have been.

If designed skillfully, the three-quarter crown can be very esthetic.[14] It is a restoration which can be used very successfully on maxillary posterior teeth, where esthetic demands are moderate and reasonable. The metal will not be totally invisible, but it will be unnoticeable in normal conversation. If the patient is one who will look at the restoration in a magnifying mirror and become apoplectic at the sight of the slightest trace of metal, or if he or she is in an occupation which precludes any display of metal, then a three-quarter crown is indeed contraindicated.

The standard three-quarter crown for a maxillary premolar or molar is one in which the facial surface is left unveneered. Because the facial surfaces of mandibular posterior teeth extend onto the functional cusps, three-quarter crown preparations of those teeth differ significantly enough to warrant a separate chapter on them (see chapter 6).

Three-quarter crowns have less retention and resistance than full veneer crowns, but more than other partial coverage restorations (Figs. 5-1 and 5-2). Step-by-step procedures for the classic three-quarter crown preparation on a maxillary premolar are shown in Figs. 5-3 through 5-49.

Clinical examples of three-quarter crowns restoring maxillary promolars and molars are shown in Figs. 5-50 through 5-58.

Maxillary posterior three-quarter crown preparation (Figs. 5-1 through 5-49)

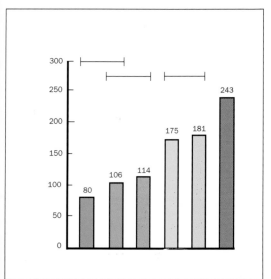

Fig. 5-1 Retention values are shown for three variations of the three-quarter crown and three other types of preparations. [13,15]

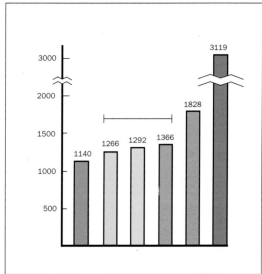

Fig. 5-2 Resistance values are compared for the three-quarter crown variations and the other three preparation designs. [13,15]

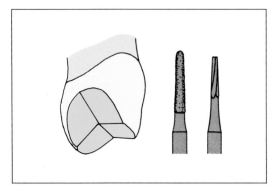

Fig. 5-3 Occlusal reduction: round-end tapered diamond and no. 171 bur.

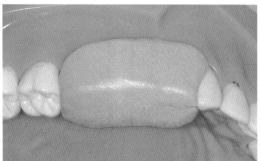

Fig. 5-4 It can be very helpful for the novice to have some type of index with which to judge the reduction for the preparation. To make one, adapt one-half scoop of silicone putty over the tooth to be prepared plus one or two adjacent teeth. This can be done in the patient's mouth while waiting for anesthesia, or it can be prepared in advance on a lubricated diagnostic cast.

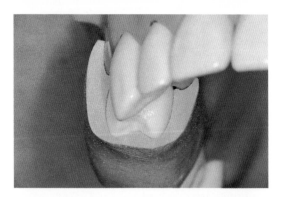

Fig. 5-5 Cut the index in half in the midsagittal plane of the tooth being prepared. Seat the distal half in the mouth to check for adaptation of the index to the unprepared tooth under it.

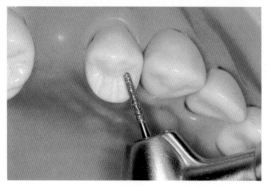

Fig. 5-6 Begin occlusal reduction by making depth orientation cuts with a round-end tapered diamond on the triangular ridges and in the major developmental grooves of the occlusal surface. The grooves should be cut to the full diameter of the tip of the diamond, which is approximately 1.0 mm. The round-end tapered diamond used for this purpose should measure 1.6 mm at the shank end, with a diameter of 1.3 at its midpoint. The diamond will need to be buried in tooth structure to its full diameter near the tip of the lingual (functional) cusp as well. This will produce occlusal reduction in the recommended range of 1.0 to 1.5 mm,[16–18] with 1.5 mm on the functional cusp.[1]

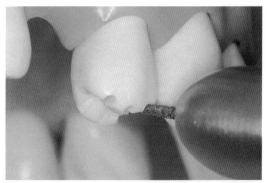

Fig. 5-7 The depth-orientation grooves must extend through the occlusofacial line angle, but to minimize the display of metal at the occlusal margin in the final restoration, the cuts will be only 0.5 mm deep at the line angle.

Fig. 5-8 Proceed with the occlusal reduction by removing the tooth structure remaining between the depth-orientation grooves with the round-end tapered diamond. The reduction is done so that it will preserve the general occlusal morphology,[19] i.e., it will reproduce the geometric inclined plane pattern of the cusps.[7,20] Reduction will be 1.5 mm on the functional cusp (the lingual cusp on maxillary teeth) and 1.0 mm on the nonfuctional cusp (here, the facial). The depth of the occlusal reduction is diminished somewhat near the facial cusp tip to minimize the display of metal.[14,21]

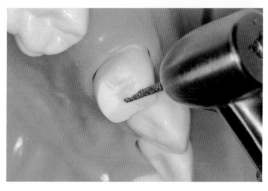

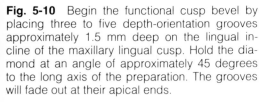

Fig. 5-9 Functional cusp bevel: round-end tapered diamond and no. 171 bur.

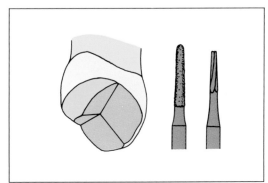

Fig. 5-10 Begin the functional cusp bevel by placing three to five depth-orientation grooves approximately 1.5 mm deep on the lingual incline of the maxillary lingual cusp. Hold the diamond at an angle of approximately 45 degrees to the long axis of the preparation. The grooves will fade out at their apical ends.

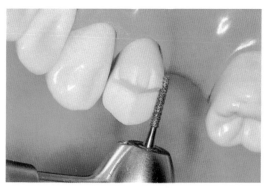

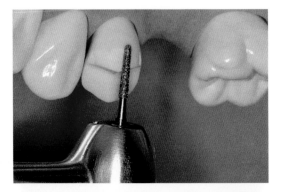

Fig. 5-11 Complete the functional cusp bevel by removing the tooth structure remaining between the grooves. The bevel should extend from the central groove on one proximal surface around to the central groove on the other proximal surface. This feature provides space for the necessary bulk of metal on the outward facing incline of the functional cusp bevel to match the space on the inward facing incline, which is provided by the occlusal reduction.

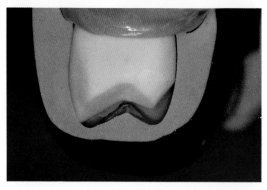

Fig. 5-12 Place the midsagittal index on the teeth to check the clearance. Notice that it is greatest on the lingual cusp and becomes progressively less near the facial cusp tip.

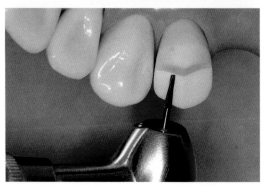

Fig. 5-13 Plane the occlusal reduction and functional cusp bevel smooth with a no. 171 bur.

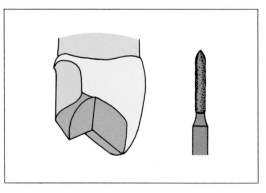

Fig. 5-14 Lingual axial reduction: torpedo diamond.

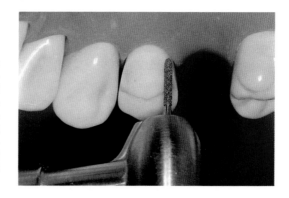

Fig. 5-15 Begin the lingual axial reduction with the torpedo diamond. Be careful not to over-incline the lingual wall. Overinclining lingual walls is a common error,[19] since those of maxillary molars, and especially premolars, have natural facial inclinations. Do not be concerned about having inadequate reduction in the occlusal one-third of the lingual wall if the lingual wall is kept upright. The functional cusp bevel has provided the needed space in that area.

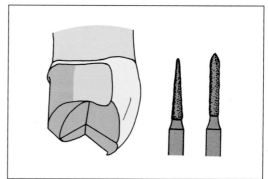

Fig. 5-16 Proximal axial reduction: short needle and torpedo diamonds.

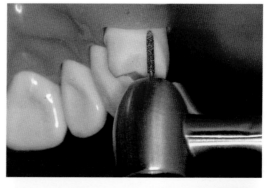

Fig. 5-17 When preparing a tooth adjacent to an edentulous space, it is possible to continue from the lingual surface around the line angle and onto the proximal surface with the same torpedo diamond.

Fig. 5-18 As the axial reduction is done, a chamfer finish line is formed. This also serves as a guide to producing adequate axial reduction. The diamond must cut into tooth structure so that the instrument tip is coincident with the finish line. This ensures the removal of an amount of tooth structure at the finish line that is equal to one-half the diameter of the diamond, or 0.5 mm. It becomes progressively greater toward the occlusal surface. Make the transition from lingual to proximal surface as smooth and continuous as possible, with no sharp angles in the axial reduction nor notches in the chamfer.

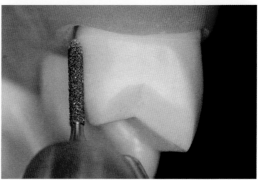

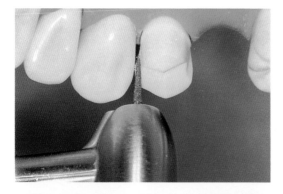

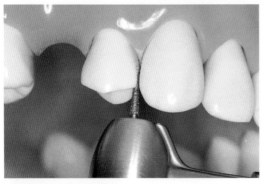

Fig. 5-19 Begin the axial reduction where there is an adjacent tooth with the short-needle diamond. This type of diamond is probably most effective in this area if it is used with an up and down "sawing" motion.

Fig. 5-20 Continue toward the facial surface until contact with the adjacent tooth is barely broken. Where a cosmetic result is important, as it is here on the mesial surface of a maxillary first premolar, make no cuts with this instrument from the facial aspect. Overextension and an unattractive display of metal will result.

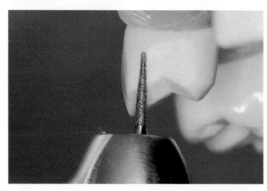

Fig. 5-21 Underextension of the proximal reduction in a facial direction can result in shortened grooves.[22] Inadequate extension in a gingival direction on the proximal surface opposite from the pontic can lead to premature failure of a fixed bridge because of poor retention and resistance.[23] Another common error is the underextension of the gingivofacial angle, shown in this figure,[19] caused by a tendency to pull occlusally with the diamond as it is pushed facially. It is important to concentrate on keeping the finish line at the same level apically throughout its entire length, since the gingivofacial angle has been identified as the most likely area of the three-quarter crown margin to fail.[24]

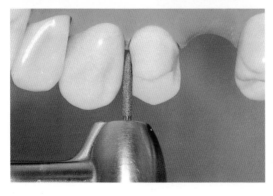

Fig. 5-22 Once enough maneuvering space has been obtained with the needle diamond, a larger instrument capable of producing a chamfer finish line, as well as axial reduction, can be used. It may be necessary to use the flame diamond as an intermediate instrument before proceeding to the torpedo diamond. Although both of them have the same diameter in the body of the diamond, the flame has a longer, thinner tip that facilitates its use where there is minimal proximal clearance. The reduction is completed with a torpedo diamond to produce a good chamfer on the proximal surface. Be sure to round the mesiolingual angle properly, to insure a continuous chamfer and adequate reduction in the angle area itself.

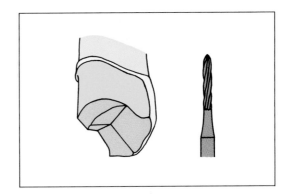

Fig. 5-23   Axial finishing: torpedo bur.

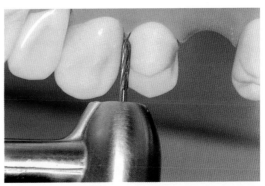

Fig. 5-24   Go over all the axial surfaces and the entire length of the chamfer with a torpedo-shaped 12-fluted carbide finishing bur. Pay special attention to the linguoproximal angles, making sure that the chamfer is distinct and continuous in these areas.

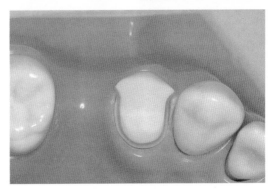

Fig. 5-25   The nearly completed preparation is seen in this occlusal view before the grooves and occlusal offset are added. Note the minimal extension at the mesiofacial corner of the tooth.

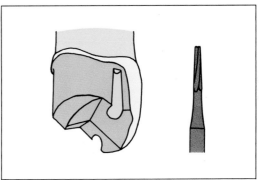

Fig. 5-26   Proximal grooves: no. 171 bur

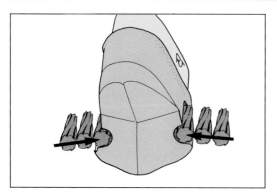

Fig. 5-27 Alignment and position are important aspects of groove placement. They have been described as forming a "lingual hook"[25] or being directed to the opposite lingual corner of the tooth.[1] Tjan and associates recommend the groove be cut along a line parallel with a line tangent to the outermost curvature of the tooth.[26] Most frequently the grooves will be placed so that the side of the bur will cut tooth structure along a line perpendicular to the *outer* surface of the enamel, at the point where the groove is placed.

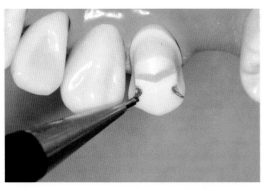

Fig. 5-28 Before attempting to start the grooves, draw the outline of the grooves on the occlusal surface of the preparation with a sharp pencil. The grooves should be placed as far facially as possible without undermining the facial surface.[27–29] On a posterior tooth, grooves should parallel the long axis of the tooth.[1,17, 27,29–31]

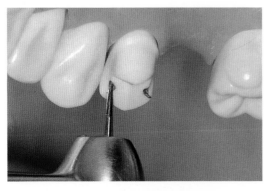

Fig. 5-29 Begin the mesial groove first by cutting a "template" in the occlusal surface with the no. 170 bur. This should follow the exact outline traced with the pencil previously and should be 1.0 mm or less in depth. The final groove will be the size of a no. 171 bur, but better results will be attained by a novice if a smaller bur is used, since it allows adjustments in direction without overcutting the groove.

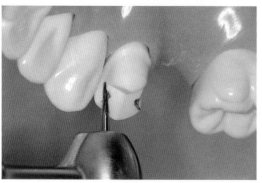

Fig. 5-30 Continue to extend the mesial groove farther apically. The distance will depend on the skill and confidence of the operator. It can be done 0.5 mm at a time, or in 2.0-mm increments by the operator who has a better sense of what he or she is trying to accomplish.

Fig. 5-31 The groove is finally extended to its full length, as far gingivally as possible, ending about 0.5 mm above the chamfer finish line.[26] It should form a definite step, rather than fading out.[1,17,24,26,32] Although V-shaped grooves were once widely used,[20,27,33,34] they provide only 68% of the retention and 57% of the resistance of rounded or concave grooves.[15] Grooves must be placed into the tooth at least to the full diameter of the bur used to prepare them. Since one of the groove's functions is to provide resistance to lingual tipping,[35] it is important that it have a definite lingual wall.[1] To prevent undermining facial enamel, and to avoid sharp unsupported "wings" of tooth structure lingual to the groove, the groove's direction toward the middle of the tooth should be at right angles to the outer surface of the tooth in the area where the groove is located.

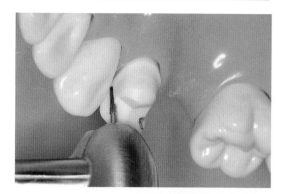

Fig. 5-32 The distal groove is cut so that it parallels the mesial groove. It may be helpful to the novice to place a cut-off tapered fissure bur in the mesial groove to provide an easily seen indicator of that groove's direction. If the distal groove is adjacent to an edentulous space as seen in this example, it should not be necessary to cut it in small increments.

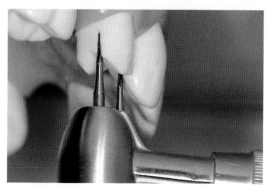

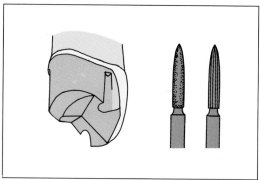

Fig. 5-33 Proximal flares: flame diamond and flame bur.

Fig. 5-34 The facial flare is cut from the groove outward to prevent overextension. It may not be possible to use any more than the tip of the flame diamond if the facial extension of the finish line is being kept conservative. The flare should be extended far enough to be reached by explorer and toothbrush, but not so far as to cause a noticeable display of metal. The actual distance will vary from tooth to tooth depending on the relative priority given to esthetics and cleansability. The flare is a flat geometric plane which is cut equally at the expense of the facial wall of the groove and the outer surface of the tooth.

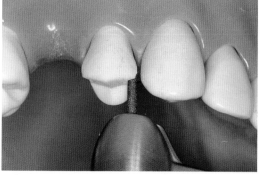

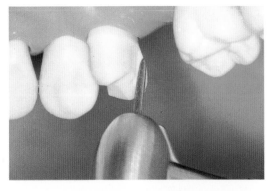

Fig. 5-35 If a flame diamond is used for creating the flare, complete the instrumentation of that flare with a flame-shaped carbide bur with the same configuration and 1.0-mm diameter as the flame diamond. Use crisp, short strokes of the handpiece and bur in one direction only. Moving the bur back and forth is likely to round over the finish line.

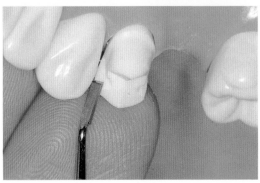

Fig. 5-36 In those areas where limiting the facial extension is critical for esthetic reasons, the flare can be formed with a just-sharpened, wide enamel chisel (1.5 to 2.0 mm).

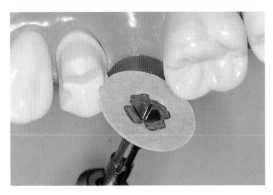

Fig. 5-37 Where access is good, a medium-grit sandpaper disk can be used to shape the flare. While this method can produce a highly desirable flat plane for the flare, it can result in a blurred or rounded finish line if the disk is used after the abrasive has worn off. Be sure to mask the lip and cheek with the fingers of the left hand to prevent injury to the patient.

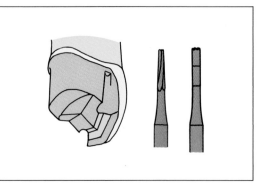

Fig. 5-38 Occlusal offset: no. 171 and no. 957 burs.

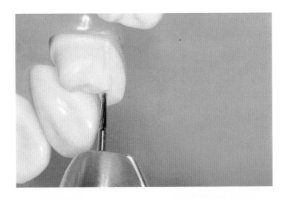

Fig. 5-39 Begin the occlusal offset with the end of a no. 171 bur. The offset is a 1.0-mm-wide ledge or flat "terrace" on the lingual incline of the facial cusp. It connects the grooves and stays a uniform distance away from the occlusofacial finish line, assuming the shape of an inverted V. This feature plays a major role in casting rigidity by tying together the proximal grooves to form a reinforcing staple.[14,16–18, 21,23,24,26,28,36]

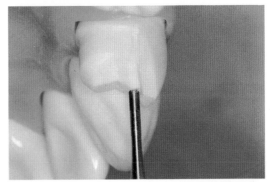

Fig. 5-40 Go over the occlusal offset with a no. 957 end-cutting bur. This will smooth the offset, insuring that it will be a flat ledge and not a V-shaped groove.

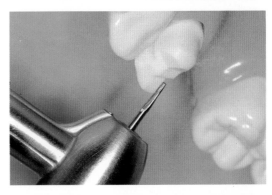

Fig. 5-41 Use a no. 170 bur to round over the angle formed between the upright wall of the offset and the lingual slope of the facial cusp.

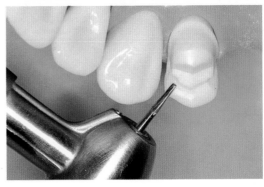

Fig. 5-42 The same bur can also be used to round any sharp corners between the lingual inclines of the facial cusp and the proximal flares.

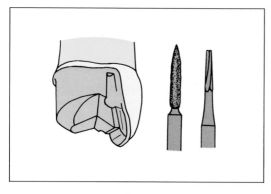

Fig. 5-43 Facial bevel: flame diamond and no. 170 bur.

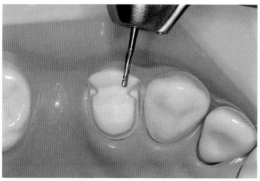

Fig. 5-44 Place a narrow occlusal finish bevel along the occlusofacial line angle, taking care to keep it perpendicular to the path of insertion. The bevel should be no more than 0.5 mm wide. Carry the bevel around the angle onto each proximal flare, keeping the outer edge of the bevel continuous with the outer edge of the flares. The bevel, both flares, and the chamfer should connect smoothly to form one continuous finish line without sharp angles.

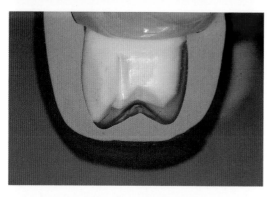

Fig. 5-45 The silicone putty index is placed over the preparation to demonstrate the depth and form of reduction, as well as the location and relative size of features such as the occlusofacial bevel, the occlusal offset, and the functional cusp bevel.

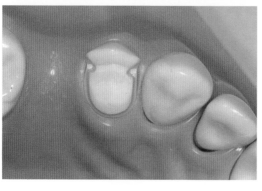

Fig. 5-46 Completed three-quarter crown preparation on a maxillary premolar.

Fig. 5-47 A common variation of the three-quarter crown preparation, employed when caries or previous restorations are present on the proximal surfaces, is one in which boxes are substituted for grooves.[14,17,27,28,31,32,34] The three-quarter crown with boxes is more retentive than the classic design with two grooves.[12,15] However, boxes are very destructive of tooth structure, so their use can be justified only when tooth structure has already been destroyed by caries or previous restorations. The box is also used to accommodate nonrigid connectors.[37]

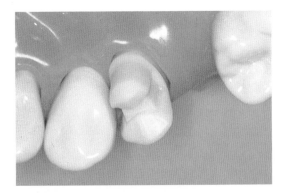

Fig. 5-48 A less destructive alternative for augmenting retention and resistance is a three-quarter crown preparation utilizing two grooves on each proximal surface.[38] There is no significant difference between the retention afforded by the four grooves and that available from two boxes.[15]

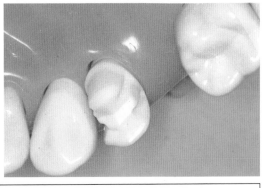

Fig. 5-49 The features of a maxillary posterior three-quarter crown and the function served by each.

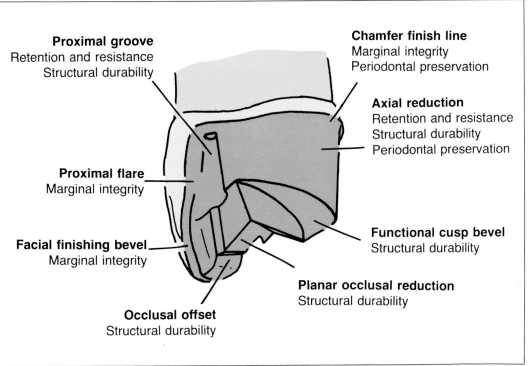

Proximal groove
Retention and resistance
Structural durability

Chamfer finish line
Marginal integrity
Periodontal preservation

Axial reduction
Retention and resistance
Structural durability
Periodontal preservation

Proximal flare
Marginal integrity

Facial finishing bevel
Marginal integrity

Functional cusp bevel
Structural durability

Occlusal offset
Structural durability

Planar occlusal reduction
Structural durability

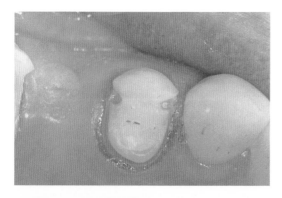

Clinical examples: Maxillary posterior (Figs. 5-50 through 5-58)

Fig. 5-50 A classic three-quarter crown preparation was done on this maxillary first premolar, which was to be used as a bridge abutment. The mesial extension was kept minimal to avoid an unnecessary display of metal.

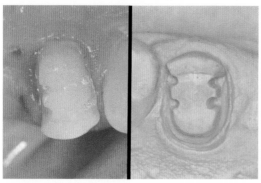

Fig. 5-51 This maxillary first premolar bridge abutment was a little shorter than ideal, so double grooves were used on each proximal surface. The fact that the proximal surfaces were free of caries or previous restorations precluded the use of boxes. The prepared tooth is seen *left,* while a stone cast of the preparation is shown *right.*

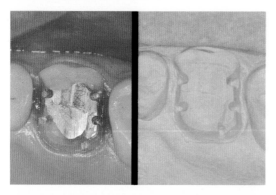

Fig. 5-52 A three-quarter crown was used to restore this maxillary first molar after completion of endodontic treatment and placement of an amalgam core *(left).* Because the tooth had a short clinical crown, multiple grooves were used to enhance retention and resistance. These can be seen in greater detail on the stone cast of the prepared tooth *(right).*

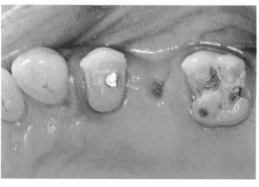

Fig. 5-53 Slightly modified three-quarter crown preparations were done on both of the periodontally involved abutment teeth for a bridge to replace a maxillary second premolar.

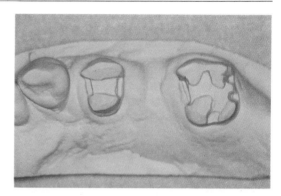

Fig. 5-54 A stone cast of the two three-quarter crowns shows more clearly the two boxes used in the first premolar preparation and the combination of a mesial box and multiple grooves used on the first molar.

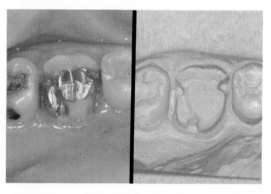

Fig. 5-55 A facial view of the bridge fabricated on the modified three-quarter crown preparations shows the extent of gingival recession around the abutments. Porcelain-fused-to-metal retainers would have been unnecessarily destructive. The patient chose partial veneer crowns when the options were explained to her. She found the minimal display of metal quite acceptable.

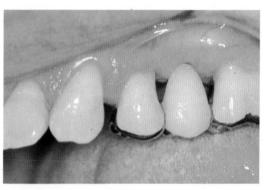

Fig. 5-56 A three-quarter crown preparation was done on this maxillary first molar after endodontic treatment and insertion of an amalgam core. The preparation is shown in the mouth *(left)* and on the stone cast *(right)*. Facial extensions were minimal on both the mesial and the distal surfaces.

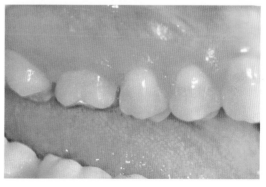

Fig. 5-57 The completed restoration is seen from the facial view. Minimal extensions on the proximal surfaces and occlusal bevel, combined with rounding of the facial occlusal line angle during intraoral finishing of the casting, have resulted in a very slight display of gold in a direct facial view.

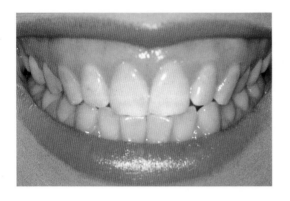

Fig. 5-58 From a conversational distance the metal ringing the facial surface of the tooth is invisible. The restoration design was more than adequate for the esthetic requirements of this 26-year-old patient.

References

1. Shillingburg, H. T., and Fisher, D. W. The partial veneer restoration. Aust. Dent. J. 17:411, 1972.
2. Kahn, A. E. Partial versus full coverage. J. Prosthet. Dent. 10:167, 1960.
3. Maxwell, E. L., and Wasser, V. E. Debate: Full vs. partial coverage as the abutment of choice in fixed bridgework. J. D. C. Dent. Soc. 36:9, 1961.
4. Miller, L. L. Partial coverage in crown and bridge prosthesis with the use of elastic impression materials. J. Prosthet. Dent. 13:905, 1963.
5. Silness, J. Periodontal conditions in patients treated with dental bridges. II. The influence of full and partial crowns on plaque accumulation, development of gingivitis and pocket formation. J. Periodont. Res. 5:219, 1970.
6. Kishimoto, M., Hobo, S., Duncanson, M. G., and Shillingburg, H. T. Effectiveness of margin finishing techniques on cast gold restorations. Int. J. Periodont. Rest. Dent. 1(5):21, 1981.
7. Shillingburg, H. T. Conservative preparations for cast restorations. Dent. Clin. North Am. 20:259, 1976.
8. Peterka, C. A modern three-quarter crown. J. Am. Dent. Assoc. 27:1175, 1940.
9. Leander, C. T. Preparation of abutments for fixed partial dentures. Dent. Clin. North Am. 3:59, 1959.
10. Grosso, F. P., and Carreno, J. A. Partial or full coverage restoration. J. Prosthet. Dent. 40:628 1978.
11. Lorey, R. E., and Myers, G. E. The retentive qualities of bridge retainers. J. Am. Dent. Assoc. 76:568, 1968.
12. Reisbick, M. H., and Shillingburg, H. T. Effect of preparation geometry on retention and resistance of cast gold restorations. Calif. Dent. Assoc. J. 3:51, 1975.
13. Potts, R. G., Shillingburg, H. T., and Duncanson, M. G. Retention and resistance of preparations for cast restorations. J. Prosthet. Dent. 43:303, 1980.
14. Ingraham, R., Bassett, R. W., and Koser, J. R. An Atlas of Cast Gold Procedures. 2nd ed. Buena Park, CA: Unitro College Press, 1969, 161–165.
15. Kishimoto, M., Shillingburg, H. T., and Duncanson, M. G. Influence of preparation features on retention and resistance. I. MOD onlays. J. Prosthet. Dent. 49:35, 1983.
16. Willey, R. E. The preparation of abutments for veneer retainers. J. Am. Dent. Assoc. 53:141, 1956.
17. Guyer, S. E. Multiple preparations for fixed prosthodontics. J. Prosthet. Dent. 23:529, 1970.
18. Abdullah, M. A., and Kumar, B. K. The principles of design of the three quarter crown. Int. Coll. Dent. Newsletter (India), Sept: 14, 1973.
19. Tjan, A. H., and Miller, G. D. Common errors in tooth preparation. Gen. Dent. 28:20, 1980.
20. Rogers, E. J. The partial veneer crown. Preparation, construction and application. Dent. Items Interest 50:397, 1928.
21. Racowsky, L. P., and Wolinsky, L. E. Restoring the badly broken-down tooth with esthetic partial coverage restorations. Comp. Cont. Educ. Dent. 11:322, 1981.
22. Tinker, E. T. Some of the fundamentals in the construction and application of crown and bridge restorations. J. Am. Dent. Assoc. 12:1374, 1925.
23. Smith, D. E. Abutment preparations. J. Am. Dent. Assoc. 18:2063, 1931.
24. Tinker, H. A. The three-quarter crown in fixed bridgework. J. Can. Dent. Assoc. 16:125, 1950.
25. Ho, G. Lecture notes. University of Southern California School of Dentistry, 1959.
26. Tjan, A. H. L., and Miller, G. D. Biometric guide to groove placement on three-quarter crown preparations. J. Prosthet. Dent. 42:405, 1979.
27. Tinker, E. T. Fixed bridgework. J. Natl. Dent. Assoc. 7:579, 1920.
28. Rhoads, J. E. Preparation of the teeth for cast restorations. pp. 34–67 In G. M. Hollenback, Science and Technic of the Cast Restoration. St. Louis: The C. V. Mosby Co., 1964.
29. Jones, W. E. The scientifically designed partial veneer crown. J. Am. Dent. Assoc. 86:1337, 1973.
30. Thom, L. W. Principles of cavity preparation in crown and bridge prosthesis. II. The three-quarter crown. J. Am. Dent. Assoc. 41:443, 1950.
31. Silberhorn, O. W. Fixed bridge retainers—Design and retention features. Ill. Dent. J. 22:641, 1953.
32. Dressel, R. P. The three-quarter crown as a bridge abutment for the posterior teeth. Dent. Cosmos 72:730, 1930.
33. Doxtater, L. W. The three-quarter crown with accessory anchorage. Dent. Items Interest 51:290, 1929.
34. Krause, O. G. Cast attachments for bridgework with special reference to vital teeth. J. Am. Dent. Assoc. 21:2104, 1934.
35. Bronner, F. J. Is there a common basis for all systems of inlay preparations? Dent. Cosmos 74:1085, 1932.
36. Klaffenbach, A. O. An analytic study of modern abutments. J. Am. Dent. Assoc. 23:2275, 1936.
37. Shillingburg, H. T., and Fisher, D. W. Nonrigid connectors for fixed partial dentures. J. Am. Dent. Assoc. 87:1195, 1973.
38. Tanner, H. Ideal and modified inlay and veneer crown preparations. Ill. Dent. J. 26:240, 1957.

Chapter 6

Mandibular Posterior Three-Quarter Crowns

The three-quarter crown preparation on mandibular premolars and molars differs from the maxillary three-quarter crown because the facial cusps of the mandibular posterior teeth are the functional cusps. The preparation on a mandibular tooth must compensate for this to protect the facial cusps and the restoration margins. Otherwise, an unprotected cusp might fracture or the crown soon wear through near the facioocclusal margin.

For this reason, early versions of three-quarter crowns for mandibular posterior teeth covered the entire facial surface, leaving the nonfunctional lingual surface unveneered.[1–6] Complete coverage of the facial surface became esthetically unacceptable, and a different design evolved for mandibular teeth.

The reverse three-quarter crown, with complete coverage of the facial surface, is used only occasionally and is usually reserved for one or two situations: (1) it is ideal for restoration of mandibular molars that are severely inclined lingually,[7] and (2) it can also be used on molars that have suffered destruction of the facial surface, but not of the lingual.[8]

The facial surface came to be left un-veneered, and the cusps themselves are capped.[7–9] The occlusal finish line can take the form of an accentuated chamfer,[9] or a shoulder with a bevel.[7,8] Either finish line will provide space for an adequate bulk of metal to reinforce the margin and tie the grooves together to form a reinforcing "truss." Because the margin and reinforcing feature are located on the facial slopes of the facial cusps, it is unnecessary to place an offset on the lingual slope of the cusps.

The mandibular first premolar is a poor candidate for use of the three-quarter crown.[10] This tooth is often too short or too small in girth to provide adequate retention and resistance to a fixed bridge retainer. In addition, its position in the arch makes the use of a standard three-quarter crown esthetically unacceptable for most patients.

The three-quarter crown is therefore restricted to use as a bridge retainer or single-tooth restoration on second premolars and molars for patients who do not object to displaying some metal. The three-quarter crown should not be used on mesially tipped molars because it is impossible to compensate for the overtapered mesial and distal walls, which inevitably occur in such situations, without involving the facial surface of the tooth. As a result, the three-quarter crown is frequently not used as a bridge retainer on mandibular second molars, even though the facial surfaces may be intact.

The steps for making a classic three-quarter crown preparation on a mandibular molar are shown in Figs. 6-1 through 6-44. It differs from the maxillary three-quarter crown (chapter 5) because the functional cusps are the facial rather than the lingual ones.

Some clinical examples of the use of mandibular three-quarter crowns are shown in Figs. 6-45 through 6-55.

Mandibular posterior three-quarter crown preparation (Figs. 6-1 through 6-44)

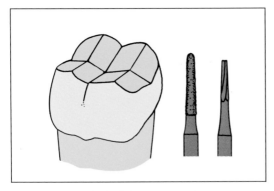

Fig. 6-1 Planar occlusal reduction: Round-end tapered diamond and no. 171 bur.

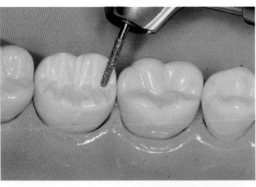

Fig. 6-2 Make depth-orientation cuts on the occlusal surface with the round-end tapered diamond. These grooves should be placed in the major developmental grooves and on the crests of triangular ridges. These bench-mark grooves should be 1.5 mm deep on the facial cusps and 1.0 mm deep on the lingual cusps.

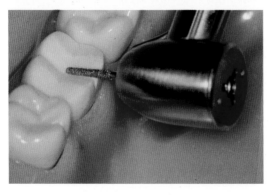

Fig. 6-3 Complete the occlusal reduction with the round-end tapered diamond by removing the tooth structure remaining between the depth-orientation grooves, maintaining the geometric planes of the occlusal surface.

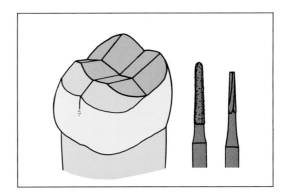

Fig. 6-4 Functional cusp bevel: round-end tapered diamond and no. 171 bur.

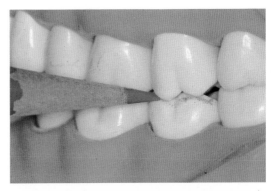

Fig. 6-5 With the patient's posterior teeth in occlusion, use a pencil to trace the outline of the opposing maxillary facial cusps onto the facial surfaces of the mandibular tooth.

Fig. 6-6 The traced outline of the maxillary facial cusps provides a pattern for the termination line of the functional cusp bevel when it is prepared.

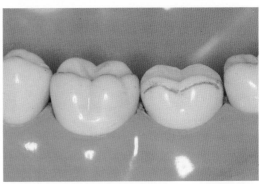

Fig. 6-7 Place depth-orientation grooves 1.5 mm deep at the occlusal line angle, roughly following the termination line traced in the previous step. Although this line usually follows an up and down path on the cusps, no special effort is made to precisely reproduce this anatomical pattern on molars. On premolars, however, it is important to reproduce the cusp pattern on the facial surfaces. There will be less metal to display in the central portion of the facial surface. The metal that is present will be less conspicuous because the remaining tooth structure will reproduce a natural cusp pattern, which will blend in better with other teeth in the arch.

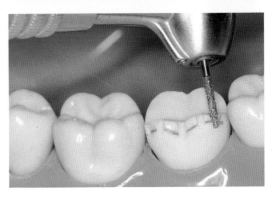

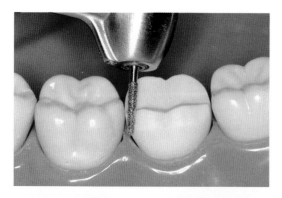

Fig. 6-8 Complete the functional cusp bevel by removing the tooth structure remaining between the depth-orientation grooves with a round-end tapered diamond.

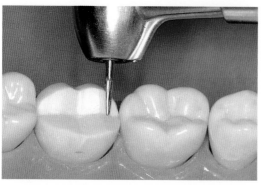

Fig. 6-9 Use a no. 171 bur to smooth the occlusal reduction and functional cusp bevel. Although the occlusal reduction should reproduce the inclined planes of the occlusal surface,[2,11,12] there should be no sharp angles on cusp tips because they will impede complete seating of the casting later.

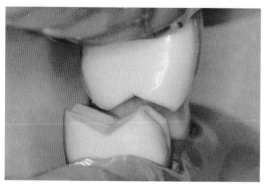

Fig. 6-10 The uniform clearance provided by the planar occlusal reduction and functional cusp bevel can be seen in this mesial view of the reduced mandibular molar and the opposing maxillary molar.

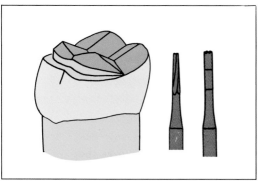

Fig. 6-11 Occlusal shoulder: no. 171 and no. 957 burs.

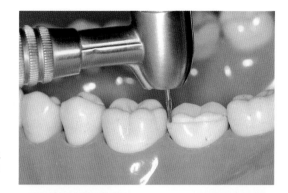

Fig. 6-12 Place the occlusal shoulder with a no. 171 bur, following the termination line drawn previously.

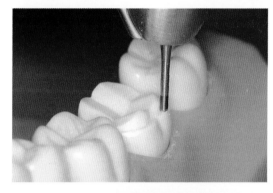

Fig. 6-13 Plane the occlusal shoulder with a no. 957 bur. Be sure that the entire shoulder is the full 1.0 mm width of the instrument.

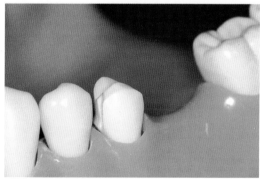

Fig. 6-14 When this preparation is used on a mandibular premolar, the extensions are kept minimal for esthetics, and there may not be space for a shoulder. In that circumstance, an accentuated chamfer should be used rather than a shoulder.

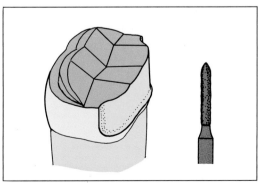

Fig. 6-15 Lingual axial reduction: torpedo diamond.

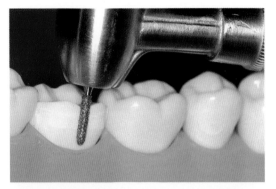

Fig. 6-16 Begin the lingual axial reduction by sweeping the torpedo diamond from mesial to distal, with the diamond aligned with the intended path of insertion of the preparation. Initially, this will result in reduction of only the occlusal portion of the lingual wall. If the novice operator becomes impatient and attempts to produce the gingival finish line at this time, the diamond will be aligned with the lingual wall of the tooth rather than with the path of insertion, and an undercut will result.

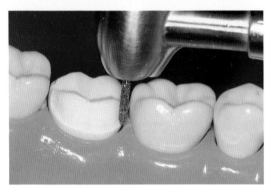

Fig. 6-17 Complete the lingual axial reduction, extending it as far into the mesial and distal embrasures as possible without nicking the adjacent teeth. When an adequate bulk of tooth structure has been removed, the end of the torpedo diamond will produce a chamfer as the lingual gingival finish line. Since the diamond is 1.0 mm in diameter, and the tip forms a sharp point, if the diamond is sunk into the tooth one-half the diameter of the instrument, the axial reduction will be 0.5 mm immediately occlusal to the chamfer. It becomes progressively greater toward the occlusal surface.

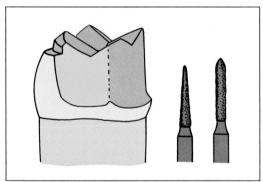

Fig. 6-18 Proximal axial reduction: short needle and torpedo diamonds.

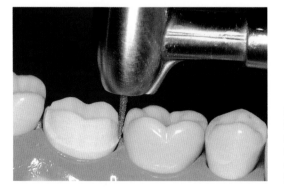

Fig. 6-19 Begin the mesial interproximal reduction with the short-needle diamond. Use an up and down sawing motion without putting excessive pressure on the tip. Avoid hitting the adjacent tooth, but do not overtaper the axial wall being prepared, either.

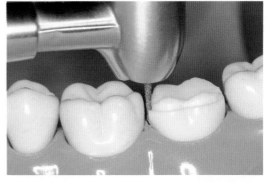

Fig. 6-20 Extend through the proximal surface from the lingual surface until contact is broken with the distal surface of the adjacent tooth. Do not be overly conservative in the facial extension, or unnecessary difficulty may be encountered in impression making, margin finishing, or home care. A 1.0 mm extension facial to the area of actual contact is acceptable.

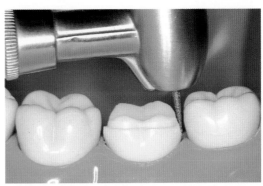

Fig. 6-21 Repeat the process on the distal surface. Be especially mindful of the mesiodistal inclination of the diamond on this surface. Access is more difficult on the distal surface, and visibility is limited. Novices have a tendency to incline the instrument mesially to accommodate limited opening and, unconciously, to avoid cutting the mesial surface of the adjacent tooth. Limited access is better compensated for by tilting the diamond *facially* or *lingually*.

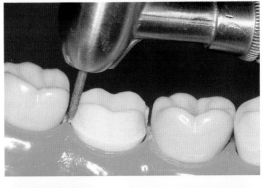

Fig. 6-22 Where access and visibility are limited, the next step may require the use of the flame diamond. Although it has the same 1.0 mm diameter as the torpedo diamond in the main body of the instrument, it has a longer, thinner tip that permits it to be used to increase the axial reduction without nicking the adjacent tooth in the gingival region.

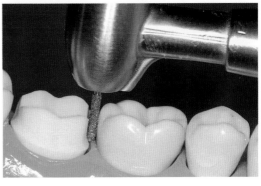

Fig. 6-23 The torpedo diamond is now used to finish the axial reduction on the proximal surfaces, insuring adequate space for the cast restoration without overcontouring it. Use the instrument to create a smooth transition from proximal to lingual surface, with equal axial depth of reduction. The chamfer finish line thus formed should be as distinct at the mesiolingual and distolingual angles as it is in the middle of any of the axial surfaces. The finish line should be at the same level gingivally throughout this transitional area.

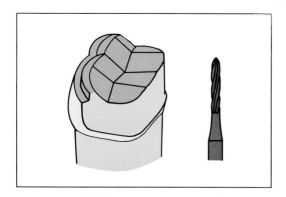

Fig. 6-24 Axial finishing: torpedo bur.

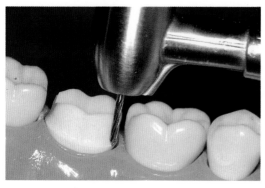

Fig. 6-25 Go over all of the axial surfaces with the torpedo bur, paying particular attention to redefining and smoothing the chamfer finish line itself.

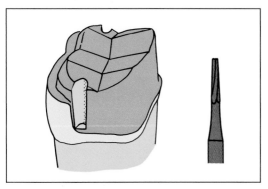

Fig. 6-26 Proximal grooves: no. 171 bur.

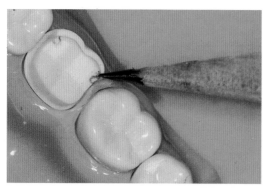

Fig. 6-27 It is a good idea for the novice to draw the outline of the grooves on the occlusal surface with a pencil. In this way, their exact position can be set before an instrument ever touches the tooth. This is an unnecessary step after an operator has gained experience with placing grooves.

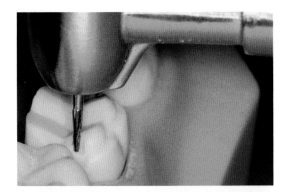

Fig. 6-28 Begin the mesial groove with a no. 170 bur, cutting it to a length of approximately 4.0 mm.

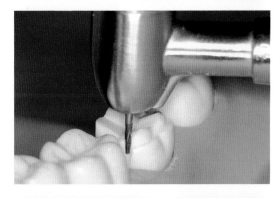

Fig. 6-29 Once you are satisfied with the outline of the groove that you have prepared, extend it gingivally in small increments (approximately 1.0 mm at a time).

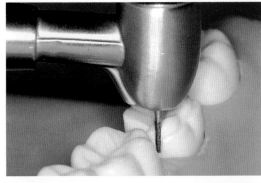

Fig. 6-30 Extend the groove to its full gingival length, ending it approximately 0.5 mm short of the chamfer finish line.

Fig. 6-31 The second groove is begun. The distal groove of a three-quarter crown preparation on a mandibular molar is one of the most difficult features to prepare properly in the mouth, owing both to difficult accessibility and poor visibility. In this example, a bur is shown in the mesial groove as an aid to visualizing the direction of the second groove. The novice may want to do this on a typodont preparation, but it is impossible to do in the mouth. It is important to keep the second groove aligned with the first, for there is a common tendency to lean it into the center of the tooth.

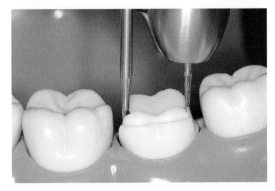

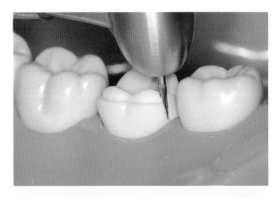

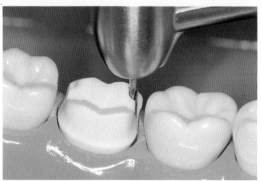

Fig. 6-32 Extend the groove to its full length in small increments.

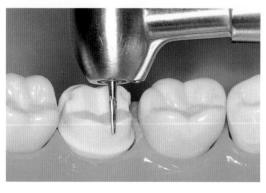

Fig. 6-33 When both grooves have been prepared to their full length in proper alignment, recut them with a no. 171 bur to insure that they are large and definite. Considering the size of the restoration and the surface area of the facial surface for which they are substituted, it is important that the grooves be of adequate size. Tjan and Miller recommend an even larger size bur than the no. 171 for molars.[13] Small, indistinct grooves serve no useful purpose.

Fig. 6-34 With either a no. 171 or no. 170 bur in the handpiece, *lightly* bevel or round over all the sharp edges on the occlusal surface of the preparation.

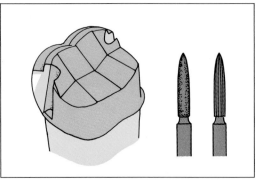

Fig. 6-35 Proximal flare: flame diamond and flame bur.

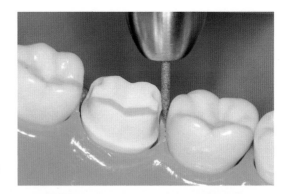

Fig. 6-36 Use the tip of the flame diamond to begin the proximal flare.

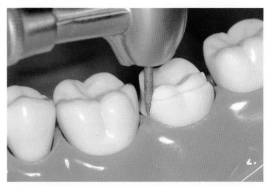

Fig. 6-37 When more maneuvering space is available, the body of the flame diamond may be brought into play, as it is not critical to keep extension minimal on a mandibular molar. The flare should form an essentially flat plane, wider at the occlusal than at the gingival, with a definite finish line. Access is too restricted in this area of the mouth to attempt the use of a sandpaper disk.

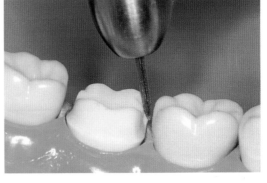

Fig. 6-38 To produce a smooth surface adjacent to the actual finish line a long flame-shaped carbide bur of the same diameter and configuration as the diamond should be used for finishing the flare.

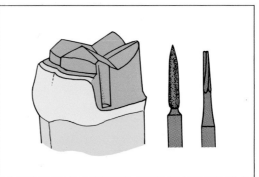

Fig. 6-39 Facial bevel: flame diamond and no. 170 bur.

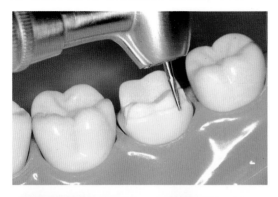

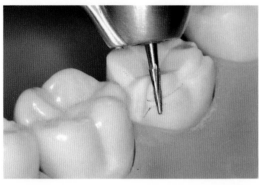

Fig. 6-40 Although a flame diamond may be used for the initial instrumentation of the bevel on the occlusal shoulder, final preparation of this 45-degree bevel should be accomplished with a no. 170 bur, or with the flame carbide bur.

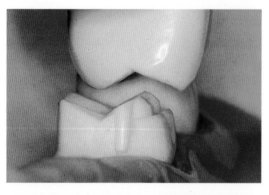

Fig. 6-41 Be sure to round over the angle between the facial occlusal bevel and the proximal flare, maintaining a smooth, unbroken finish line from one to the other.

Fig. 6-42 A proximal view of the finished preparation shows the continuity of finish line from occlusal bevel to flare to chamfer, as well as the adequacy of the occlusal reduction.

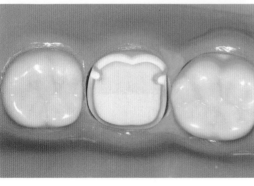

Fig. 6-43 An occlusal view of the complete preparation.

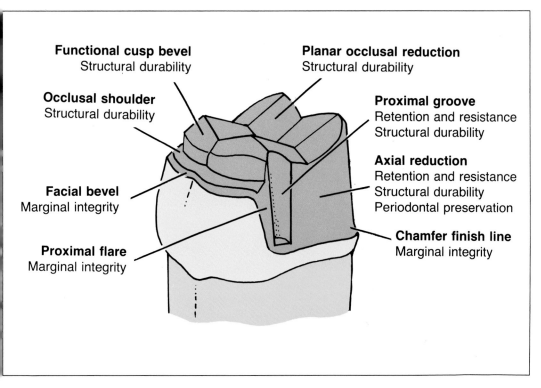

Functional cusp bevel
Structural durability

Occlusal shoulder
Structural durability

Facial bevel
Marginal integrity

Proximal flare
Marginal integrity

Planar occlusal reduction
Structural durability

Proximal groove
Retention and resistance
Structural durability

Axial reduction
Retention and resistance
Structural durability
Periodontal preservation

Chamfer finish line
Marginal integrity

Fig. 6-44 The features of a three-quarter crown preparation on a mandibular molar, and the function served by each.

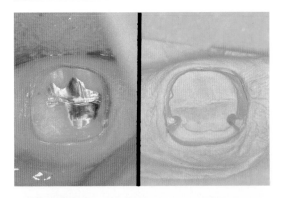

Clinical examples: Mandibular posterior (Figs. 6-45 through 6-55)

Fig. 6-45 A three-quarter crown preparation was made on this mandibular second molar to accommodate a bridge retainer. A stone cast of this typical preparation is shown on the right.

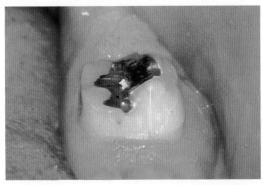

Fig. 6-46 A mesial view of the three-quarter crown preparation shows groove placement and the occlusal shoulder in detail.

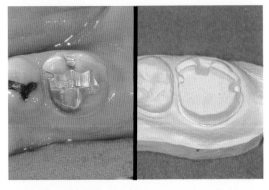

Fig. 6-47 A three-quarter crown design was selected for a single tooth restoration on this mandibular first molar after placement of a rather large amalgam core. The small box form added to incorporate a defective facial groove can be seen clearly in the stone cast on the right.

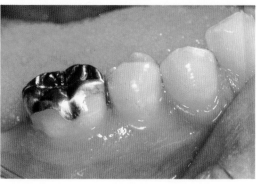

Fig. 6-48 A facial view of the completed three-quarter crown, the preparation for which was seen in Fig. 6-47. The small projection in the occlusofacial margin covers the box form in the preparation, which was added to take care of a carious facial groove.

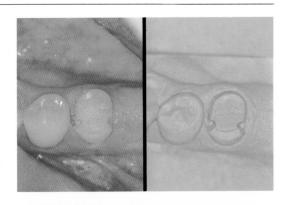

Fig. 6-49 A three-quarter crown preparation on a mandibular premolar to be used as a bridge abutment. It is seen in the mouth *(left)* and on the cast *(right)*.

Fig. 6-50 A modified three-quarter crown preparation was done on this mandibular first premolar, utilizing two grooves on each proximal surface to enhance resistance *(left)*, and an accentuated chamfer occlusofacial finish line with minimal extension onto the facial surface *(right)*.

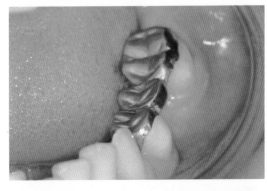

Fig. 6-51 A mesiofacial view of the completed bridge for which the premolar abutment preparation is seen in Fig. 6-50.

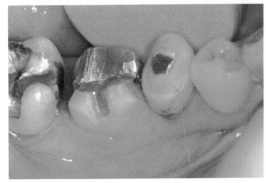

Fig. 6-52 This three-quarter crown preparation for a single-tooth restoration of a mandibular first molar makes use of an accentuated chamfer for the occlusofacial finish line, with a narrow box form for the facial groove.

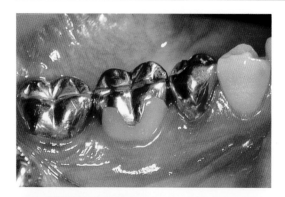

Fig. 6-53 A facial view of the finished three-quarter crown on the previous preparation.

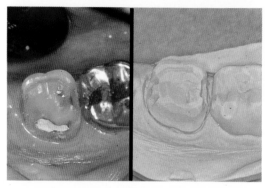

Fig. 6-54 A reverse three-quarter crown preparation was used on this mandibular right second molar with facial caries and an unblemished lingual surface *(left)*. The stone cast *(right)* shows more clearly the box used on the mesial surface and the two grooves placed on the distal.

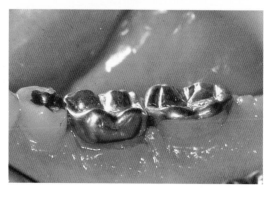

Fig. 6-55 A lingual view is shown of the reverse three-quarter crown on the second molar.

References

1. Tinker, E. T. Fixed bridgework. J. Natl. Dent. Assoc. 7:579, 1920.
2. Rogers, E. J. The partial veneer crown. Preparation, construction and application. Dent. Items Interest 50:397, 1928.
3. Smith, D. E. Abutment preparations. J. Am. Dent. Assoc. 18:2063, 1931.
4. Potter, H. R., and Smith, D. E. Practical bridgework. III. Non-vital teeth in bridgework. Pac. Dent. Gaz. 40:519, 1932.
5. Dressel, R. P. The three-quarter crown as a bridge abutment for the posterior teeth. Dent. Cosmos 72:730, 1930.
6. Dietz, W. H. Modified abutments for removable and fixed prosthodontics. J. Prosthet. Dent. 11:1112, 1961.
7. Schwartz, J. R. The basic or structural character of abutment preparations. Dent. Items Interest 56:897, 1934.
8. Shillingburg, H. T., and Fisher, D. W. The partial veneer restoration. Aust. Dent. J. 17:411, 1972.
9. Ingraham, R., Bassett, R. W., and Koser, J. R. An Atlas of Cast Gold Procedures. 2nd ed. Buena Park, CA: Unitro College Press, 1969, 161–165.
10. Thom, L. W. Principles of cavity preparation in crown and bridge prosthesis. II. The three-quarter crown. J. Am. Dent. Assoc. 41:443, 1950.
11. Shillingburg, H. T. Conservative preparations for cast restorations. Dent. Clin. North Am. 20:259, 1976.
12. Tjan, A. H., and Miller, G. D. Common errors in tooth preparation. Gen. Dent. 28:20, 1980.
13. Tjan, A. H., and Miller, G. D. Biometric guide to groove placement on three-quarter crown preparations. J. Prosthet. Dent. 42:405, 1979.

Chapter 7

Anterior Three-Quarter Crowns

The first true anterior three-quarter crown was developed by Carmichael from wire, foil, and solder before the advent of an accurate casting technique for dentistry.[1] In that technique, foil was adapted over the completed preparation and an iridioplatinum wire staple was fitted into the grooves of the preparation. Wax was added to attach the staple to the foil, and these were withdrawn from the mouth and invested. Solder was then melted over the foil to form the restoration. From these humble beginnings use of the restoration grew. For many years it offered the only means of making an esthetic retainer for a fixed bridge.

The three-quarter crown preparation design currently employed is a direct descendant of that early restoration. This type of preparation is not used nearly as frequently today as it once was. A retainer with a suitable esthetic veneer has replaced it in those situations where greater retention and restoration stability are needed. Improperly executed three-quarter crowns, with ugly and frequently unnecessary displays of gold, have given the restoration a bad name with both the general public and the dental profession. Coupled with the ease with which a tooth can be prepared for a porcelain-fused-to-metal restoration, this has led to the near total demise of the anterior three-quarter crown, a most unfortunate development.

Porcelain-fused-to-metal restorations have been a boon to dentistry because they exhibit a strength, durability, and esthetic potential lacking in all other anterior full veneer restorations. Unquestionably there are numerous clinical situations in which porcelain-fused-to-metal crowns are the restorations of choice: caries or previous restorations that have affected the facial or incisal edges of the tooth, excessive destruction of coronal tooth structure, unsightly discolorations of enamel from systemic conditions, and short clinical crowns on bridge abutments, to name some of the more frequently occurring indications. Some unblemished anterior teeth are destroyed in the name of esthetics when a partial veneer crown could have been used. Obtaining a natural appearance and contour in porcelain is difficult, and creating a natural texture is impossible. Tinker's 1920 admonition that " . . . conservation of tooth structure is all important," is still worth remembering.[2]

Well-executed three-quarter crowns can avoid an objectionable display of metal and can be quite esthetic.[3] However, they require more time and skill than do full veneer restorations[4] and are not for every tooth nor every patient. Successful anterior use of a three-quarter crown will depend upon careful evaluation of each case prior to treatment. Anterior three-quarter crowns are well suited for short-span bridges with abutments that are relatively restoration- and caries-free.[5,6]

The morphology of the tooth in question must also be taken into account. A thick, square anterior tooth with an adequate faciolingual bulk of structure is the best candidate for a three-quarter crown.[7] Thin tapering teeth prohibit the proper placement of grooves or pins. To preserve esthetics and facilitate parallelism of abutment preparations, the teeth must be well aligned. A deep overbite complicates the use of this retainer design by requiring excessive lingual reduction. A final prerequisite is that the patient should demonstrate immaculate oral hygiene.

Like its posterior counterpart, the anterior three-quarter crown is more likely to exhibit improved marginal integrity over a full-coverage restoration because it is open to visual inspection.[8] Christensen demonstrated that clinicians are much more demanding in their assessment of visible margins than they are of those which can be evaluated by tactile sensation alone.[9] In addition, the margins of a cemented partial veneer crown are likely to fit well. A full veneer crown acts as a closed hydraulic chamber during cementation,[10] while the open-faced partial veneer crown will not confine the cement to produce the pressure that will prevent complete seating during cementation.

As with all other preparations for cast restorations, the fundamental component of retention of an anterior partial veneer crown is the presence of opposing walls.[11,12] In these preparations, one or more surfaces will be left uncovered, so the partial veneer crown is not as retentive as the full veneer crown.[13–15] Features such as pins, grooves, and boxes must be substituted for the unveneered axial wall.[16] These features increase the surface area of the preparation, which increases the retention of the casting.[13]

In the standard three-quarter crown for an anterior tooth, the most commonly used retentive and resistance feature is the proximal groove. The path of insertion, determined in large part by the placement of the grooves, must be correct to guarantee an esthetic restoration.[17] It is just as imperative that the extensions be minimal.[18] The three-quarter crown, used in carefully selected cases, can be both esthetic and conservative.

Figures 7-1 through 7-46 illustrate the steps in the preparation for a three-quarter crown on a maxillary canine tooth. The preparation for an incisor differs only in that the lingual surface incisal to the cingulum would be a single, slightly concave surface. Mandibular anterior three-quarter crown preparations closely resemble their maxillary counterparts.

Clinical examples of maxillary anterior three-quarter crowns are shown in Figs. 7-47 through 7-55.

Maxillary canine three-quarter crown preparation (Figs. 7-1 through 7-46)

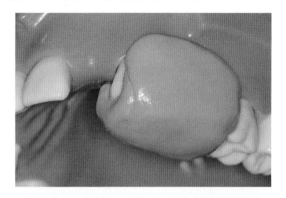

Fig. 7-1 A silicone index can be most helpful in gauging reduction for one who is inexperienced with this preparation. Before starting the preparation for a three-quarter crown, adapt one-half scoop of condensation-reaction silicone putty on the facial and lingual aspects of the tooth to be prepared and one tooth distal to it.

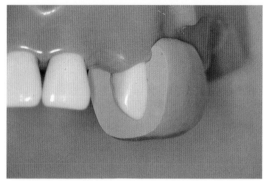

Fig. 7-2 A midsagittal index is very helpful in judging lingual reduction. Make it by cutting the index into mesial and distal segments and aligning the cut with the midline of the tooth from faciocervical to facioincisal to linguocervical.

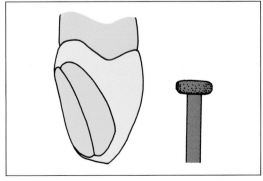

Fig. 7-3 A wrap-around horizontal index can be used on bridge abutments, such as the one illustrated here. A horizontal cut is made in the putty at the incisogingival midpoint of the tooth to be prepared.

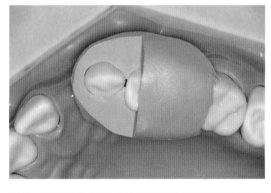

Fig. 7-4 Lingual reduction: small wheel diamond.

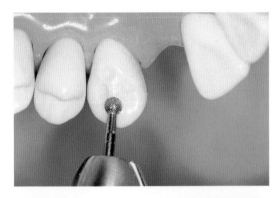

Fig. 7-5 Before beginning the lingual reduction, make at least four depth-orientation cuts on the lingual surface to insure that an adequate amount of tooth structure will be removed.

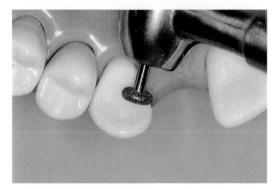

Fig. 7-6 Use a small round diamond with a head 1.4 mm larger in diameter than the shaft of the instrument. When buried in the enamel to the shaft, the depth of the cut will be approximately 0.7 mm.

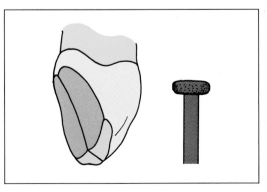

Fig. 7-7 Use the small round-edged diamond wheel to create a concave surface over the lingual surface of the tooth incisal to the cingulum. A slight ridge is left on a maxillary canine, resulting in two concave depressions on the lingual surface. The lingual surfaces of incisors and mandibular canines are uninterrupted. The reduction should be made to the depth of the orientation cuts, and should remove all tooth structure remaining between them. Avoid cutting excessive tooth structure from the vertical wall of the cingulum.

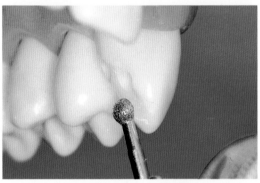

Fig. 7-8 Incisal reduction: small wheel diamond.

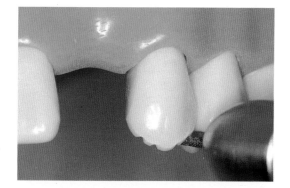

Fig. 7-9 Make depth orientation cuts on the incisal edge. They should barely break through the facioincisal line angle.

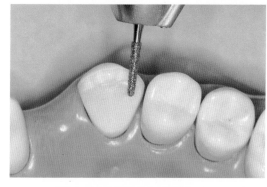

Fig. 7-10 Toward the junction between the incisal edge and the lingual surface, the depth orientation grooves should be about 0.7 mm deep.

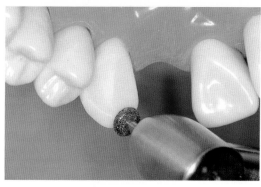

Fig. 7-11 The actual incisal reduction, which parallels the inclination of the uncut incisal edge, is made with the small round-edged wheel diamond. On a canine tooth this reduction follows the natural mesial and distal inclines of the incisal edge. On an incisor the incisal reduction will be in a straight line.

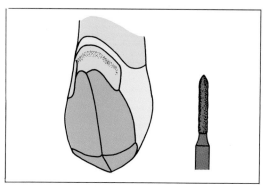

Fig. 7-12 Lingual axial reduction: torpedo diamond.

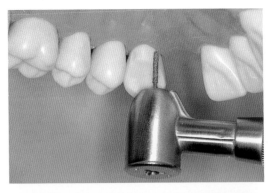

Fig. 7-13 Begin the reduction of the vertical wall of the cingulum with the torpedo diamond, creating a definite chamfer finish line as you do.

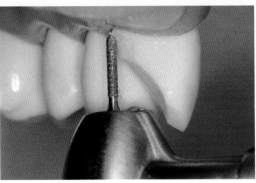

Fig. 7-14 Concentrate on keeping the diamond parallel with the incisal two-thirds of the tooth, which will ultimately become the path of insertion for the preparation. In conjunction with the grooves, which will be added shortly, this vertical lingual wall plays an essential role in restoration retention.[3,19–21] If the cingulum is short, it may be necessary to make a beveled shoulder finish line on the lingual surface, in order to move the wall farther into the center of the tooth where it will be longer. To compensate for a grossly insufficient lingual wall, a pin may be added.[2,4,5,19] Lorey and Meyers found that a cingulum pin increased the retention of an anterior three-quarter crown by 31%.[13] The cingulum pin should be placed halfway between the outer surface of the tooth and the pulp. Lorey et al.[22] and Dilts et al.[23] found that cemented pins are most retentive when placed to a depth of 4.0 mm.

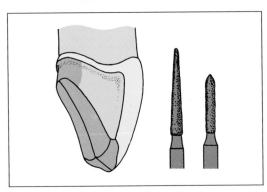

Fig. 7-15 Proximal axial reduction: long needle and torpedo diamonds.

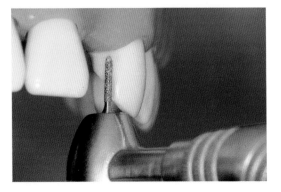

Fig. 7-16 On the proximal surface adjacent to any edentulous spaces, the axial reduction is extended with the same torpedo diamond used on the lingual surface. Bring it facially to the line angle in most circumstances.

Fig. 7-17 On the axial surface adjacent to other teeth, use the long needle diamond to produce the initial reduction. Take care to neither nick the adjacent tooth, nor lean the instrument too far over to the center of the tooth being prepared. Do not be overly concerned with the smoothness or roughness of the prepared surface or the gingival finish line at this time. Once a little maneuvering space has been achieved, the axial surface can be smoothed.

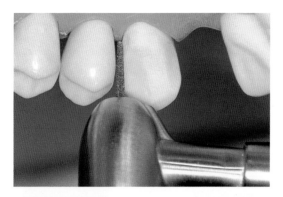

Fig. 7-18 A particular problem to be alert for is the underextension of the faciogingival angle, which will produce a critical shortening of the proximal wall and groove. This problem is due in part to two factors. One is the tendency to pull the instrument incisally (where the diamond is, in fact, thinner) to avoid cutting the adjacent tooth. The other is the widening of the tooth in the contact area. If the operator concentrates on maintaining a uniform depth of reduction centrally, using the incisalmost portion (which is most visible) of the axial reduction as an indicator, the diamond will produce a slice through the thickest part of the tooth and will not extend gingivally to the cervical region where the tooth is narrower.

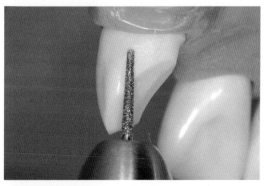

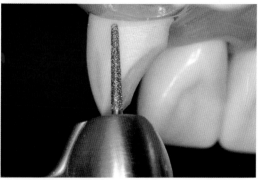

Fig. 7-19 Only by extending the diamond facially and gingivally, while simultaneously carring the axial reduction farther into the center of the tooth, can the correct extension be achieved at the faciogingival angle of the preparation.

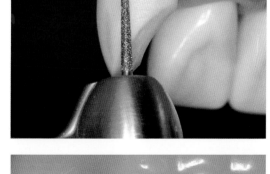

Fig. 7-20 Extension in a facial direction should just barely break contact with the adjacent tooth. The preparation must be instrumented from the lingual to avoid overextension. More extension is permissible on the distal of a canine than anywhere else in the anterior portion of the mouth, because the distal aspect of maxillary canines are not visible in a normal, "conversational" view in most patients.[24]

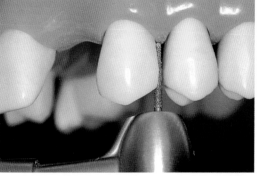

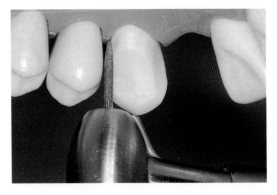

Fig. 7-21 Once space has been created with the long needle diamond, it is possible to introduce the flame diamond into the interproximal area without binding between the tooth preparation wall and the proximal surface of the adjacent tooth. After instrumenting the proximal surface with the flame diamond, switch to the torpedo diamond to insure a definite chamfer finish line interproximally.

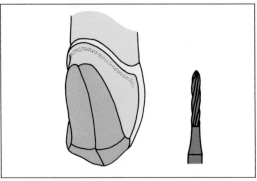

Fig. 7-22 Axial finishing: torpedo bur.

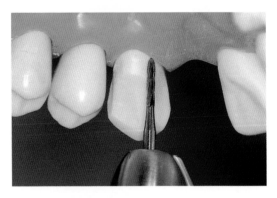

Fig. 7-23 Now use the torpedo carbide bur to create a smooth, definite finish line along the entire gingival extension of the preparation.

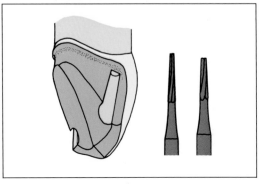

Fig. 7-24 Proximal grooves: nos. 169L and 170 bur.

Fig. 7-25 To facilitate proper placement of the grooves, it is a good idea to draw their outline on the lingual incisal area of the preparation. This simple step will do a great deal to insure that the grooves will not be placed in some undesirable location, farther either facially or lingually than their intended positions.

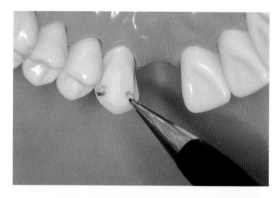

Fig. 7-26 Begin the first groove, usually on the mesial surface, with a shallow "template." This is cut with a no. 170 bur to a depth of 1.0 mm, following exactly the outline penciled on the tooth. The groove should progress gingivally in small increments until it reaches its full length. Although the final groove will be the size of a no. 170 bur, the inexperienced operator would do well to use a no. 169L bur for the initial placement. This allows some adjustment of groove direction without overcutting the groove. To assure maximum retention, the proximal grooves must meet several criteria. Unlike the grooves in the posterior three-quarter crown, which parallel the long axis of the tooth, the grooves of the three-quarter crown preparation for an anterior tooth must parallel the incisal one-half to two-thirds of the facial surface.[2,7,8,19,25–27] This slight lingual inclination enables a much longer groove to be made. It also decreases the likelihood of

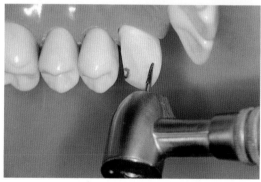

overcutting the facio-incisal corners, which would result in an unsightly display of metal.

Enhancement of retention (Fig. 7-27)

For maximum effectiveness, the proximal grooves must be distinct, be as nearly parallel as possible, and have definite gingival seats (see Fig. 7-27).[12,20] These grooves, which replace the facial surface of the preparation, provide a "lock" to the tooth.[8] The locking effect of the grooves provides resistance to torquing and is accomplished by forming a definite lingual wall in the groove.[7,16] This form has been described as a "lingual hook."[28] It is made by directing the upright bur in a diagonal direction toward the opposite corner of the tooth.

The grooves should be placed as far facially as possible.[2,29] This facial placement will result in the longest possible groove, and it will improve marginal integrity by allowing space for a bulk of metal near the acute edge of the margin.

Occasionally, boxes will be substituted for grooves. This is the best way of handling existing restorations or caries.[3,8,30] Well-defined narrow boxes will also increase the retention of the preparation.[12] However, the boxes must remain narrow to preserve resistance form, since the lingual wall of the box becomes shorter as it is moved lingually.

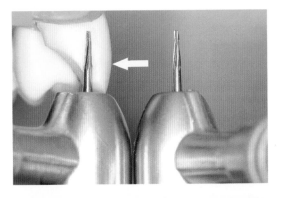

Fig. 7-27 When the groove has been extended to its full length, evaluate its direction and size. Place the bur back in the groove, and then move the handpiece facially, keeping your wrist rigid to prevent any change in the bur's angulation.

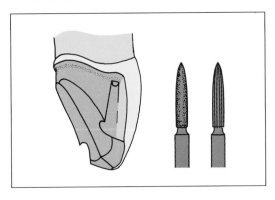

Fig. 7-28 Position the bur against the uncut proximal surface and cut the second groove. Again, the best results are obtained by cutting the groove in increments. Refer back to the inclination of the first groove frequently. Sometimes it is helpful, especially in laboratory exercises, to secure a tapered fissure bur in the first groove with utility wax. It will serve as a benchmark against which the direction of the second groove can be checked.

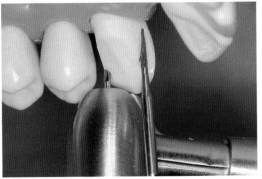

Fig. 7-29 Proximal flares: flame diamond and flame bur.

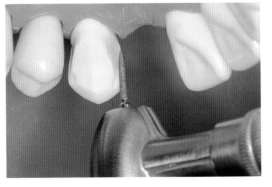

Fig. 7-30 Use the flame diamond to create the flare on the facial aspect of the groove. The flare is a flat plane which is wider at the incisal that it is at the gingival end. The side of the entire instrument can be used adjacent to an edentulous space such as shown here. Where access is restricted interproximally, the thin tip of the flame diamond is used to start the flare at its gingival end. Then the diamond is brought up the line angle formed by the facial wall of the groove and the outside of the tooth.

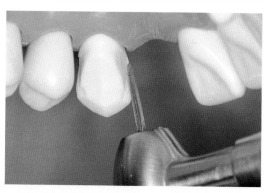

Fig. 7-31 Follow up with the flame carbide bur to obtain a smooth flare and a sharp, definite finish line. Again, as with the flame diamond, it may be possible to use only the tip of this instrument on the flare adjacent to another tooth.

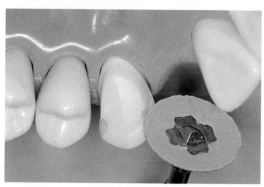

Fig. 7-32 In the anterior region of the mouth it is possible to use a sandpaper disk to form the flare. This technique is more certain to create a flat surface on the flare. It is possible that it may cause rounding of the actual finish line, though, and it does represent some hazard to the patient unless caution is exercised.

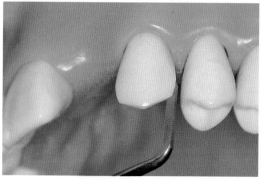

Fig. 7-33 Where an absolute minimal extension of the flare is desired, most commonly the case on incisors, use either a 1.5 or 2.0 mm wide enamel chisel (either a hatchet, as shown here, or a binangle chisel). Esthetically, the distal finish line of a canine is the least critical area of the anterior segment of the arch.

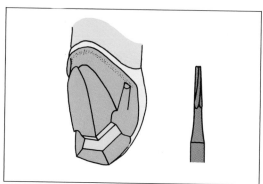

Fig. 7-34 Incisal offset: no. 171 bur.

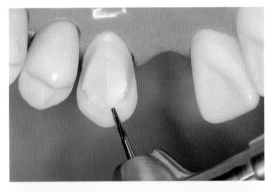

Fig. 7-35 The incisal offset, cut with the no. 171 bur, stays a uniform distance from the incisal edge. It is placed as close to the incisal edge as possible without undermining the enamel, providing space for the bulk of metal necessary for the integrity of the margin of gold overlying the narrow finishing bevel placed on the incisal edge. On a canine the incisal offset forms an inverted V, but on an incisor it follows a straight line across the incisal edge. Although some operators omit it, the incisal offset does enhance both the structural durability and the marginal integrity;[29] it reinforces the restoration in a fragile area, and completes the reinforcing staple or "truss."[3,8,30-34]

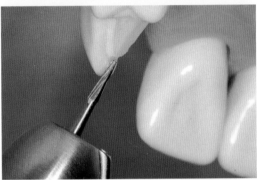

Fig. 7-36 Round over the sharp angle between the vertical wall of the offset and the incisal reduction with a no. 171 bur. This allows space for a little more metal near the margin, and it removes sharp angles that might prevent the casting from seating.

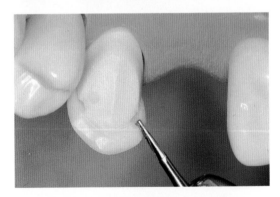

Fig. 7-37 Use the same nondentate tapered fissure bur to round over the angle between the incisal reduction and each flare.

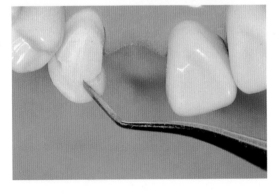

Fig. 7-38 The offset can be instrumented with a 1.0 mm wide enamel chisel, such as the binangle chisel shown here. If finishing is needed on the offset, it is more often accomplished with a no. 957 end-cutting bur.

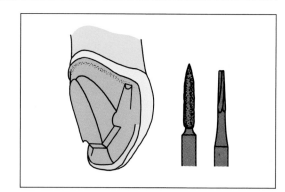

Fig. 7-39 Incisal bevel: flame diamond and no. 170 bur.

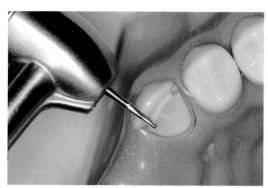

Fig. 7-40 Hold the no. 170 bur at right angles to the path of insertion of the preparation and move it lightly from one incisoproximal angle to the other, creating a finishing bevel about 0.5 mm wide. A flame diamond and bur can be used for the same purpose, but the final bevel should be done with a carbide bur to produce the sharpest finish line. Do *not* drop the handpiece over to the faciogingival, or this will create a "reverse bevel." An unnecessary display of metal would result.

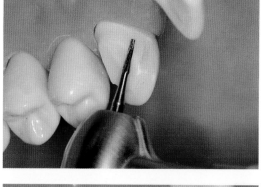

Fig. 7-41 Round over any other sharp internal angles with the no. 170 bur. This will make the seating of the casting easier.

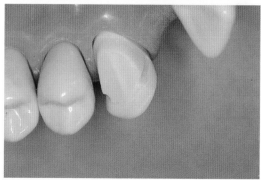

Fig. 7-42 A lingual incisal view of the completed preparation.

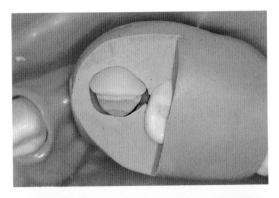

Fig. 7-43 The wrap-around horizontal-cut index gives a clear view of the amount of lingual reduction accomplished in the middle of the preparation incisogingivally.

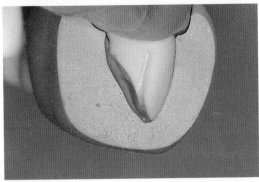

Fig. 7-44 The vertically cut midsagittal index shows the quantity of lingual reduction done in the middle of the preparation mesiodistally.

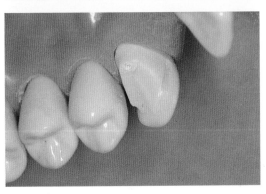

Fig. 7-45 A common variation of the anterior three-quarter crown utilizes a cingulum pin, to enhance retention in a tooth with little or no cingulum, or for a tooth which will serve as an abutment for a fixed bridge.

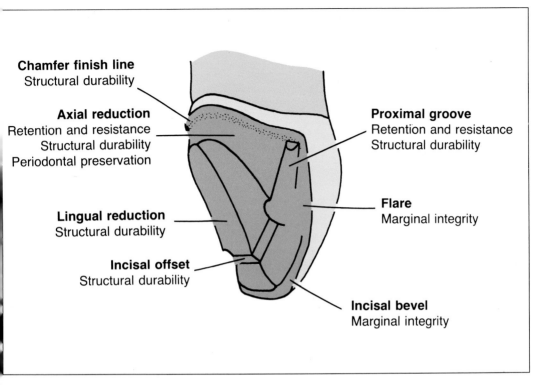

Chamfer finish line
Structural durability

Axial reduction
Retention and resistance
Structural durability
Periodontal preservation

Proximal groove
Retention and resistance
Structural durability

Lingual reduction
Structural durability

Flare
Marginal integrity

Incisal offset
Structural durability

Incisal bevel
Marginal integrity

Fig. 7-46   The features of an anterior three-quarter crown and the function served by each.

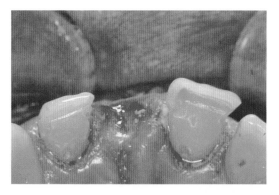

Clinical examples: Maxillary anterior (Figs. 7-47 through 7-55)

Fig. 7-47 Three-quarter crown retainers were selected for this bridge to replace a maxillary central incisor. The bridge was removed, with some difficulty, after 21 years of service because of an irreparably fractured pontic facing. The only preparation done at this time was retouching the flares and chamfers to correct any minor damage done during the removal of the old restoration.

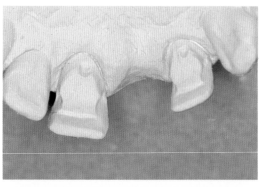

Fig. 7-48 A lingual view of the preparations on the stone casts.

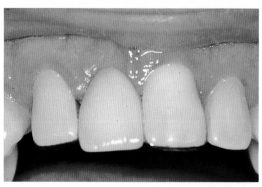

Fig. 7-49 A facial view of the completed bridge shows the very minimal extensions of the mesial and distal finish lines on both abutments. Conservative extension and careful finishing of the incisal margin insure that light is reflected downward, making the incisal edges appear dark rather than metallic to the viewer.[3] As a result, they blend in with the dark background of the oral cavity.

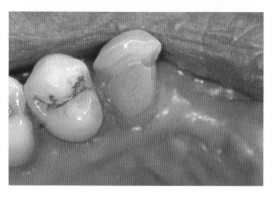

Fig. 7-50 A three-quarter crown was used as the retainer for this canine bridge abutment. Because of the large tooth size and the relative shortness of the pontic span, an unmodified preparation design was employed.

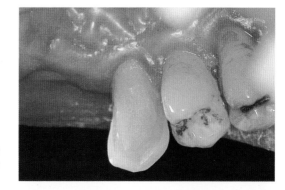

Fig. 7-51 A lingual view of the same canine preparation displays more detail, as well as the length of the tooth.

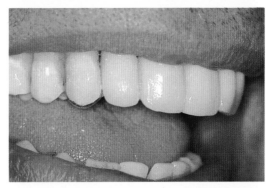

Fig. 7-52 A facial view of the completed bridge. The display of metal on the incisal edge is minimal, while the proximal metal margins are completely hidden from view.

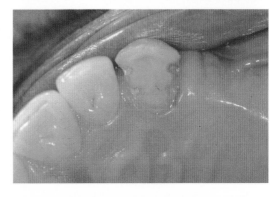

Fig. 7-53 The three-quarter crown preparation on this maxillary canine bridge abutment employed double grooves on the large proximal surfaces to provide additional retention for a posterior bridge replacing two teeth. Notice the minimal mesial extension.

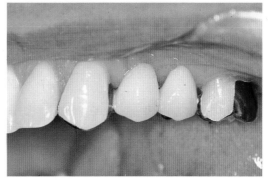

Fig. 7-54 This direct facial view of the completed bridge reveals no metal display on the mesial margin. The metal seen on the distal of the canine in this view would not be readily seen in a normal mesiofacial "conversational" view. The distal retainer is a seven-eighths crown.

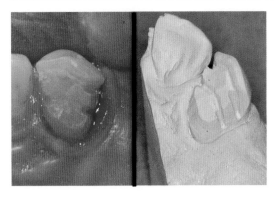

Fig. 7-55 Two views of another canine abutment three-quarter crown preparation. The incisal view of the preparation in the mouth *(left)* shows a minimal mesial extension. A distal view of the preparation on a stone cast *(right)* shows the length of the grooves and the way in which the grooves in each set are joined together by an offset to increase retainer rigidity.

References

1. Carmichael, J. P. Attachment for inlay and bridgework. Dent. Rev. 15:82, 1901.
2. Tinker, E. T. Fixed bridgework. J. Natl. Dent. Assoc. 7:579, 1920.
3. Ingraham, R., Bassett, R. W., and Koser, J. R. An Atlas of Cast Gold Procedures. 2nd ed. Buena Park, CA: Unitro College Press, 1969, 161–165.
4. Pruden, K. C. Abutments and attachments in fixed partial dentures. J. Prosthet. Dent. 7:502, 1957.
5. Hughes, H. J. Are there alternatives to the porcelain fused to gold bridge? Aust. Dent. J. 15:281, 1970.
6. Leander, C. T. Preparation of abutments for fixed partial dentures. Dent. Clin. North Am. 3:59, 1959.
7. Cowger, G. T. Retention, resistance, and esthetics of the anterior three-quarter crown. J. Am. Dent. Assoc. 62:167, 1961.
8. Gade, E. Function and esthetics of anterior bridges. Int. Dent. J. 12:18, 1962.
9. Christensen, G. J. Marginal fit of gold inlay castings. J. Prosthet. Dent. 16:297, 1966.
10. Jorgensen, K. D. Structure of the film thickness of zinc phosphate cements. Acta Odontol. Scand. 18:491, 1960.
11. Dressel, R. P. The three-quarter crown applied to anterior teeth. Dent. Cosmos 72:565, 1930.
12. Prime, J. M. A plea for conservatism in operative procedures. J. Am. Dent. Assoc. 15:1234, 1928.
13. Lorey, R. E., and Myers, G. E. The retentive qualities of bridge retainers. J. Am. Dent. Assoc. 76:568, 1968.
14. Reisbick, M. H., and Shillingburg, H. T. Effect of preparation geometry on retention and resistance of cast gold restorations. J. Calif. Dent. Assoc. 3:51, 1975.
15. Potts, R. G., Shillingburg, H. T., and Duncanson, M. G. Retention and resistance of preparations for cast restorations. J. Prosthet. Dent. 43:303, 1980.
16. Shillingburg, H. T., and Fisher, D. W. The partial veneer restoration. Aust. Dent. J. 17:411, 1972.
17. Doxtater, L. W. The three-quarter crown with accessory anchorage. Dent. Items Interest 51:290, 1929.
18. Crispin, B. J. Conservative alternative to full esthetic crown. J. Prosthet. Dent. 42:392, 1979.
19. Rogers, E. J. The partial veneer crown. Preparation, construction and application. Dent. Items Interest 50:397, 1928.
20. Tinker, H. A. The three-quarter crown in fixed bridgework. J. Can. Dent. Assoc. 16:125, 1950.
21. McEwen, R. A. Anterior three-quarter crown. Ga. Dent. J. 24:11, 1951.
22. Lorey, R. E., Embrell, K. A., and Myers, G. E. Retentive factors in pin-retained castings. J. Prosthet. Dent. 17:271, 1967.
23. Dilts, W. E., Welk, D. A., and Stovall, J. Retentive properties of pin materials in pin-retained silver amalgam restorations. J. Am. Dent. Assoc. 77:1085, 1968.
24. McAdam, D. B. A maxillary cuspid three-quarter crown preparation of increased retentive form. J. Can. Dent. Assoc. 28:291, 1962.
25. Fisch, G. M. The three-quarter crown as a filling for anterior teeth. J. Am. Dent. Assoc. 18:2393, 1931.
26. Rudin, B. M. A conservative abutment restoration for anterior fixed partial dentures. J. Prosthet. Dent. 11:272, 1961.
27. Silberhorn, O. W. Fixed bridge retainers—Design and retention features. Ill. Dent. J. 22:641, 1953.
28. Ho, G. Lecture notes. University of Southern California School of Dentistry, 1959.
29. Rhoads, J. E. Preparation of the teeth for cast restorations. pp. 34–67 In G. M. Hollenback, Science and Technic of the Cast Restoration. St. Louis: The C. V. Mosby Co., 1964.
30. Thom, L. W. Principles of cavity preparation in crown and bridge prosthesis. II. The three-quarter crown. J. Am. Dent. Assoc. 41:443, 1950.
31. Smith, D. E. Abutment preparations. J. Am. Dent. Assoc. 18:2063, 1931.
32. Willey, R. E. The preparation of abutments for veneer retainers. J. Am. Dent Assoc. 53:141, 1956.
33. Guyer, S. E. Partial veneer crowns: Preparation alignment. Wa. Univ. Dent. J. 26:72, 1960.
34. Tjan, A. H. L., and Miller, G. D. Biometric guide to groove placement on three-quarter crown preparations. J. Prosthet. Dent. 42:405, 1979.

Chapter 8

Pin-Modified Three-Quarter Crowns

The pin-modified three-quarter crown is recognized as both an esthetic and a conservative restoration.[1-3] It relies heavily upon substitution of pinholes for axial walls that are left unveneered, and it is unquestionably the most conservative of the partial veneer crowns in percentage of axial enamel that is left undisturbed.

However, the retention is gained internally by placement of pinholes into the dentin. Depending on morphology, tooth size, and operator skill, this could bring the pinhole in close proximity with or even cause penetration into the pulp. For this reason, it is contraindicated for small teeth,[4] those that are thin faciolingually,[5,6] teeth with large pulps,[7] and those which are malpositioned.

The pin-modified three-quarter crown has been considered the retainer of choice when an unblemished tooth is to be used as an abutment for a bridge in an esthetically critical area.[8] More recently, acid-etched resin-bonded retainers (see chapter 17) have become increasingly popular in these situations. With less proximal surface coverage, the pin-modified three-quarter crown is an excellent restoration for the repair of severe lingual abrasion.[8-11] It was used at one time for restoring Class IV fractures on incisors,[8,9,12,13] but it is more likely that this type of damage would be restored with an acid-etch composite resin restoration or a porcelain veneered crown today.

It is best reserved for use on maxillary central incisors and canines,[14] although it can be utilized on maxillary lateral incisors with enough bulk to safely accommodate the pinholes. Because it is an esthetic restoration that avoids subgingival marginal placement totally, or nearly so, it is periodontally preferable to any type of full porcelain crown.[15]

The pin-modified three-quarter crown is an old type of restoration that received a boost from improved technology in relatively recent years. Forms of pinledges, utilizing pins placed through metal backings or "wings" extending from the pontic onto the lingual surfaces of abutment teeth, were described in 1880 by Litch,[16] and in 1896 by Gabriel.[17] A more typical form of pinledge crown was presented by Burgess[1] who flowed gold solder over a foil matrix adapted around the pins.[18] Another modification, named the "pit ledge," used "pits" cut with a no. 560 bur to a depth of 1.0 mm for retention.[19] It was not until 1960, however, that the restoration was made popular by the development of twist drills and nylon bristles which enabled the dentist to drill precise pinholes and accurately reproduce them in an impression.[20]

Because the pin-modified three-quarter crown depends so heavily on pins for its retention, many authors have turned their attention to various aspects of this retentive device. Retention can be increased by using larger-diameter or longer pins.[21,22] Retention can also be enhanced by increasing the number of pins.[22] As few as two[23] and as many as four[8,24–26] have been suggested as the optimum number of pins, with three pins recommended most often.[3,20,26–28] In fact, it takes a large tooth to accommodate three pins while meeting the requirements of positioning them at least 1.0 mm apart[25] (or, stated in another way, of placing them so there will be at least 0.5 mm of dentin around each pinhole).[10] The pinholes should also be kept 1.5 mm from the dentino-enamel junction[25,28] to avoid crazing of the enamel and discoloration arising from oxidized opaque metal showing through the enamel.

Because serrated pins have been found to produce better retention than smooth pins,[21,22,29] serrated iridioplatinum pins are preferred instead of small nylon bristles for fabricating the wax pattern and casting.

The most commonly recommended pin diameter has been 0.6 mm (0.024 in.),[4,10,20,24,30] although 0.7-mm pins (0.028 in.) are occasionally used.[4,24,31] Recommended pin length in the literature has varied, with earlier clinicians, using inefficiently cutting steel burs, tending to settle for shallow pinholes of 1.0 mm[19,32,33] or 1.5 mm.[34] This was increased to 2.0 to 3.0 mm by later authors.[3,4,13,20,24,25,28,31,35–37] Lorey recommended 4.0 mm,[21] and Hughes, 3.0 to 5.0 mm.[5]

Longer pins produce more retention, and it would be a shame to cause the failure of a conservative bridge by having pins that were too short to retain the prosthesis. These are especially destructive failures, since the other re-

tainer seldom fails at the same time. The pinholes become access points for oral fluids and microorganisms to penetrate deep into the tooth. This process often goes on for some time before it is detected. Therefore, if pinholes of adequate depth cannot be made for any reason, a different retainer design should be selected.

Not all pins used for the retention of pin-modified three-quarter crowns are of the parallel-sided variety. Tapered pins the diameter and configuration of 700 burs have also been used extensively for casting retention.[12,38–40] This type of pin has been described as being five times as rigid as a 0.55-mm (0.022 in.) parallel-sided pin.[41] Lorey and Myers reported a pinledge three-quarter crown with three tapered pins on a canine to be equal in retention to a standard three-quarter crown with a cingulum pin.[42] A hard, plastic tapered pin of the size and taper of a 700 bur is used for picking up the pinhole in the impression and then for fabricating the pin in the casting.

The pinholes in the preparation are too small to be accurately reproduced by any impression material. Therefore, a nylon or plastic bristle, slightly smaller in diameter than the drill, is placed in a pinhole.[20,24,43] A metal pin has also been used for this purpose.[44] The impression is made around the pin and, when the impression is withdrawn, the pin whose head has become embedded in the impression material is "picked up" or "captured" by the impression. When the impression is poured, the pinholes are reproduced by the plastic bristles protruding from the impression. The bristles usually remain embedded in the stone when the impression and cast are separated, making it impossible to make more than one complete pour of the impression.

Reproduction of the pinholes is difficult,[45] and if it cannot be done accurately, the restoration cannot be successfully completed.

Paralleling the pinholes can also be a difficult task.[44] If very many are used on multiple abutment preparations, a better result will be obtained by using a paralleling device* to aid their accurate orientation and placement.[25,28,46,47]

Some techniques make deliberate use of nonparallelism of the pins for retention. Timmermans and Courtade employed a short, parallel guide pinhole in each preparation.[48] These were augmented by at least two nonparallel pinholes in each preparation. The parallel pins are created with iridioplatinum pins in the wax pattern, while the nonparallel pinholes are established in the wax pattern and maintained with nickel silver pins during investing and casting. They are removed after casting, and the nonparallel pinholes are enlarged in the preparation. Upon cementation of the restoration, threaded pins are inserted through the holes in the crown into tooth structure.[49]

The castings for mandibular anterior periodontal splints can be retained by horizontal nonparallel pins. A threaded pin extends through the tooth from the facial surface, with a countersink on the facial surface to accommodate the head of the pin when it is threaded. First described by Weissman,[50] the technique was subsequently modified by Courtade by adding a short, parallel guide pin in the cingulum.[51]

Periodontal splints can also be made with parallel horizontal pins providing the retention. The pinholes are drilled with a paralleling device, with the pins entering the tooth from the lingual surface and passing all the way through the facial surface of the tooth, where they are ground flush with the outer surface of the enamel.[52]

Another interesting variation of the pin-retained restoration described in the literature utilizes a sleeve in the casting that fits over a threaded pin previously screwed into the preparation, which is 0.1 mm smaller than the sleeve.[53] Retention provided in this manner is superior to the retention obtained from cemented pins that are an integral part of the casting.[54] The technique is not widely used at this time, however.

The technique sequence shown in Figs. 8-1 to 8-45 demonstrates the method of preparing an incisor for a pin-modified three-quarter crown, which is a modified pin-ledge design adapted for use as a bridge retainer by covering the axial surface immediately adjacent to the edentulous space.

Examples of clinical cases treated with pin-modified three-quarter crowns are shown in Figs. 8-46 through 8-51.

*Paramax, Whaledent International, New York, N.Y.

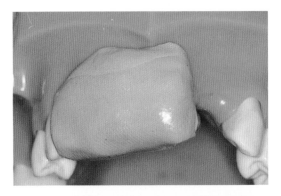

Pin-modified three-quarter crown preparation (Figs. 8-1 through 8-45)

Fig. 8-1a One-half scoop of condensation reaction silicone putty is adapted to the facial surface of the tooth to be prepared, and at least two other adjacent teeth.

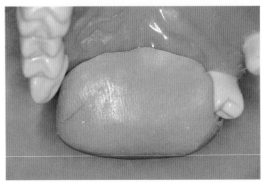

Fig. 8-1b The silicone putty adapted to the lingual surface.

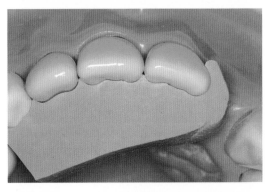

Fig. 8-2 The putty index is cut into facial and lingual halves along the incisal edges of the teeth. Then the lingual half is cut evenly into incisal and gingival halves. Place the linguogingival portion back onto the teeth to insure that it is well adapted.

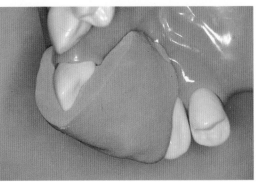

Fig. 8-3 An index can also be made by cutting the adapted putty in a midsaggital plane along the midline of the tooth to be prepared.

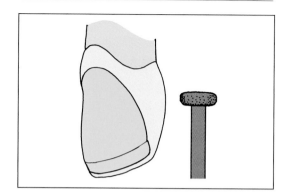

Fig. 8-4 Lingual reduction: small wheel diamond.

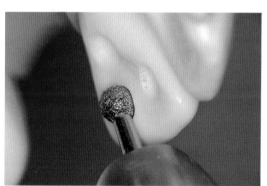

Fig. 8-5 Make depth-orientation cuts on the lingual surface of the tooth to assist in removing adequate tooth structure. Use a small round diamond whose head diameter exceeds the shaft diameter by 1.4 mm. When sunk into enamel to the shaft as shown here, the depth of the cut will be approximately 0.7 mm.

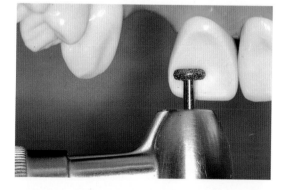

Fig. 8-6 Create a concave surface over the lingual aspect of the tooth to the depth of the orientation cuts, using the small diamond wheel. Avoid cutting any more off the vertical wall of the cingulum than is absolutely necessary.

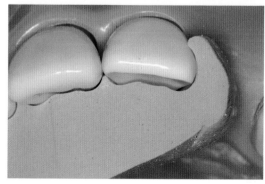

Fig. 8-7 Use a linguogingival silicone reduction index to insure that the depth of reduction is both sufficient and uniform.

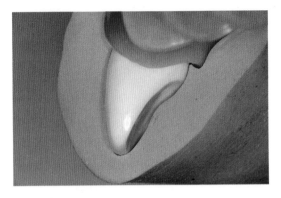

Fig. 8-8 As an alternate measure, you may prefer to use a midsagittal index, which will permit you to judge reduction from the incisal edge to the gingival crevice in the midline of the lingual surface. For the novice who wants both, it is necessary to adapt two mixes of putty and trim each appropriately.

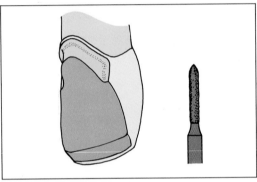

Fig. 8-9 Lingual axial reduction: torpedo diamond.

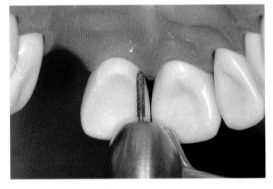

Fig. 8-10 Reduction of the vertical lingual wall and formation of the lingual chamfer finish line is accomplished with a torpedo diamond. End the extension far enough lingually to the proximal contact with the adjacent tooth that the margin will be in the lingual embrasure where it can be finished at the time of insertion and maintained by the patient. If the cingulum is extremely short, it may be necessary to use a shoulder with a bevel in order to move the lingual wall further into the center of the tooth, thus lengthening it.

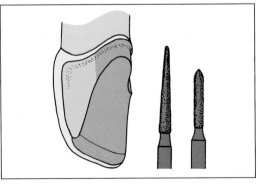

Fig. 8-11 Proximal axial wall reduction: long-needle and torpedo diamonds.

Fig. 8-12 Use the same torpedo diamond to extend the axial reduction around to the facial extension, thinning the reduction to a flare at the actual finish line. This extension is critical. If underextended, it could lead to a poor connector, undersized and weak.[10] The connector would come right up to the margin, making it impossible to finish properly. If this preparation is done on a tooth that is not a bridge abutment, where interproximal access is difficult, a long-needle diamond would produce the initial reduction necessary to allow access for the larger torpedo diamond.

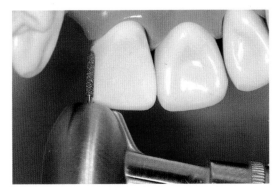

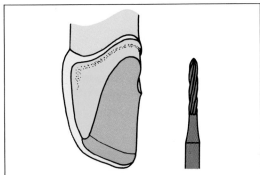

Fig. 8-13 Axial finishing: torpedo bur.

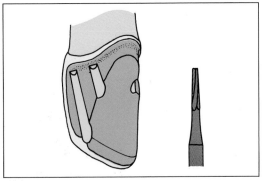

Fig. 8-14 Smooth the axial reduction and the chamfer finish line with a torpedo carbide bur.

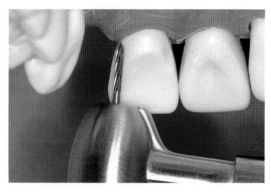

Fig. 8-15 Proximal grooves: nos. 169L and 170 burs.

Retention and resistance features

Figure 8-16 shows that the primary retention/resistance features for the axial surfaces are placed adjacent to the edentulous space. If the proximal surface of the tooth has been restored previously, or if it has caries on that surface, the feature will be a box form instead of a groove. The box is too destructive a feature to use if the proximal surface is unblemished.

Kishimoto et al. demonstrated that two grooves are equal to a box on a premolar.[55] On an anterior tooth they are almost certainly superior. Since the lingual surface slopes drastically to the linguogingival, moving the lingual wall just a short distance in a lingual direction will shorten it and decrease its resistance markedly.[56] By using two grooves instead, there will be *two* lingual walls, with the one for the more facially positioned groove being much longer and providing more resistance than could be provided by the single, shorter lingual wall of a box.

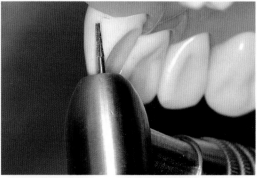

Fig. 8-16 The first, more facial groove is placed with a no. 170 bur. An inexperienced operator may want to start the grooves with a no. 169L bur to avoid overcutting. If the no. 169L bur is used, shallow grooves are made and checked for position and direction. If they are satisfactory, a no. 170 bur is sunk into the track of the trial groove to the full diameter of the bur.

Fig. 8-17 Place the second, more lingual groove, taking care that it is parallel with the first. A bur is shown in the facial groove to illustrate the parallelism of the instrument placement. If desired, the shank can be cut off a discarded no. 170 bur so the novice can place it in the facial groove with a little soft wax to see the parallelism more clearly.

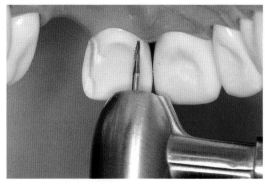

Fig. 8-18 A third and much shorter groove is placed on the opposite side of the cingulum than the first two grooves. It is placed at the facial-most extension of the axial reduction on that surface.

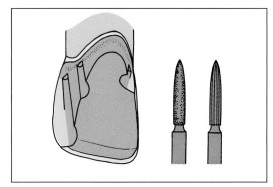

Fig. 8-19 Proximal flares: flame diamond and flame bur.

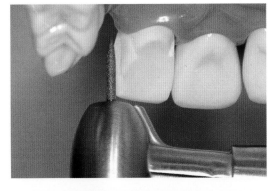

Fig. 8-20 Proximal flares are most easily formed with the flame diamond. A flare must be wider incisally than it is gingivally if it is to draw. It will practically eliminate the facial wall of the groove at its incisal end.

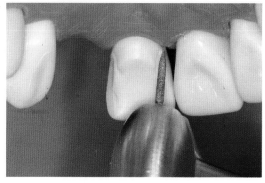

Fig. 8-21 The flare on the shorter cingulum groove is made with the tip of the flame diamond.

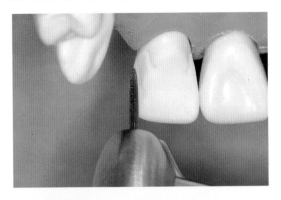

Fig. 8-22a Go over the distal flares again with the matching flame-shaped carbide finishing bur. Be careful not to round over the actual finish line.

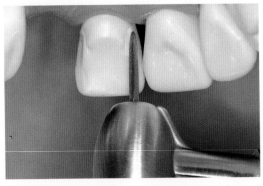

Fig. 8-22b Go over the mesial flares again.

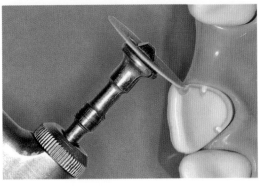

Fig. 8-23 When access is good, as it usually is on an anterior tooth adjacent to an edentulous space, a small sandpaper disc can be used for making the flare. When using a disc in this area, it is extremely important to securely retract the lip to protect it from being lacerated by the disk.

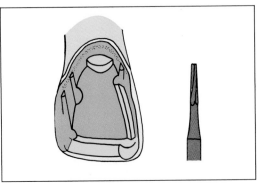

Fig. 8-24 Ledges and offsets: no. 171 bur.

Fig. 8-25 Make a ledge or countersink in the incisal corner opposite the site of the proximal groove with the no. 171 bur. It must be far enough gingival to the incisal edge that it can be cut into dentin and end lingual to the incisal finish line. There should also be a ledge in the middle of the cingulum. These ledges provide level starting points for the pinholes. This will allow for starting them accurately without the instrument skidding on a sloping surface. They also provide space for a bulk of metal surrounding the base of the pins, which helps resist shearing stress on the pins.[57]

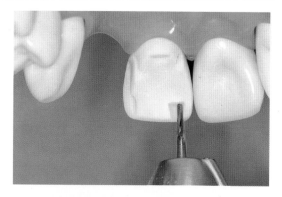

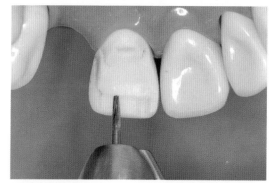

Fig. 8-26 Connect the incisal ledge and the facialmost proximal groove with an incisal offset. Cut it with the no. 171 bur.

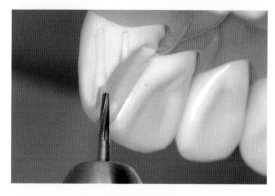

Fig. 8-27 Seen from a proximal view, the offset is a narrow flat shelf perpendicular to the preparation's path of insertion.

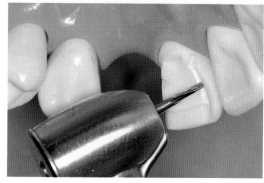

Fig. 8-28 Connect the incisal and cingulum edges with a V- shaped trough. The metal in this area of the casting will help to reinforce the linguoproximal margin of the restoration.

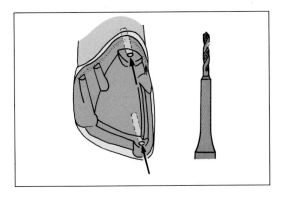

Fig. 8-29 Pinholes: no. 1/2 bur and 0.6-mm drill.

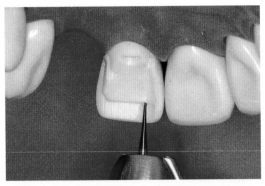

Fig. 8-30 Start the pinhole in the incisal ledge by cutting a shallow hole with a no. 1/2 round bur. This pilot hole makes it much easier to start the pinhole exactly where desired.

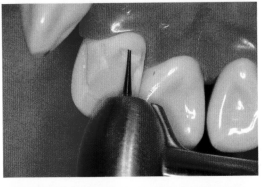

Fig. 8-31 Make another shallow hole on the cingulum ledge with the no. 1/2 round bur.

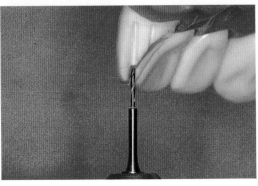

Fig. 8-32 Carefully align a 0.6-mm (0.024 in.) drill with the grooves and other vertical features of the preparation in a faciolingual direction.

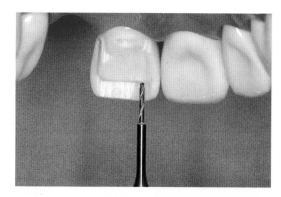

Fig. 8-33 Repeat the process in a mesiodistal direction, being careful not to change the orientation in the faciolingual plane. It is usually necessary to do this by looking in a mouth mirror. Recheck the orientation of the faciolingual plane before proceeding with the pinhole.

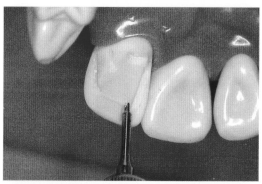

Fig. 8-34 Start the handpiece before touching the tooth with the instrument, and place the pinhole to a depth of 3.0 mm or more. The optimum depth for cemented pins was found by Dilts et al.[58] to be 3.0 to 4.0 mm. Under no circumstances should you stop the handpiece with the drill in the pinhole. To do so almost guarantees breaking it off.

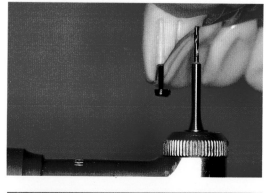

Fig. 8-35 Place a nylon pin in the first pinhole, and use it as a guide for aligning the drill for the second or any other pinhole to be placed. Make sure it is aligned in a faciolingual plane first.

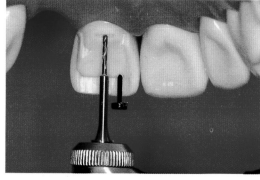

Fig. 8-36 Check the direction of the drill mesiodistally. It may be helpful to the inexperienced operator to observe the drill's orientation in one plane while an assistant checks it in the other.

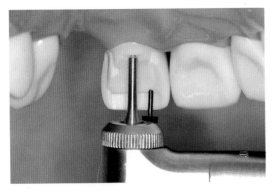

Fig. 8-37 Drill a pinhole in the middle of the cingulum ledge to a minimum depth of 3.0 mm.

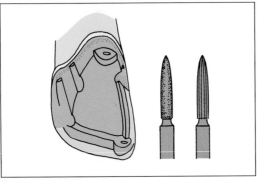

Fig. 8-38 Incisal bevel: flame diamond and flame bur.

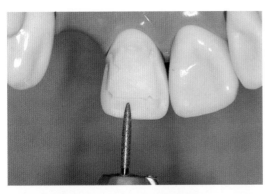

Fig. 8-39 Use the flame diamond to bevel the angle between the facial wall of the incisal offset and the incisal edge of uncut tooth structure. Be careful not to extend this bevel far enough facially that there will be a display of metal on the facial surface.

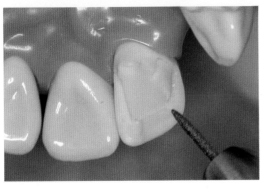

Fig. 8-40 Round over the angle between the flare and the incisal bevel with the flame diamond.

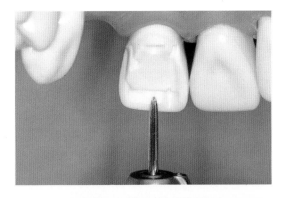

Fig. 8-41 Repeat the instrumentation of the incisal angles just rounded with a flame diamond, using the flame bur. It is best not to use this instrument for the initial cutting. The tip of it is not as effective at bulk removal as the diamond, and it is easily dulled, as well.

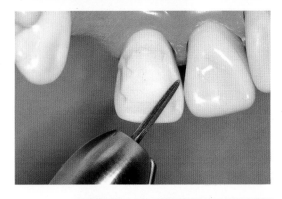

Fig. 8-42 The flame bur is utilized to bevel or blunt any sharp line angles between the lingual and proximal surface. Pay particular attention to eliminating sharp angles at the incisal ends of the grooves.

Fig. 8-43 Use the flame bur to redefine the bevel running on the marginal ridge of the tooth alongside the incisocingulum trough.

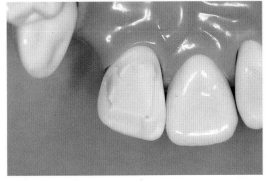

Fig. 8-44 The completed pin-modified three-quarter crown preparation on a maxillary central incisor.

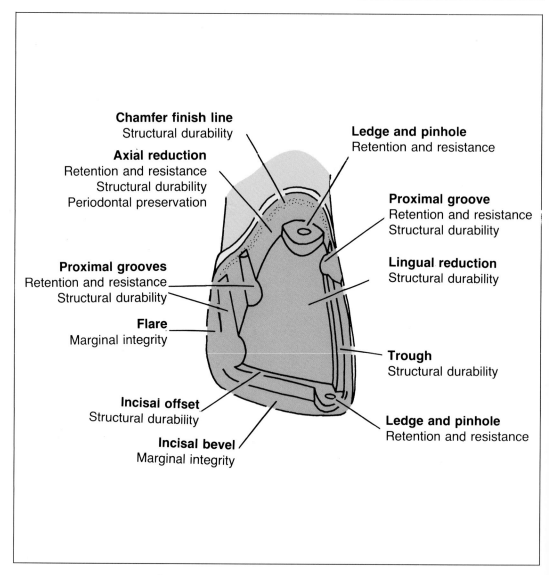

Fig. 8-45 The features of a pin-modified three-quarter crown and the function served by each.

Clinical examples: Pin-modified three quarter crown (Figs. 8-46 through 8-51)

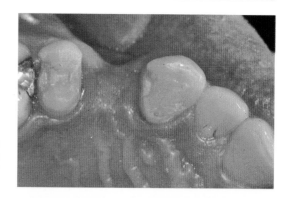

Fig. 8-46 A pin-modified three-quarter crown preparation was done on this maxillary canine bridge abutment. A box form was substituted for grooves because of preexisting caries.

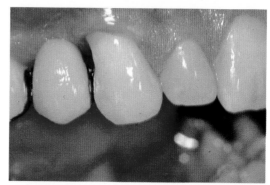

Fig. 8-47 The completed bridge in place on the prepared teeth seen in Fig. 8-46.

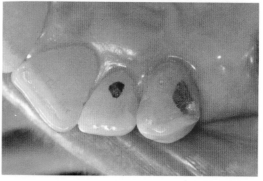

Fig. 8-48 A similar pin-modified three-quarter crown was selected as the retainer design for this bridge abutment. The carious lesion in the distal aspect of this tooth was large enough to warrant the placement of an amalgam core with a groove as the proximal resistance feature.

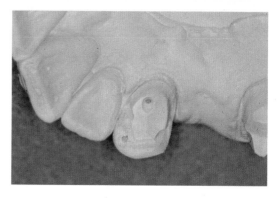

Fig. 8-49 A photograph of the stone cast shows more of the detail of this conservative bridge preparation.

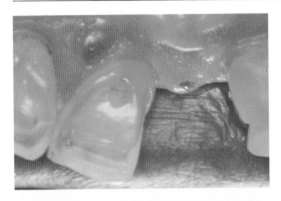

Fig. 8-50 A pin-modified three-quarter crown on a bulky maxillary central incisor. (Photograph courtesy of Dr. Sumiya Hobo, Tokyo, Japan.)

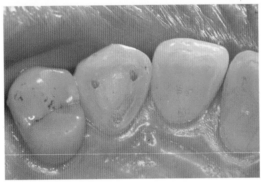

Fig. 8-51 A pinledge preparation done on a maxillary canine prior to restoring lost canine rise in the occlusion caused by abrasion.

References

1. Burgess, J. K. Modern attachments for bridgework and stabilizers for loose teeth. Dent. Cosmos 57:1335, 1915.
2. Johnston, J. F. The application and construction of the pinledge retainer. J. Prosthet. Dent. 3:559, 1953.
3. Morrant, G. A. The pinlay preparation as a bridge abutment. Dent. Pract. 2:328,1952.
4. Baum, L., and Contino, R. M. Ten years of experience with cast pin restorations. Dent. Clin. North Am. 14:81, 1970.
5. Hughes, H. J. Are there alternatives to the porcelain fused to gold bridge? Aust. Dent. 15:281, 1970.
6. Crispin, B. J. Conservative alternatives to full crowns. J. Prosthet. Dent. 42:392, 1979.
7. Bruce, R. W. Parallel pin splints for periodontally involved teeth. J. Prosthet. Dent. 14:738, 1964.
8. Baum, L. New cast gold restorations for anterior teeth. J. Am. Dent. Assoc. 61:15, 1960.
9. Arbo, M. A. A simple technique for castings with pin retention. Dent. Clin. North Am. 14:19, 1970.
10. Clyde, J. S., and Sharkey, S. W. The pin ledge crown. A reappraisal. Br. Dent. J. 144:239, 1978.
11. Doxtater, L. W. The pinledge attachment. Dent. Items Interest 50:800–807, Oct 1928.
12. Chechik, M. M. Employing prefabricated tapered gold pins. Dent. Digest 61:38, 1955.
13. Lawrence, K. E. Restoration of fractured anterior teeth for the young patient. Northwest Dent. 44:269, 1965.
14. Iwansson, R. The pin-ledge attachment and its use for fixed bridges. Dent. Items Interest 96:202, 1934.
15. Alpert, C. C. The anterior pin-ledge abutment. J. D. C. Dent. Soc. 34:11, 1959.
16. Litch, W. F. Some methods for the permanent attachment of artificial teeth in the mouth. Dent. Cosmos 22:396, 1880.
17. Gabriel, W. M. An improved method of making a pin-bridge. Br. Dent. J. 17:740, 1896.
18. Burgess, J. K. The preparation of abutments and construction of pinlay and pinledge attachments for bridgework. Pac. Dent. Gaz. 24:559, 1916.
19. Kabnick, H. H. The "pitledge" as a cast bridge attachment. Dent. Items Interest 53:376, 1931.
20. Shooshan, E. D. A pin-ledge casting technique—Its application in periodontal splinting. Dent. Clin. North Am. 4:189, 1960.
21. Lorey, R. E., Embrell, K. A., and Myers, G. E. Retentive factors in pin-retained castings. J. Prosthet. Dent. 17:271, 1967.
22. Moffa, J. P., and Phillips, R. W. Retentive properties of parallel pin restorations. J. Prosthet. Dent. 17:387, 1967.
23. Brigadier, L. R. The anterior one-half pin-lay. Dent. Digest 45:448, 1939.
24. Mosteller, J. H. Parallel pin castings. pp. 5–29 In Practical Dental Monographs. Chicago: Year Book Medical Publ., Inc., 1963.
25. Mann, A. W., Courtade, G. L., and Sanell, C. The use of pins in restorative dentistry. I. Parallel pin retention obtained without using paralleling devices. J. Prosthet. Dent. 15:502, 1965.
26. Rosen, H. The incisal insertion pin inlay. J. Prosthet. Dent. 19:263, 1968.
27. Manning, E. A. Tooth conservation in anterior bridge construction. Pinlay attachments. Dent. Surv. 30:31, 1954.
28. Courtade, G. L., Sanell, C., and Mann, A. W. The use of pins in restorative dentistry. II. Paralleling instruments. J. Prosthet. Dent. 15:691, 1965
29. Courtade, G. L., and Timmermans, J. J. Pins in Restorative Dentistry. St. Louis: The C. V. Mosby Co., 1971, 6.
30. Burns, B. B. Pin retention of cast gold restorations. J. Prosthet. Dent. 15:1101, 1965.
31. Sanell, C. Vertical parallel pins in occlusal rehabilitation. Dent. Clin. North Am. 7:755, 1963.
32. Klaffenbach, A. O. An analytic study of modern abutments. J. Am. Dent. Assoc. 23:2275, 1936.
33. Burgess, J. K. Further consideration of the pinlay (posterior) and the pinledge (anterior) bridge abutments. Dent. Cosmos 14:681, 1917.
34. Skinner, J. A. Pinledge attachments as aids in bridge retention. Dent. Surv. 24:1577, 1948.
35. Carpenter, E. E. Pinledge attachments for anterior bridgework. Dent. Items Interest 72:132, 1950.
36. Rudin, B. M. A conservative abutment restoration for anterior fixed partial dentures. J. Prosthet. Dent. 11:272, 1961.

37. Nealon, F. H., and Sheakley, H. G. An extra-oral pin technique. J. Prosthet. Dent. 22:638, 1969.
38. Steen, P. M. Positive pin retention. Dent. Surv. 30:757, 1954.
39. Wagner, A. W. Pin retention for extensive posterior gold onlays. J. Prosthet. Dent. 15:719, 1965.
40. Willmott, J. T. Pin retention for indirect inlays utilizing rubber base impression material. Br. Dent. J. 102:359, 1957.
41. Guthrie, J. D. *Cited in* M. A. Johnson, Anterior castings retained by pins: A direct method. Oper. Dent. 5:149, 1980.
42. Lorey, R. E., and Myers, G. E. The retentive qualities of bridge retainers. J. Am. Dent. Assoc. 76:568, 1968.
43. Mosteller, J. H. Pin castings by a paralleling device and hydrocolloid technique. Dent. Clin. North Am. 14:53, 1961.
44. Mollersten, L. An impression technique for teeth prepared for parallel pin. J. Prosthet. Dent. 18:579, 1967.
45. Kahn, A. E. Partial vs. full coverage. J. Prosthet. Dent. 10:167, 1960.
46. Sobel, S. L. A technique for using parallel pins. J. Prosthet. Dent. 20:526, 1968.
47. Sanell, C., Mann, A. W., and Courtade, G. L. The use of pins in restorative dentistry. III. The use of paralleling instruments. J. Prosthet. Dent. 16:286, 1966.
48. Timmermans, J. J., and Courtade, G. L. Nonparallel threaded pin retention of fixed prosthesis. J. Prosthet. Dent. 19:381, 1968.
49. Perry, G. D. Pins in crown and bridge for retention and venting. Quint. Int. 13:153, 1982.
50. Weissman, B. A nonparallel universal horizontal pin splint. J. Prosthet. Dent. 15:339, 1965.
51. Courtade, G. L. Methods for pin splinting the lower anterior teeth. Dent. Clin. North Am. 14:3, 1970.
52. Sanell, C., and Feldman, A. J. Horizontal pin splint for lower anterior teeth. J. Prosthet. Dent. 12:138, 1962.
53. Chan, K. C., Khera, S. C., and Torney, D. L. Cast gold restoration with self-threading pins. J. Prosthet. Dent. 41:296, 1979.
54. Chan, K. C., Boyer, D. B., and Reinhardt, J. W. Comparison of the retentive strength of two cast gold pin techniques. J. Prosthet. Dent. 42:527, 1979.
55. Kishimoto, M., Shillingburg, H. T., and Duncanson, M. G. Influence of preparation features on retention and resistance. II. Three-quarter crowns. J. Prosthet. Dent. 49:188, 1983.
56. Welk, D. A. Personal communication, May 1976.
57. Pruden, W. H. Partial coverage retainers: A critical evaluation. J. Prosthet. Dent. 16:545, 1966.
58. Dilts, W. E., Welk, D. A., and Stovall, J. Retentive properties of pin materials in pin-retained silver amalgam restorations. J. Am. Dent. Assoc. 77:1085, 1968.

Chapter 9

Seven-Eighths Crowns

The seven-eighths crown is an especially useful variation of the partial veneer crown that can be employed successfully on many maxillary and mandibular premolars and molars.[1] It is suitable for use on teeth having an intact mesiofacial cusp but restoration, caries, decalcification, or fracture of the distofacial cusp.[2] If conservatively prepared, it is an acceptably esthetic restoration, even on an occasional maxillary premolar.

The classic indication for its use is the maxillary first molar, in which a large distal or distofacial restoration precludes the use of three-quarter crown. If the preparation is carefully and skillfully done, the contours of the mesiofacial cusp will obscure the view of metal covering the distofacial cusp.[3,4] This advantage, coupled with the fact that no porcelain-fused-to-metal restoration will duplicate the surface smoothness of unprepared enamel, makes this an excellent restoration for many patients.

Because the seven-eighths crown covers the distofacial surface of the tooth, it has significantly better retention and resistance than does the three-quarter crown.[5] The seven-eighths crown should be considered for a bridge retainer on an abutment whose short crown length might make the retention or resistance of a three-quarter crown insufficient. It is also useful as a retainer for bridges whose span exceeds one pontic, when the greater retention of a full-coverage retainer is not needed but esthetics is a consideration.

While the seven-eighths crown may seem exotic and difficult at first, a second look will show that the preparation is actually a simple and practical modification of the standard three-quarter crown. Tooth preparation is actually easier for the seven-eighths crown than for the standard three-quarter crown, because the mesial extension of the vertical distofacial finish line provides better access for groove placement and margin finishing by the dentist. It is also easier for the patient to maintain.

The steps in preparing a maxillary molar for a seven-eighths crown are shown in Figs. 9-1 through 9-43.

Figures 9-44 through 9-52 show clinical examples of maxillary and mandibular molars restored with seven-eighths crowns.

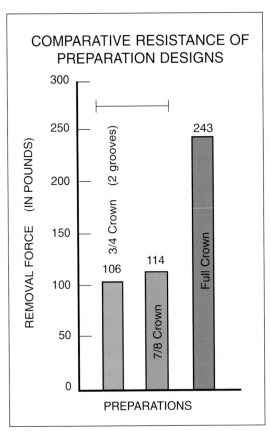

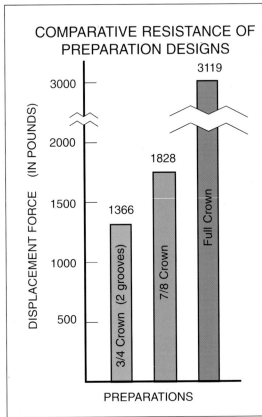

Fig. 9-1 Comparison of the retention values for the seven-eighths crown, the three-quarter crown, and the full veneer crown.[5]

Fig. 9-2 Resistance values for the seven-eighths crown, the three-quarter crown, and the full veneer crown.[5]

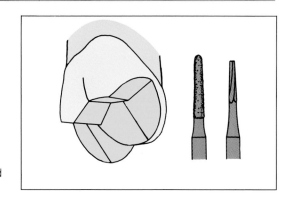

Fig. 9-3 Planar occlusal reduction: round-end tapered diamond and no. 171 bur.

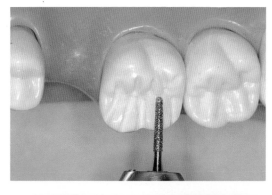

Fig. 9-4 Depth-orientation grooves are placed to a depth of 1.5 mm on the triangular ridges and in the major developmental grooves of the lingual cusps with the round-end tapered diamond. The grooves on the facial cusps are 1.0 mm deep in most areas, but they are made shallower as they approach the occlusofacial line angle of the mesiofacial cusp.

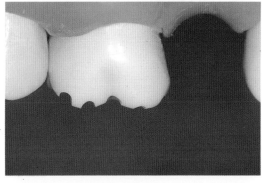

Fig. 9-5 A facial view of the depth-orientation grooves shows the difference in depth of penetration of the grooves at the occlusofacial line angle. The grooves on the distofacial cusp are the full diameter of the diamond at the line angle, while those on the mesial cusp make a less prominent indentation in the line angle.

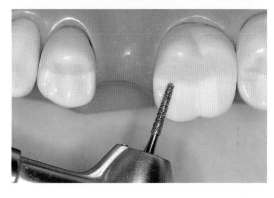

Fig. 9-6 The actual occlusal reduction consists of removing the tooth structure remaining between the orientation grooves and smoothing the reduced surfaces to inclined planes. The reduction is 1.0 mm on the nonfunctional cusps, with slightly less near the occlusofacial line angle of the mesiofacial cusp. The functional cusp reduction is approximately 1.5 mm.

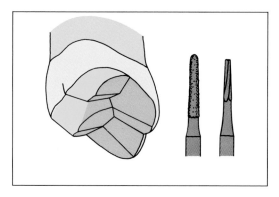

Fig. 9-7 Functional cusp bevel: round-end tapered diamond and no. 171 bur.

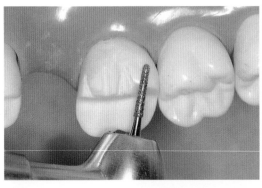

Fig. 9-8 Depth-orientation grooves are also made on the lingual inclines of the lingual cusps with the round-end tapered diamond.

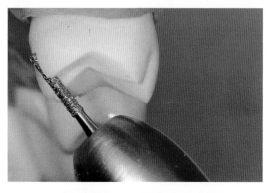

Fig. 9-9 The diamond is oriented so that it parallels the inclination of the opposing cusps.

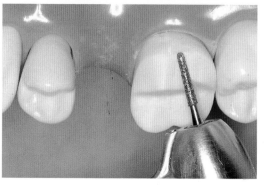

Fig. 9-10 The functional cusp bevel is produced by removing the "islands" of tooth structure isolated by the orientation grooves. It extends around to the central groove, becoming narrower as it does. Be sure that there is ample reduction in the vicinity of the distolingual groove, or the thickness of the wax pattern will be compromised in this area.

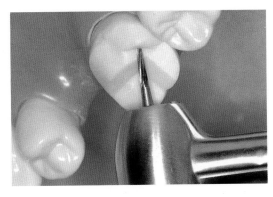

Fig. 9-11 The occlusal reduction and functional cusp bevels are finished with a no. 171 bur, to remove rough areas that could impede the complete seating of the casting.

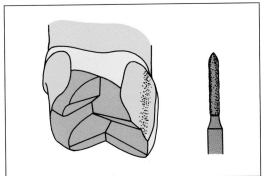

Fig. 9-12 Facial and lingual axial reduction: torpedo diamond.

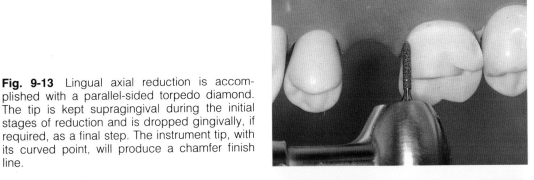

Fig. 9-13 Lingual axial reduction is accomplished with a parallel-sided torpedo diamond. The tip is kept supragingival during the initial stages of reduction and is dropped gingivally, if required, as a final step. The instrument tip, with its curved point, will produce a chamfer finish line.

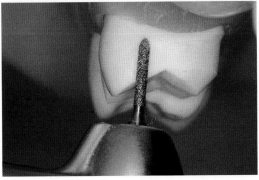

Fig. 9-14 When the tooth being prepared is a bridge abutment, extend the axial reduction onto the mesial surface with the torpedo diamond. It should terminate in the vicinity of the mesiofacial line angle. Be sure to keep the diamond upright and parallel with the path of insertion of the preparation. There is a tendency to lean it mesially to place the entire length of the diamond in contact with the mesial wall starting with the very first stroke to the instrument. This should be avoided, because it will produce an undercut mesial wall.

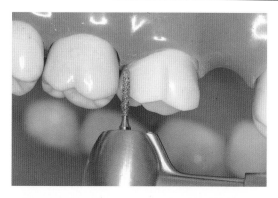

Fig. 9-15 Perform the distofacial axial reduction with the same torpedo diamond. This reduction should end about 1.0 mm mesial to the facial groove. Extend it as far as possible into the interproximal area without nicking the adjacent tooth.

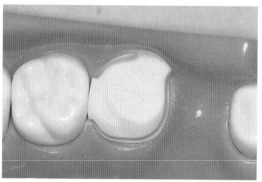

Fig. 9-16 An occlusal view of the tooth preparation at this point reveals an intact distal contact area, with facial and lingual axial reduction ending just short of contact with the adjacent tooth.

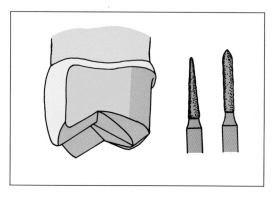

Fig. 9-17 Complete axial reduction: short-needle and torpedo diamonds.

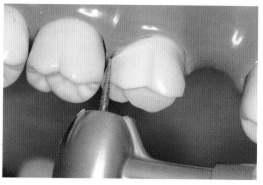

Fig. 9-18 The remaining interproximal tooth structure is removed with the tip of the short-needle diamond. Enter the facial or lingual embrasure with the instrument parallel with the path of insertion of the preparation, moving the instrument occlusally and gingivally as it is pushed through the contact area.

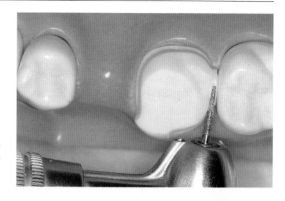

Fig. 9-19 It may prove helpful to lay the diamond horizontally, parallel with the distal surface of the tooth being prepared. Then draw the instrument across the marginal ridge.

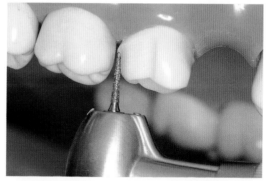

Fig. 9-20 Once there is space for the diamond to enter the interproximal area, pass it lightly faciolingually, smoothing the distal wall and finish line as you do.

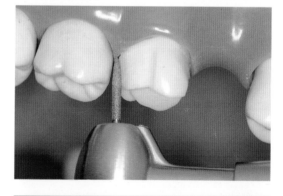

Fig. 9-21 If the contact extends very far gingivally, as it sometimes does between maxillary molars, it may be necessary to employ the flame diamond before the torpedo diamond. Although both instruments have the same diameter in the body, the flame diamond has a longer, thinner tip, which can be used to gain access near the interdental papilla.

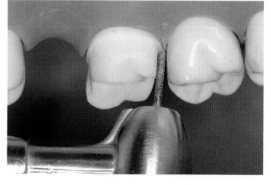

Fig. 9-22 When there is sufficient space to permit it, change to the torpedo diamond to complete the axial reduction. Be sure to round the corners between the proximal surfaces and the facial and lingual surfaces. There is a tendency to leave them "squared off," and inadequate reduction at the angles of the tooth is one of the leading causes of overcontouring in cast restorations.[6] The chamfer should be smooth and without interruptions where it passes from one surface to another.

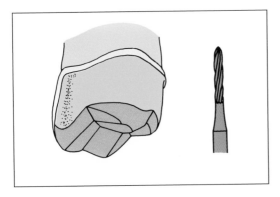

Fig. 9-23 Axial finishing: torpedo bur.

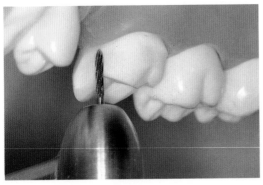

Fig. 9-24 Smooth the axial surface, and, most importantly, the chamfer finish line with the carbide finishing bur, which matches the size and configuration of the torpedo diamond.

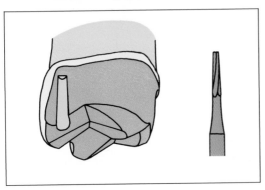

Fig. 9-25 Grooves: no. 171 bur.

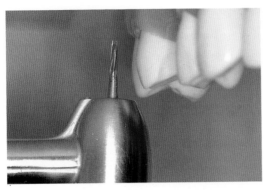

Fig. 9-26 Align a tapered fissure bur with the long axis of the preparation. Although the grooves will be the size of a no. 171 bur, the novice may wish to begin the groove with a no. 169L bur, since it permits the groove to be realigned or repositioned slightly without over cutting it if the initial alignment was incorrect. It can be enlarged once you are satisfied with its position and direction.

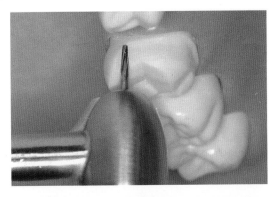

Fig. 9-27 Make the mesial groove with the no. 171 bur. On a bridge abutment, the entire groove can be done simultaneously. When there is a tooth adjacent to the groove site, the groove should be cut in 1- or 2-mm increments, starting from the occlusal surface (see page 104). The groove should be made to the full diameter of a no. 171 bur, parallel with the path of insertion of the preparation and extending to within 0.5 mm of the gingival finish line. The bottom of the groove should have a definite, flat seat, and not fade out to the finish line.

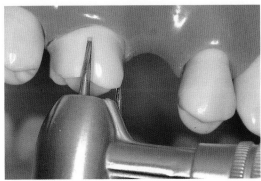

Fig. 9-28 Use the same bur to prepare the facial groove. This groove must be correctly aligned with the path of insertion. Many novices concentrate so hard on aligning it correctly faciolingually that they forget to check it mesiodistally.

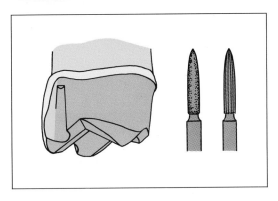

Fig. 9-29 Flares: flame diamond and carbide bur.

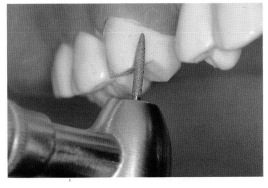

Fig. 9-30 The mesial flare is formed with a flame diamond. It will be narrow at its gingival end, becoming progressively wider occlusally. It will be prepared equally at the expense of the facial wall of the groove and the outer wall of the tooth. Because of the convexity of the mesial surface of the tooth, the difference in width should be quite noticeable.

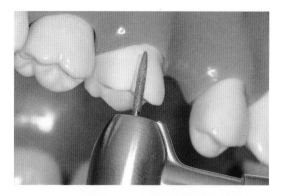

Fig. 9-31 The flame diamond is also used to make the facial flare. Since the facial surface does not exhibit a marked convexity, this flare will be only slightly wider at the occlusal end than at the gingival end.

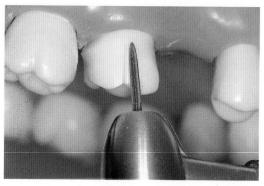

Fig. 9-32 A flame-shaped bur whose size and shape match the flame diamond should be used to finish the flares.* This will produce a smooth flare with a distinct finish line.

*No. H48L-010, Brasseler USA Inc., Savannah, Ga.

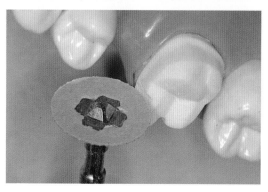

Fig. 9-33 A paper- or plastic-backed abrasive disk can be used to form and finish the flares when there is adequate access. Take extreme care when using this technique in the mouth, or the patient's lip can be cut. The flare should be flat and the finish line crisp. If the flare assumes a convex shape with a "rounded" finish line, the disk has worn out. Replace it and retouch the flare.

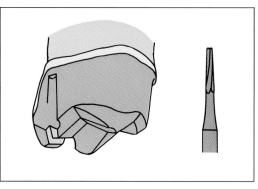

Fig. 9-34 Occlusal offset: no. 171 bur.

Fig. 9-35 The occlusal offset is placed with a no. 171 bur. Its floor is perpendicular to the path of insertion and forms a level "terrace" on the lingual slope of the mesiofacial cusp. One of its functions is to provide space for a bulk of metal which will reinforce the margin. The offset should connect the lingual walls of the grooves. In this way the metal in the corresponding area of the casting will connect the bulk of metal in the grooves to provide the "truss effect" described by Willey.[7]

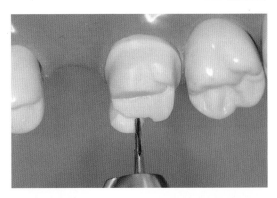

Fig. 9-36 Round over the angle between the occlusal edge of the offset and the inclined planes of the mesiofacial cusp with a no. 171 bur. Continue this rounding onto the mesial and facial flares so there will be no sharp line angles between the occlusal surface of the mesiofacial cusp and its two flares.

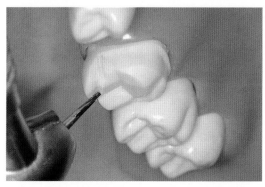

Fig. 9-37 Use the no. 170 bur to blunt any sharp angles on the occlusal surface. Recheck the occlusal reduction of the distofacial cusp at this time to insure that it is sufficient. There is a common tendency not to reduce it enough, which will cause severe problems when the wax pattern is fabricated.

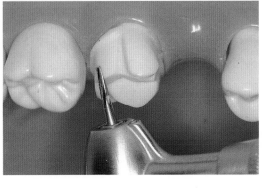

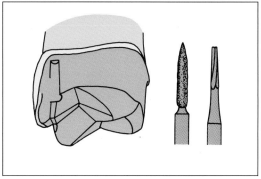

Fig. 9-38 Occlusal finishing bevel: flame diamond and no. 170 bur.

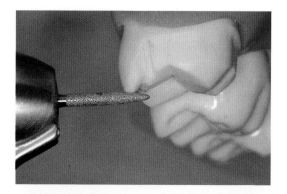

Fig. 9-39 The occlusal finishing bevel can be placed with one of several instruments. A fine-grit flame diamond can be used for creating an occlusofacial finishing bevel. It will produce a coarse finish, however, and should be followed by a carbide bur.

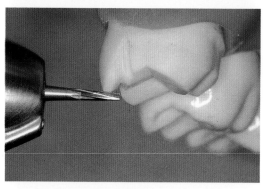

Fig. 9-40 The instrument of choice, however, is the no. 170 bur or the long-flame carbide bur, since a carbide bur will produce the smoothest surface and the clearest finish line. The bevel is made at a right angle to the path of insertion and is 0.5 mm or slightly more in width.

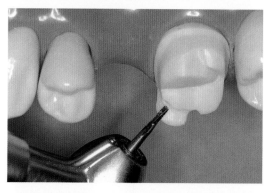

Fig. 9-41 The bevel is rounded over the proximal occlusal line angle to blend in with the proximal flares. Be sure that the outer edge of the bevel is continuous with the the edge of the flare, in order to produce a continuous finish line. Sharp corners in the finish line of a preparation are likely to cause voids in the corresponding angle of the stone die.

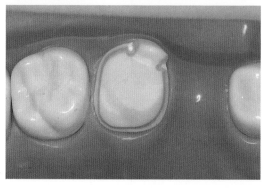

Fig. 9-42 An occlusal view of the seven-eighths crown preparation on a maxillary first molar. Notice that after the addition of the facial flare, the distal finish line is far mesial to the anatomical facial groove.

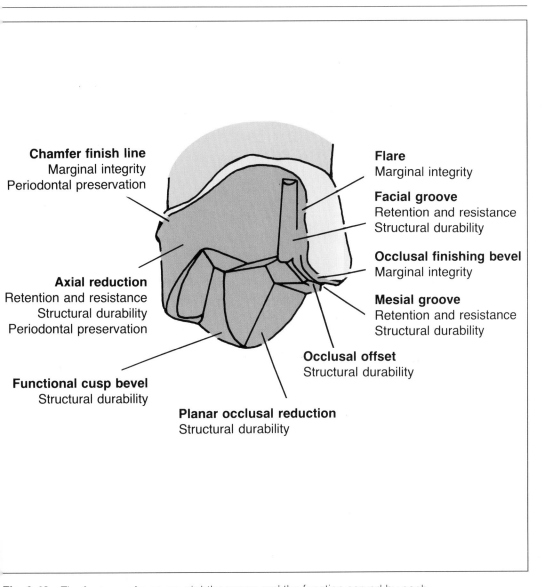

Chamfer finish line
Marginal integrity
Periodontal preservation

Flare
Marginal integrity

Facial groove
Retention and resistance
Structural durability

Occlusal finishing bevel
Marginal integrity

Axial reduction
Retention and resistance
Structural durability
Periodontal preservation

Mesial groove
Retention and resistance
Structural durability

Occlusal offset
Structural durability

Functional cusp bevel
Structural durability

Planar occlusal reduction
Structural durability

Fig. 9-43 The features of a seven-eighths crown and the function served by each.

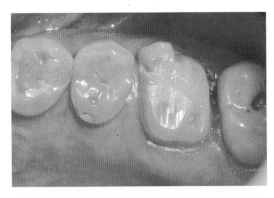

Fig. 9-44 A seven-eighths crown preparation was done on this severely abraded maxillary first molar.

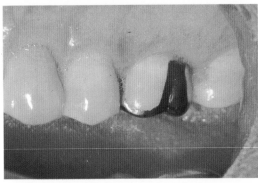

Fig. 9-45 The completed seven-eighths crown is shown cemented on the prepared tooth.

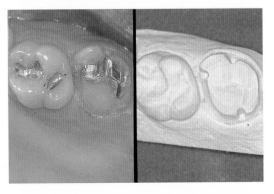

Fig. 9-46 A seven-eighths crown was selected for this second molar because the linguoversion of the first molar makes the second molar more visible than usual. The prepared tooth is shown in the mouth *(left)* and on the stone cast *(right)*. A groove was placed on the distolingual aspect of the tooth for added resistance and for relief for the distolingual groove in the wax pattern.

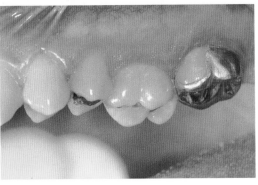

Fig. 9-47 The finished seven-eighths crown is shown in the mouth.

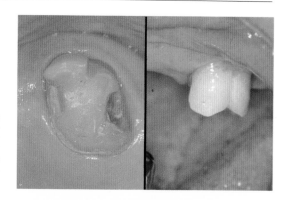

Fig. 9-48 An occlusal view of a seven-eighths crown preparation on a maxillary first molar bridge abutment shows the inclusion of mesial and distal boxes to accommodate caries and a previous restoration *(left)*. A facial view of the preparation is seen on the right.

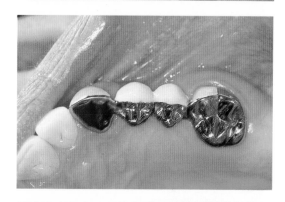

Fig. 9-49 This is a facial view of the finished bridge, retained on the molar abutment by a seven-eighths crown.

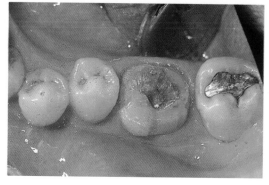

Fig. 9-50 An occlusal view of the same bridge replacing two missing maxillary premolars.

Fig. 9-51 Destruction of central tooth structure had been severe in this mandibular first molar, and a seven-eighths crown design was selected to take advantage of the sound facial tooth structure. The use of a full crown would have destroyed much of the remaining facial tooth structure, necessitating the placement of a core before proceeding.

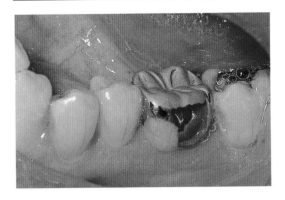

Fig. 9-52 The cemented seven-eighths crown is shown on the mandibular first molar.

References

1. Kessler, J. C., and Shillingburg, H. T. The seven-eighths crown. Gen. Dent. 31:132, 1983.
2. Ingraham, R., Bassett, R. W., and Koser, J. R. An Atlas of Cast Gold Procedures. 2nd ed. Buena Park, CA: Unitro College Press, 1969, 165.
3. Shillingburg, H. T., and Fisher, D. W. The partial veneer restoration. Aust. Dent. J. 17:411, 1972.
4. Crispin, B. J. Conservative alternatives to full esthetic crowns. J. Prosthet. Dent. 42:392, 1979.
5. Potts, R. G., Shillingburg, H. T., and Duncanson, M. G. Retention and resistance of preparations for cast restorations. J. Prosthet. Dent. 43:303, 1980.
6. Higdon, S. J. Tooth preparation for optimum contour of full coverage restorations. Gen. Dent. 26:47, 1978.
7. Willey, R. E. The preparation of abutments for veneer retainers. J. Am. Dent. Assoc. 53:141, 1956.

Chapter 10

Proximal Half-Crowns

An especially perplexing problem for the dentist is that of the tilted mandibular molar abutment. In most preparation designs the path of insertion for the preparation more or less parallels the long axis of the tooth, while being perpendicular to the plane of occlusion. This permits adequate resistance to occlusal loading while facilitating the seating of the restoration.

When the prospective abutment tooth has tipped toward the edentulous space, it is no longer possible for the path of insertion of the abutment preparation to be both parallel to the long axis of the tooth and perpendicular to the plane of occlusion.

Several solutions have been offered for this problem. Whenever possible, the tooth is uprighted orthodontically to permit a favorable path of insertion with optimum preparation retention and to eliminate uncleanable periodontal defects on the mesial aspect of the root. Brown reported a decrease of 3.1 mm in pocket depth by uprighting mesially inclined molars.[1]

If orthodontic treatment is not feasible for any reason, other solutions may be used. A telescopic crown retainer on the bridge may be fitted over a cast coping on the tooth if the clinical crown of the tooth has suffered moderate to severe destruction.[2,3] This approach, utilizing two crowns, telescope, and coping on the abutment, requires the destruction of considerable tooth struc-

ture and should not be used to restore minimally damaged teeth.

Another, less destructive retainer design for the tilted abutment is the proximal half-crown,[4-7] which is a three-quarter crown variant.[8-10] In concept it is a three-quarter crown which has been rotated 90 degress so that a proximal surface, rather than the facial, is left unveneered.[11] It can be employed if the tooth has been damaged only slightly. Two criteria must be met, however:

1. The distal surface must be caries-free.
2. There should be minimal interproximal caries throughout the rest of the mouth.

There is some risk in leaving the interproximal surface of a bridge abutment unrestored. The risk can be minimized by using this retainer design only in those mouths where there is little history of interproximal caries and therefore less likelihood of future occurrence.

The proximal half-crown has also been described for use as a retainer on mandibular premolars, especially when the tooth is somewhat malpositioned. In such applications it minimizes the display of metal.[4]

The sequence for preparing a tipped mandibular second molar for a proximal half-crown is shown in Figs. 10-1 through 10-39. Clinical examples are shown in Figs. 10-40 through 10-48.

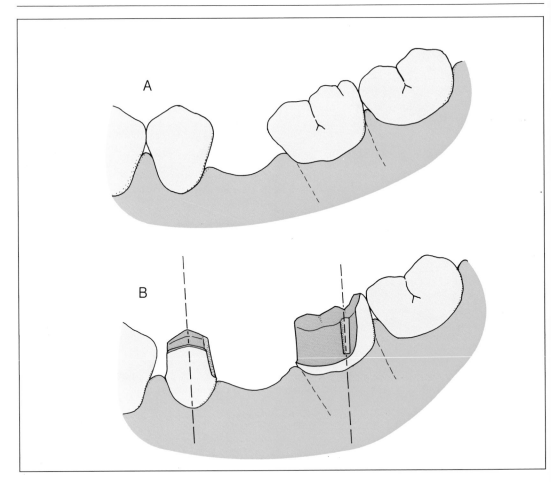

Fig. 10-1 In this typical situation, a mandibular molar bridge abutment is tipped mesially, creating an exaggerated curve of Spee (A). It would not be possible to prepare this molar for a full crown with a path of insertion paralleling that of the premolar abutment preparation. In mouths where conditions are favorable, a proximal half-crown can be utilized as a retainer on the molar, allowing the distal surface of the tooth to remain untouched (B).

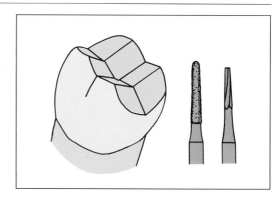

Fig. 10-2 Planar occlusal reduction: round-end tapered diamond and no. 171 bur.

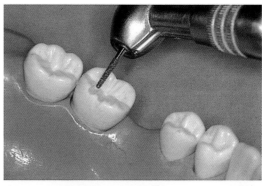

Fig. 10-3 Begin the occlusal reduction by placing depth-orientation grooves on the occlusal surface with the round-end tapered diamond.

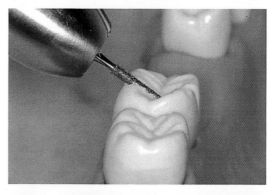

Fig. 10-4 On the distal aspect of the occlusal surface the occlusal reduction, and therefore the depth-orientation grooves, will be the normal depth.

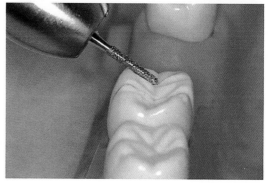

Fig. 10-5 The grooves and the reduction that will follow may not be as deep in the mesial portion of the occlusal surface, since this segment of the tooth has dropped below the occlusal plane.

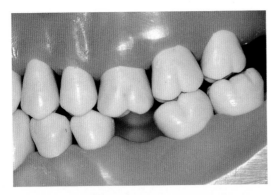

Fig. 10-6 The normal occlusal reduction will be required if the tooth opposing the edentulous space has supererupted into the space. Correction of the occlusal plane to prevent occlusal disharmony often will require placement of a restoration with occlusal coverage on that opposing tooth.

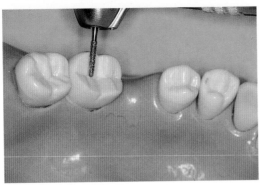

Fig. 10-7 Using the round-end tapered diamond, remove the tooth structure remaining between the depth-orientation grooves to reproduce the geometric planes of the occlusal surface.

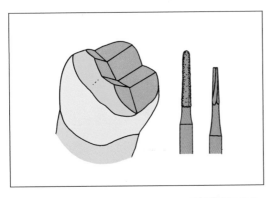

Fig. 10-8 Functional cusp bevel: round-end tapered diamond and no. 171 bur.

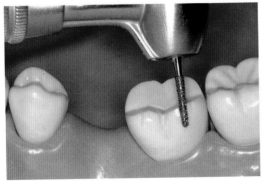

Fig. 10-9 Begin the functional cusp bevel by placing depth-orientation grooves with the round-end tapered diamond. These grooves, as well as the bevel which will follow, often will be shorter and shallower on the mesial cusp than on the distal. There will be less need for the bevel where the tooth has tipped below the occlusal plane, providing the opposing tooth has either not supererupted or has been restored back to the proper occlusal plane.

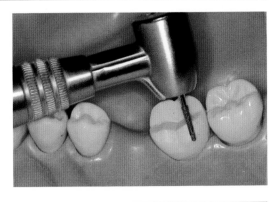

Fig. 10-10 Complete the functional cusp bevel with the round-end tapered diamond, removing the tooth structure between the depth-orientation grooves.

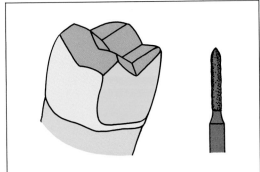

Fig. 10-11 Mesial axial reduction: torpedo diamond.

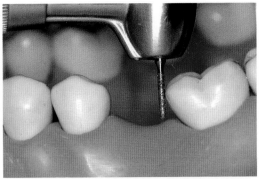

Fig. 10-12 Begin the axial reduction by making the path of insertion of the mesial surface parallel with the long axis of the premolar abutment. At this point the diamond instrument will make contact with only a small area of the mesial surface just apical to the marginal ridge. Do not attempt to produce a mesial gingival finish line at this point, or an undercut will be produced.

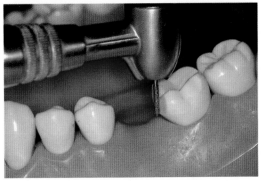

Fig. 10-13 Continue cutting the mesial surface with the torpedo diamond oriented with the eventual path of insertion of the preparation. Enough tooth structure will be removed so that the end of the diamond will eventually make contact with the tooth and produce a chamfer finish line in the gingival area of the mesial surface.

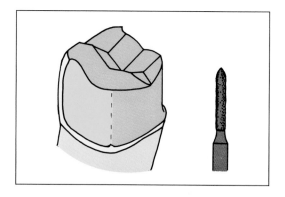

Fig. 10-14 Facial and lingual axial reduction torpedo diamond.

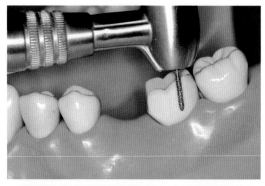

Fig. 10-15 Use the same diamond to produce axial reduction with a chamfer finish line on the facial surface. End the extension 1.0 mm or more mesial to the distofacial embrasure. Overextension distally will leave the vertical finish line in a position where it will be difficult to capture in the impression, hard to finish, and impossible for the patient to keep clean.

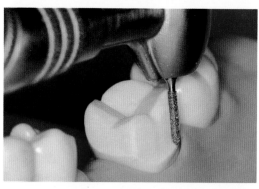

Fig. 10-16 Since mesially tipped molars also frequently exhibit some lingual inclination as well, take care to keep the diamond as upright as possible to avoid excessive facial wall inclination and resultant loss of retention.

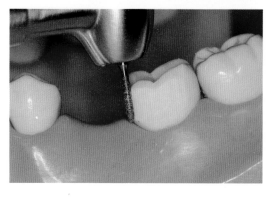

Fig. 10-17 Often there will be a sharp angle where the facial and mesial reductions meet. Round this angle from facial to mesial, and make sure that the chamfer does not have a "scallop" or a rise occlusally at the angle.

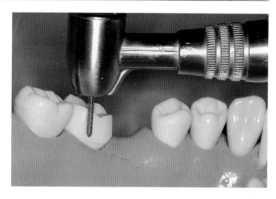

Fig. 10-18 Repeat the process on the lingual surface, creating a definite chamfer finish line, and keeping the surface as upright as possible. Again, do not extend the vertical distal finish line too far into the distolingual embrasure.

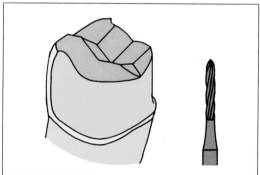

Fig. 10-19 Axial finishing: torpedo bur.

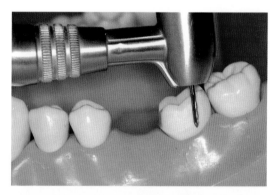

Fig. 10-20 Go over all three axial surfaces with a torpedo-shaped carbide finishing bur to produce a precise, well-defined chamfer finish line.

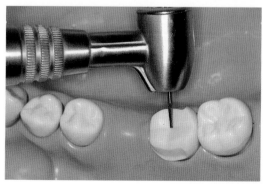

Fig. 10-21 Smooth the planes and angles of the occlusal surface with a no. 171 bur at this time.

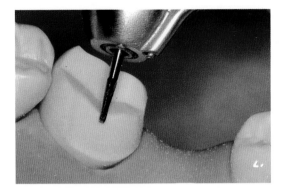

Fig. 10-22 Now finish the functional cusp bevel with the same carbide bur. This finishing step is delayed to this time because of the large quantities of tooth structure removed during the uprighting of the mesial surface. Going over the functional cusp bevel now enables the operator to better blend it with the other occlusal and axial features of the preparation.

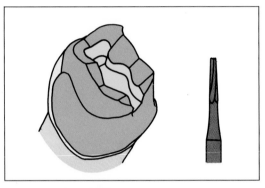

Fig. 10-23 Occlusal isthmus and countersink: no. 171 bur.

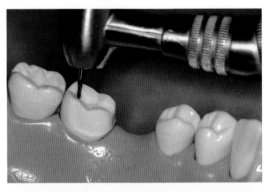

Fig. 10-24 The addition of an occlusal isthmus increases bulk and rigidity in the casting as well as providing much needed retention. This feature is usually "automatic" inasmuch as most prospective abutments will have either an old restoration or caries in the central groove.

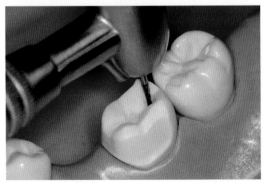

Fig. 10-25 A countersink is added to the distal fossa with the no. 171 bur. This feature not only supplements retention and resistance, but it also provides greater bulk to the casting in the critical area near the distal occlusal margin.

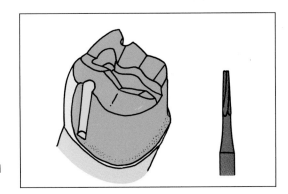

Fig. 10-26 Facial and lingual grooves: no. 171 bur.

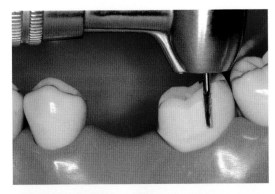

Fig. 10-27 Place a groove on the facial surface within 1.0 mm of the vertical distal extension of the preparation. The groove should parallel the mesial surface of the tooth and the long axis of the other abutment tooth. The groove must also be upright faciolingually and should not lean to the lingual.

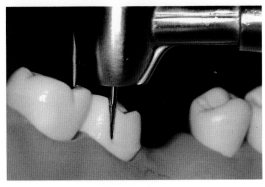

Fig. 10-28 Repeat the process on the lingual surface, paralleling that groove with the one on the facial surface. Be careful not to place it too far distally. The groove may be started with a no. 170 bur and finished with the no. 171 to prevent its becoming too large.

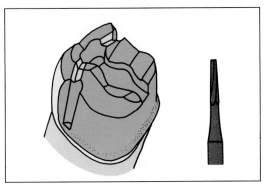

Fig. 10-29 Distal occlusal offset: no. 171 bur.

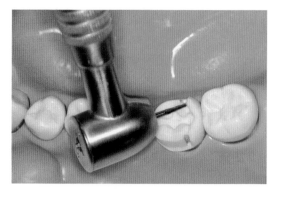

Fig. 10-30 Create a V-shaped offset 0.5 to 1.0 mm from the distal occlusal finish line, connecting the lingual groove to the countersink to the facial groove. It will produce a rigid staple with the grooves to reinforce the distal marginal area of the casting.

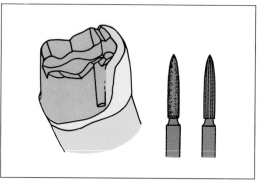

Fig. 10-31 Flares and occlusal bevel: flame diamond and flame bur.

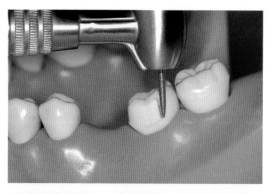

Fig. 10-32 Place a flare distal to the facial groove with the flame diamond. The flare will be a flat plane, wider at the occlusal end than at the gingival.

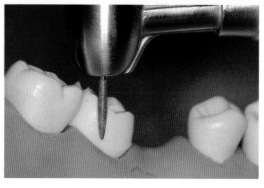

Fig. 10-33 Repeat the process on the lingual surface, creating a flare distal to the lingual groove, tying it in with the gingival chamfer.

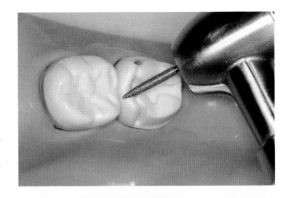

Fig. 10-34 Cut a bevel along the distal marginal ridge with the flame diamond, taking care not to extend into the distal occlusal embrasure, where the compromised location of the finish line would jeopardize the success of the restoration.

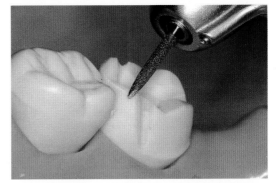

Fig. 10-35 Round over the angles between the distal occlusal bevel and the facial and lingual flares. Sharp angles in these areas will cause severe problems in the restoration margin.

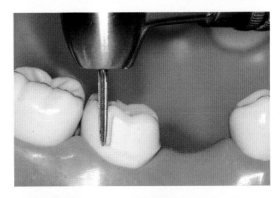

Fig. 10-36 Go over both of the flares with the flame carbide bur to produce the sharpest finish line possible.

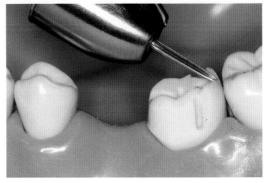

Fig. 10-37 Redo the occlusal bevel with the flame carbide bur.

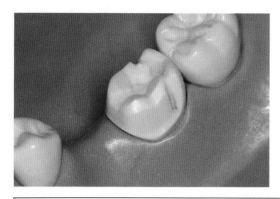

Fig. 10-38 The completed preparation for a proximal half-crown on a tilted mandibular second molar.

Fig. 10-39 The features of a proximal half-crown preparation on a mandibular molar, and the function served by each.

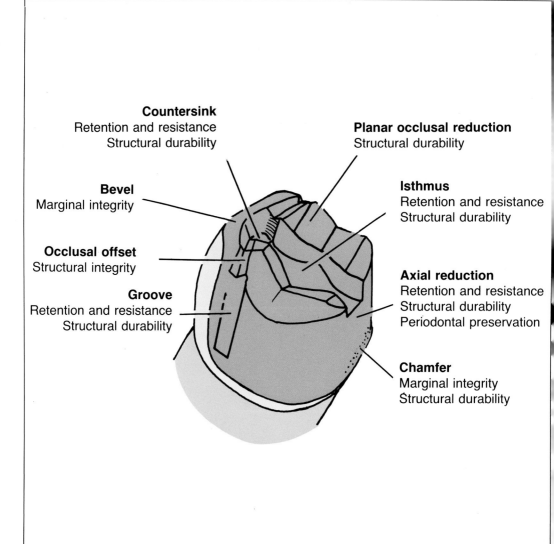

Countersink
Retention and resistance
Structural durability

Planar occlusal reduction
Structural durability

Bevel
Marginal integrity

Isthmus
Retention and resistance
Structural durability

Occlusal offset
Structural integrity

Groove
Retention and resistance
Structural durability

Axial reduction
Retention and resistance
Structural durability
Periodontal preservation

Chamfer
Marginal integrity
Structural durability

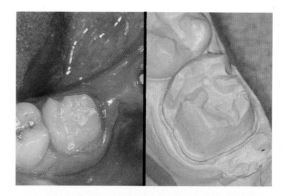

Fig. 10-40 A proximal half-crown was used on this tipped mandibular second molar as a retainer for a fixed bridge. This bridge was a remake of one that had been in the mouth for fourteen years. The original proximal half-crown on this tooth was still intact and had to be sectioned to be removed. The retainer on the *other* abutment failed. An occlusal view is seen in the mouth *(left)*, and the cast is seen from a mesiofacial angle *(right)*.

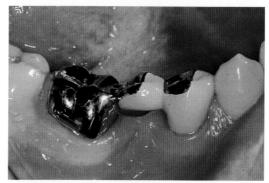

Fig. 10-41 A facial view of the completed bridge.

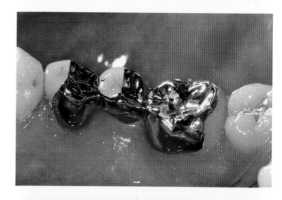

Fig. 10-42 An occlusolingual view of the bridge shows the conservative extensions of the occlusal and distolingual margins.

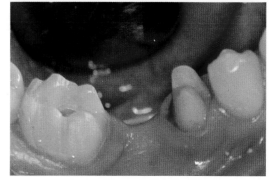

Fig. 10-43 A proximal half-crown was used on this mandibular second molar to compensate for its mesial inclination. A full veneer crown was utilized as a retainer on the second premolar.

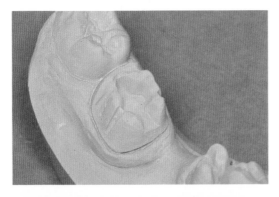

Fig. 10-44 In this mesiofacial view of the cast, the two grooves on each of the facial and lingual surfaces are clearly evident.

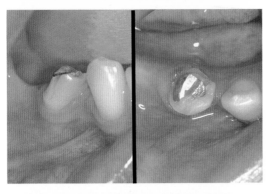

Fig. 10-45 This is the completed all-metal bridge fabricated for the preparations seen in Figs. 10-43 and 10-44.

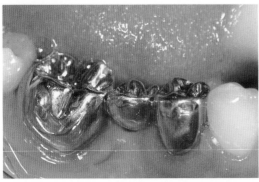

Fig. 10-46 A proximal half-crown was selected as a retainer for this tipped mandibular premolar. The preparation is seen here from the facial side *(left)* and the occlusal side *(right)*.

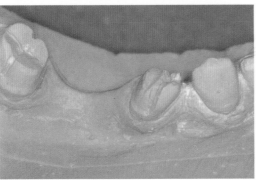

Fig. 10-47 A stone cast of the half crown preparation on the first premolar.

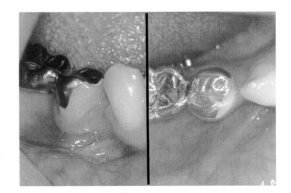

Fig. 10-48 Mesiofacial *(left)* and occlusal *(right)* views of the cemented retainer on the premolar reveal less metal display than one might expect. It is less than that of a standard three-quarter crown on this tooth.

References

1. Brown, I. W. The effect of orthodontic therapy on certain types of periodontal defects. I. Clinical findings. J. Periodontol. 44:742, 1973.
2. Eisenbrand, G. F. A method for constructing a fixed bridge with an extremely tipped abutment. Dent. Digest 68:514, 1962.
3. Shillingburg, H. T., and Fisher, D. W. Bridge retainers for tilted abutments. N. M. Dent. J. 22:16, 1972.
4. Smith, D.E. Abutment preparations. J. Am. Dent. Assoc. 18:2063, 1931.
5. Potter, H. R., and Smith, D. E. Practical bridgework. III. Non-vital teeth in bridgework. Pac. Dent. Gaz. 40:519, 1932.
6. Klaffenbach, A. O. An analytic study of modern abutments. J. Am. Dent. Assoc. 23:2275, 1936.
7. Ingraham, R., Bassett, R. W., and Koser, J. R. An Atlas of Cast Gold Procedures. 2nd ed. Buena Park, CA: Unitro College Press, 1969, 164.
8. Smith, D. E. Fixed bridge restorations with the tilted mandibular second or third molar as an abutment. J. South. Calif. Dent. Assoc. 6:131, 1939.
9. Schwartz, J. R. The basic or structural character of abutment preparations. Dent. Items Interest 56:897, 1934.
10. Willey, R. E. The preparation of abutments for veneer retainers. J. Am. Dent. Assoc. 53:141, 1956.
11. Shillingburg, H. T., and Fisher, D. W. The partial veneer restoration. Aust. Dent. J. 17:411, 1972.

Chapter 11

Inlays

The cast metal inlay has its roots in crude restorations that were in use before an accurate casting technique existed in dentistry. The first inlay in dentistry is credited to John Murphy of London, who was fabricating porcelain inlays in 1835.[1] In 1880, Ames and Swasery used a burnished foil technique for fabricating inlays. After adapting gold or platinum foil into a cavity preparation, they lifted it out, invested it, and then flowed molten solder or gold into the cavity form reproduced in foil.[2] The technique was still in use near the end of the first decade of this century.[3]

The first cast inlay is attributed to Philbrook, who reported the technique to the Iowa State Dental Society in 1897.[4] It is Taggart, however, who is credited with introducing the ancient lost wax technique to dentistry in 1907. He described the inlay as "an honest filling: it is either in the tooth saving it from decay, or it is in the appendix."[5] The restoration grew in popularity from that time, aided by the contributions of Lane, Van Horn, Weinstein, Souder, Scheu, and Hollenback, who improved the materials and techniques of fabricating the restoration.[6]

Inlays have required an extensive destruction of tooth structure, which was recognized by one of their early proponents, Bodecker.[7] The large preparations in vogue in the early part of this century were due partly to the concept of "extension for prevention," and partly to the large, easily dulled instruments in use at the time.[8] Bodecker, practicing in Berlin, introduced the slice preparation for inlays, which was brought to the United States by Rhein, where it was further developed by Gillett.[9]

The slice inlay utilized a disk cut to flatten the proximal surface. Extensions were wide but shallow. The slice inlay could be made with a box form of near normal size;[10] a groove;[11] a dovetail, or "lock;"[12,13] or a wide dovetail, or "channel,"[14] similar to a narrow box. Considered by its proponents to be a truly conservative restoration,[10,15] the slice inlay was thought to be less likely to fracture the tooth supporting it.[16] It was even promoted at one time as a retainer for fixed bridges.[17–19]

Inlays have been described as the weakest of retainers, however,[20] weakening the tooth[21] and exerting inadequate resistance to accomplish their task.[22] Smith described them as being "the most outstanding of all causes in abutment failures of fixed bridgework."[23] With the possible exception of bridges with nonrigid connectors, inlays are no longer advocated as retainers for fixed bridges. The slice inlay was inferior to the conventional box inlay in resistance,[24,25] and it was overextended as well.[25] Photoelastic stress analysis showed that the restoration placed in a slice preparation exhibited greater stress than did one placed in a box preparation.[26]

Use of the cast metal inlay has declined markedly in recent years. At one time considered the mark of quality restorative care, it is used far less now than in the past. In a survey of practitioners conducted in the southeastern United States in 1980, only 8% of the respondents fabricated as many as ten Class II inlays per year.[27] A survey of dental educators published in 1984 indicated that 8% of North American dental schools do not teach the use of inlays, while 25% teach only two surface inlays.[28]

A meeting of dental educators representing eight schools in six states of the southeastern United States in 1979 reached the following conclusion: "Cast gold restorations should be limited to those teeth which need cusp coverage for protection and reinforcement of the tooth. The true cast gold inlay is no longer a reasonable consideration in the conservative treatment of unrestored teeth."[29]

What has happened to the cast gold restoration to bring it to this nadir of esteem? The answer lies in the ascendancy of its primary alternative, the silver amalgam restoration. This material has been greatly improved in recent years, resulting in restorations with higher early strength and lower dynamic creep. Concurrent with the improvements in strength, which permit less bulk, preparations for this restoration have become more conservative. In addition, it is not necessary to make as large a preparation for the amalgam to allow finishability, resulting in amalgam being a more conservative restoration.

Stress analysis has shown greater stress when the preparation for an intracoronal restoration is wide.[30,31] The indications for the use of an inlay have become progressively more conservative as clinicians and researchers have tied marginal failures to weakened cusps and preparation walls bending [32,33] or springing away from the restoration.[25] The recognition that a wider isthmus could lead to failure[33–35] has caused a change in the recommended extensions of the restoration. In 1926 Ward suggested an isthmus width that was one-half the intercuspal distance faciolingually.[36] That width has now shrunk to from one-third[37] to one-fourth the intercuspal distance.[38]

Vale found that the strength of a maxillary premolar with a two-surface preparation mesio-occlusal or disto-occlusal (MO or DO) was diminished by 35% merely by increasing the isthmus width from one-fourth the intercuspal distance to one-third.[39] Mondelli et al. did a similar study, looking at three isthmus widths: one-quarter, one-third, and one-half the intercuspal distance. These isthmus variations were tested in Class I, Class II (MO), and Class II (MOD) preparations. The greatest percentage decreases in resistance to fracture seen in that study occurred in widening the isthmus of a Class I preparation from one-fourth to one-third the intercuspal distance, and in converting an MO preparation with a narrow isthmus to an MOD preparation.[40] These results tend to confirm the clinical observation that an inlay one-third the faciolingual width of the occlusal surface may act to wedge the cusps apart.[41]

In separate studies, Blaser and associates[35] and Re et al.[42] found depth, in conjunction with width, produced a significant decrease in fracture strength of the tooth. This corroborates the observations of astute clinicians who have described the inlay as acting like a wedge between the facial and lingual cusps of the tooth.[23,25] The early practice of using a deep isthmus to increase resistance,[43] or to increase inlay strength,[44] clearly should be avoided.

Not too surprisingly, the majority of schools teaching the use of three-surface inlays today restrict them to situations in which the isthmus can be kept narrow.[28]

Class II inlays

The Class II inlay should be used on those premolars or molars with minimal caries or previous restoration that need a two-surface restoration (MO or DO) made of a long-lasting material. A small, usually acceptable amount of metal will be seen. MOD inlays with *no* occlusal coverage, which can be kept narrow (one-quarter of the faciolingual width of the tooth), can be employed on molars, but their use on premolars is highly questionable.

Figures 11-1 through 11-35 show the techniques for preparing a maxillary molar for a proximo-occlusal inlay. Preparations for Class I, Class III, and Class V inlays are then demonstrated.

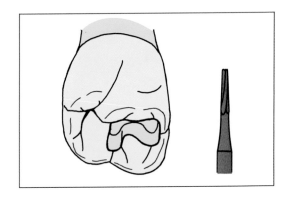

Fig. 11-1 Occlusal outline: no. 170 bur.

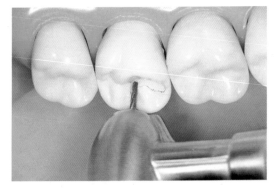

Fig. 11-2 Initial penetration into the enamel is done in a fossa with the *edge* of the tip of a non-dentate tapered fissure bur. Once a cut has been started, drag the bur through the central groove of the occlusal surface, leaning the instrument in the direction the handpiece is moving.

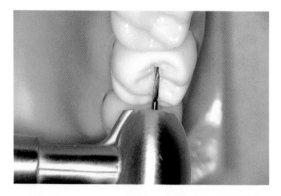

Fig. 11-3 Follow any defective developmenta grooves, making the isthmus approximately 1.5 mm deep. The penetration should end at leas 1.0 mm from the nearest occlusal contact. I there is any doubt about the location of these contacts, mark them with articulating paper.

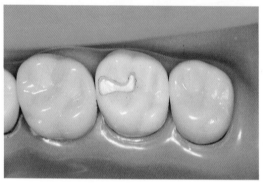

Fig. 11-4 The completed occlusal outline is quite narrow at this time. It will be extended farther when the occlusal bevel is added. There is a distinct dovetail extending into the facia groove, which is placed to enhance resistance and retention.[34,45-47] In order to provide max imum resistance, the pulpal floor should be flat at an even depth, and perpendicular to the path of insertion of the preparation.[18,25]

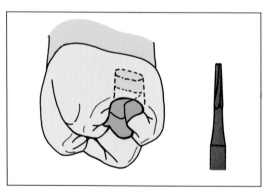

Fig. 11-5 Undermining marginal ridge: no 169L bur.

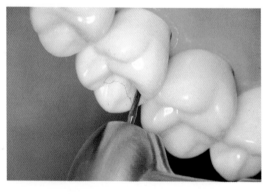

Fig. 11-6 Begin the proximal box by running a no. 169L bur just inside the cemento-ename junction interproximally.

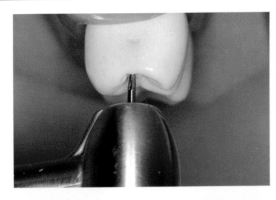

Fig. 11-7 In this proximal view, with the adjacent tooth removed for better vision, it is possible to see how far gingivally the bur has been extended.

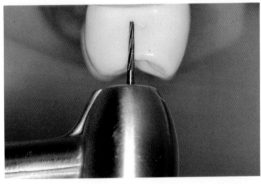

Fig. 11-8 The bur has been removed from the preparation and has been superimposed over the proximal surface to the full gingival length to which the preparation was extended. It would normally end supragingivally if caries did not dictate otherwise. Do not be too conservative with the gingival extension, since box length is an important factor in inlay retention.[38]

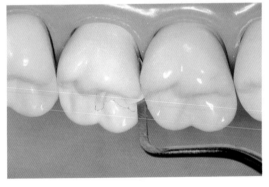

Fig. 11-9 A sharp enamel chisel, such as the hatchet shown here, can be used to break out the undermined tooth structure and expedite the preparation of the proximal box. A hand instrument will break this enamel out very cleanly in the mouth. However, it doesn't always work as it should in laboratory exercises, because resin is not as brittle as enamel. As a result, the fracture will sometimes extend far enough to damage the walls of the proximal box on a typodont tooth.

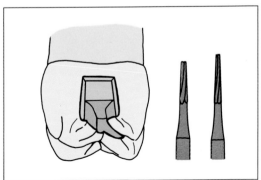

Fig. 11-10 Proximal box: nos. 169L and 170 burs.

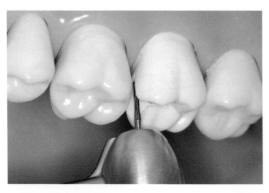

Fig. 11-11 Use a no. 169L bur to extend the box facially and lingually to the point where the box breaks contact with the adjacent tooth. Create facial and lingual line angles to give definition to the box.

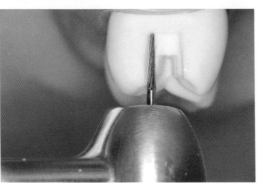

Fig. 11-12 A no. 169L bur can also be used to form the facial and lingual walls of the box. Although parallel walls were advocated by some early authors,[34,43,48] nearly parallel walls were presented as a more likely attainable goal.[49,50] Ward was one of the first to recommend a taper as such. He prescribed a 5% to 20% taper per inch (3 to 12 degrees).[36] Gillett, a leading proponent of inlays, was in favor of a 5% taper per inch (3 degrees).[10] A 5-degree divergence has also been suggested.[18,51] More recently, Gilmore has recommended a more practical 8 to 12 degrees.[37] As the taper increases from 7 to 15 degrees, stress rises and retention decreases.[31]

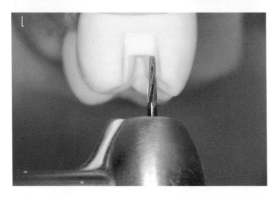

Fig. 11-13 Widen the isthmus where it joins the proximal box, rounding any angle that may have formed in the area where they meet.

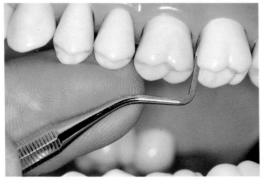

Fig. 11-14 Use an enamel chisel, such as the hatchet shown here, or a binangle chisel, to smooth and define the facial and lingual walls of the box. It is the box walls and not the angles that resist displacement.[38]

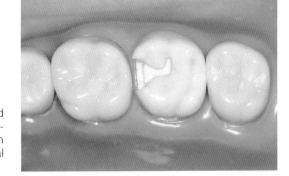

Fig. 11-15 The completed proximal wall should just barely break contact with the proximal surface of the adjacent tooth. The final extension will be achieved when the facial and lingual flares are placed.

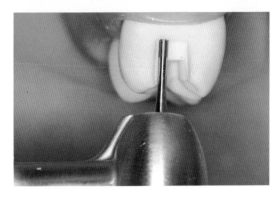

Fig. 11-16 Plane the pulpal floor of the isthmus with a no. 957 endcutting bur. The gingival floor of the box should likewise be flat.[25,52,53]

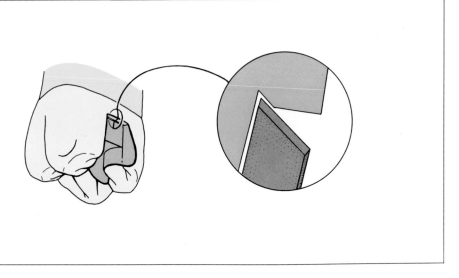

Fig. 11-17 Gingivo-axial groove: gingival margin trimmer.

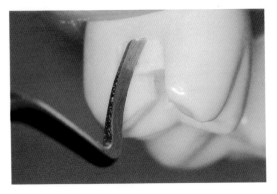

Fig. 11-18 Use a sharp gingival margin trimmer to create a V-shaped groove at the junction of the axial wall and the gingival floor of the box. This groove, sometimes referred to as the "Minnesota ditch,"[54] is placed to enhance resistance to displacement by occlusal forces.[39,55,56]

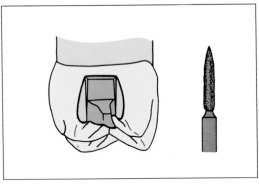

Fig. 11-19 Flare: flame diamond.

Fig. 11-20 The flare is a flat plane cut across the curving proximal surface of the tooth. The flare leans into the center of the tooth slightly, as the surface of the tooth is curving outward in the proximal contact area. It is cut equally at the expense of the facial or lingual wall of the box and the outer enamel surface of the tooth. As a result, a flare is narrow at its gingival end and much wider at its occlusal end. To start the flare, place the sharp-tipped flame diamond in the proximal box and use the small-diameter tip to cut the cavosurface angle of the box from the gingival floor up.

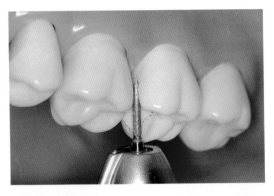

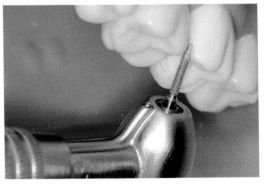

Fig. 11-21 Continue the occlusalward sweep of the diamond without changing the angle or direction of the instrument. You should still be using the tip of the flame diamond. If your wrist is locked and you move your entire hand, it is possible to cut a flat plane in this manner. The diamond should be cutting only when you are moving it toward the occlusal end. If you move it back and forth, you are likely to round over the actual finish line.

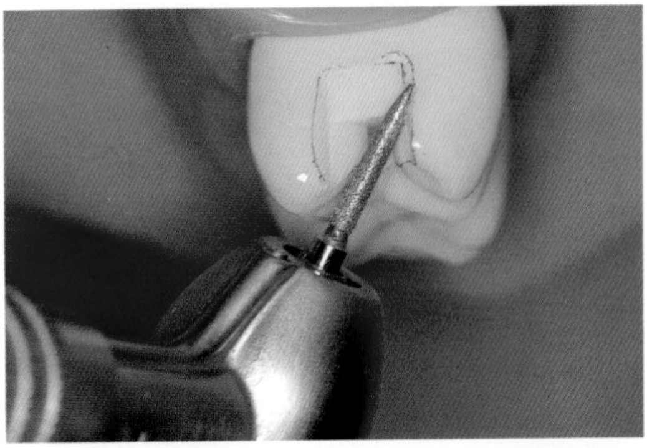

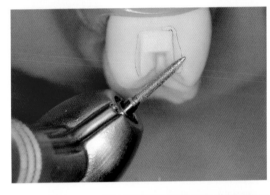

Fig. 11-22 With the adjacent tooth removed, you can see the narrow flare produced up to this point.

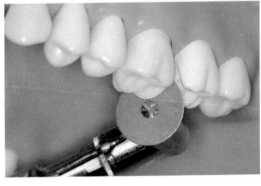

Fig. 11-23 With the space created by the first passes of the diamond tip, it is now possible to use a larger portion of the instrument, which can remove tooth structure more efficiently.

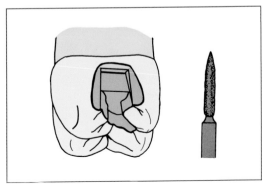

Fig. 11-24 A sandpaper disk can be used for shaping the flares, but extreme caution must be used to prevent accidental laceration of soft tissues. This technique is best reserved for those cases in which a rubber dam has been employed.

Fig. 11-25 Gingival bevel: flame diamond.

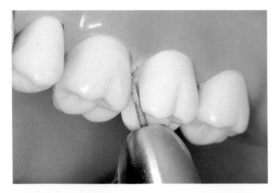

Fig. 11-26 Lean the flame diamond over against the pulpal axial line angle to produce a proper bevel on the gingival floor. A butt joint has long been recognized as an inferior finish line in this area.[57] Metzler and Chandler have recently confirmed the bevel as the finish line of choice for inlays.[58] The marginal bevel should lie between 30 and 45 degrees to provide an optimum blend of strength and marginal fit.[59,60] Although many operators use a gingival margin trimmer for this feature,[28] it is likely to produce a ragged finish line (see page 77).

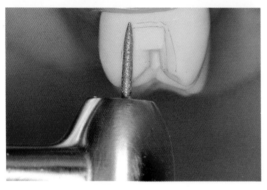

Fig. 11-27 Take care to blend the gingival bevel with the facial and lingual flares to avoid a scooped-out area, which would result in an undercut.

Fig. 11-28 Occlusal bevel: flame diamond.

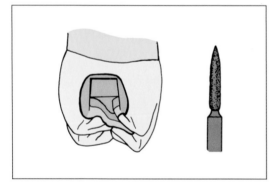

Fig. 11-29 A bevel is placed around the entire periphery of the occlusal portion of the preparation. Varying degrees of taper have been recommended for this bevel. Generally, if the bevel is at too shallow an angle and does not extend far down the isthmus wall, it will produce an occlusal finish line that is very difficult to trace when the wax pattern is fabricated. On the other hand, a substantial bevel extending far down the isthmus wall can increase stress.[31] Ingraham et al. recommend using a bevel of 15 to 20 degrees, beginning at the junction of the occlusal one-third and the pulpal two-thirds of the isthmus wall.[61] It is likely to produce some stress, but it is a necessary risk to produce a finishable casting. If the convex part of the diamond is used for producing the bevel, the bevel will be "hollow ground" or slightly concave, as suggested by Tucker.[4] This results in a much more easily read finish line.

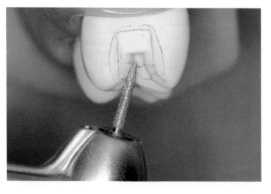

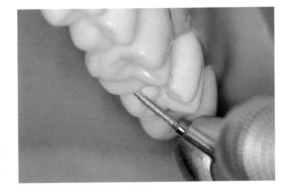

Fig. 11-30 Carefully blend the proximal flares with the occlusal bevel to produce a smooth, continuous finish line.

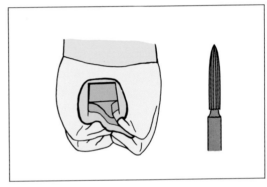

Fig. 11-31 Bevel and flare finishing: flame bur.

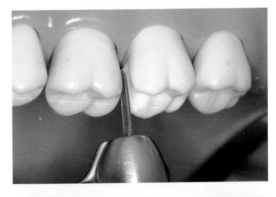

Fig. 11-32 Use a flame-shaped carbide finishing bur to go over the flares and the gingival bevel. The flame bur produces the most consistent bevel.[62] The finish line is the most vulnerable area of the preparation, and a smooth finish line diminishes that vulnerability. Carbide finishing burs will produce the smoothest finish lines.[63]

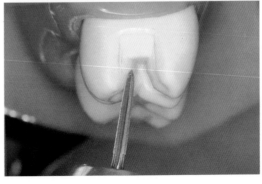

Fig. 11-33 The flame-shaped carbide finishing bur is also used to refine the occlusal bevel. The resultant concave bevel with a distinct finish line is easily identified in the impression, and the inlay is easily waxed and finished against it.

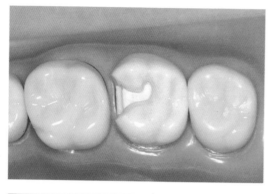

Fig. 11-34 An occlusal view of the completed Class II inlay preparation on a maxillary molar.

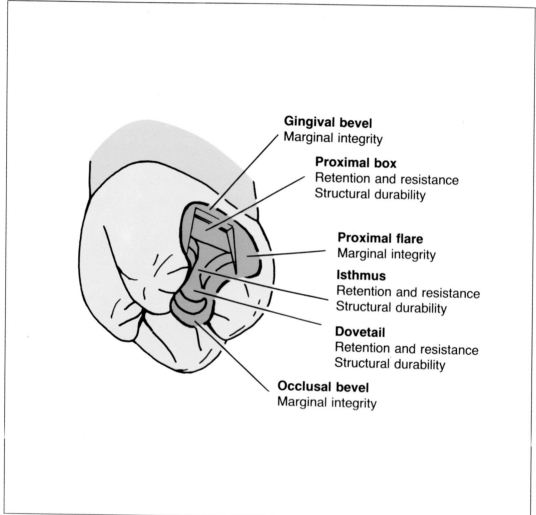

Gingival bevel
Marginal integrity

Proximal box
Retention and resistance
Structural durability

Proximal flare
Marginal integrity

Isthmus
Retention and resistance
Structural durability

Dovetail
Retention and resistance
Structural durability

Occlusal bevel
Marginal integrity

Fig. 11-35 The features of a Class II inlay preparation and the function served by each.

Class I inlays

Probably the best indication for a Class I inlay occurs when restoring a moderate-sized carious lesion in the occlusal surface of a patient with predominantly gold restorations. It consists of the occlusal portion of the Class II inlay, following the central groove and any defective developmental grooves. The technique for making a Class I inlay preparation on a mandibular molar is shown in Figs. 11-36 through 11-47.

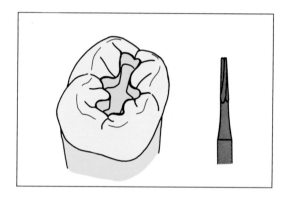

Fig. 11-36 Occlusal outline: no. 170 bur.

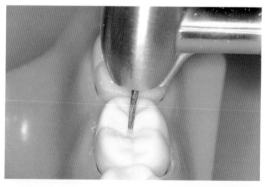

Fig. 11-37 Make the initial cut in the defective central groove with a no. 170 bur to an approximate depth of 1.5 mm. Lean the handpiece mesially or distally, since the edge and side of the tip will cut more efficiently than the end itself.

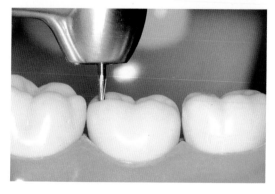

Fig. 11-38 Straighten up the handpiece to avoid encroaching on the marginal ridges. Extending too far into them will remove all dentinal support and excessively weaken them. Holding the tapered fissure bur upright now will produce the desired minimal taper on the "end walls" of the preparation.

217

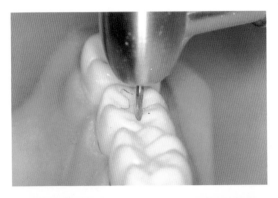

Fig. 11-39 Continue extending the cut along the central groove to the other marginal ridge or transverse ridge (if the tooth being restored has an intact one). The isthmus should be approximately 1.0 mm wide.

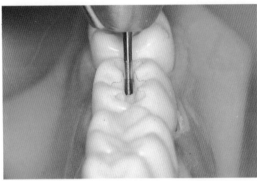

Fig. 11-40 Flatten the pulpal floor with a no. 957 endcutting bur.

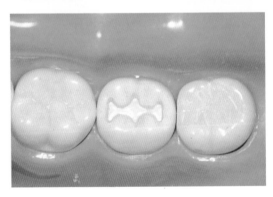

Fig. 11-41 An occlusal view of the outline form reveals moderate extensions into the facial and lingual grooves, with small "barbell" dovetails at each end. In addition to providing additional retention and resistance, these extensions move the finish line up the slopes of the respective triangular and marginal ridges where the inlay margin will be more accessible for finishing.

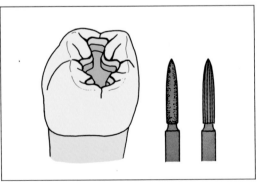

Fig. 11-42 Occlusal bevel: flame diamond and bur.

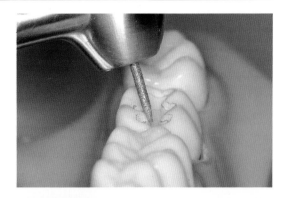

Fig. 11-43 The occlusal bevel is initially placed with a flame diamond. It extends one-third of the way down the sides of the isthmus wall and has a 15- to 20-degree inclination.[61] Do not overextend this bevel laterally onto the occlusal surface. Not only will it make the restoration too wide, but the finish line will form such an obtuse angle with the enamel surface that it will be difficult to identify during margin finishing in wax or gold.

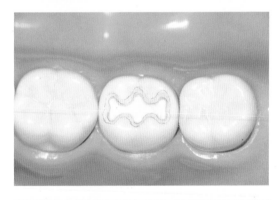

Fig. 11-44 Finish the occlusal bevel with a flame carbide finishing bur. The resultant finish line is more distinct and more easily identified than a bevel produced by a diamond alone.

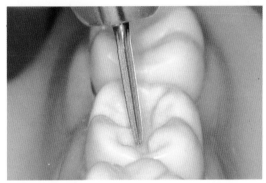

Fig. 11-45 An occlusal view of a Class I inlay preparation.

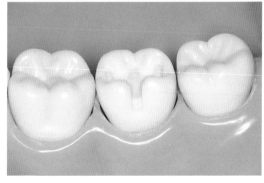

Fig. 11-46 A variation of the Class I inlay preparation has a small beveled box which follows the facial or lingual groove onto the respective axial surface.

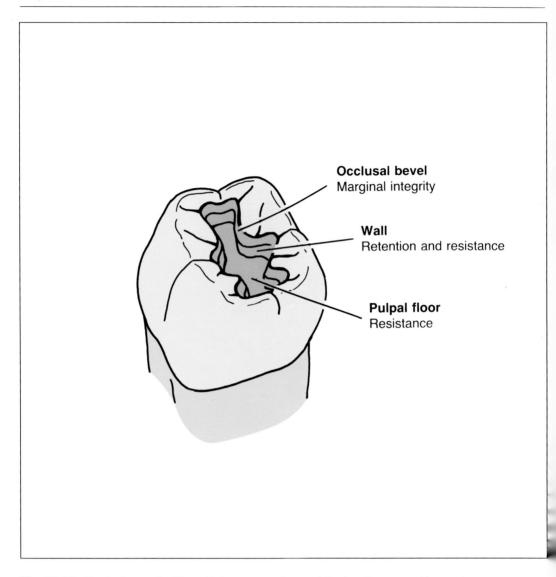

Occlusal bevel
Marginal integrity

Wall
Retention and resistance

Pulpal floor
Resistance

Fig. 11-47   The features of a Class I inlay preparation and the function served by each.

Class III inlays

The Class III inlay has drastically diminished in use, to the point of near extinction. Because it inevitably displays some metal, it is contraindicated for use on incisors. Conzett, in 1910, stated that Class III inlays were contraindicated for use on any tooth because of the extent of tooth destruction required for its cavity preparation.[43] Redfern, however, recommends it for teeth with extensive caries, or for the replacement of failed resin restorations.[64] It is an excellent restoration for the distal surface of canines.

The slight display of metal on the facial aspect of the tooth is not objectionable to many patients. A well done inlay in this situation will look better than an amalgam restoration, will last longer than an amalgam or composite resin restoration, and will be much less destructive than a full veneer porcelain crown of any sort. Its indications are not numerous, but the restoration has its place. The stages of a preparation for a Class III inlay on the distal of a maxillary canine are shown in Figs. 11-48 through 11-65.

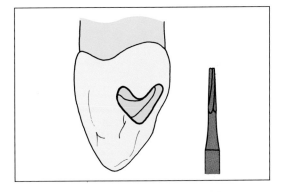

Fig. 11-48 Lingual outline: no. 170 bur.

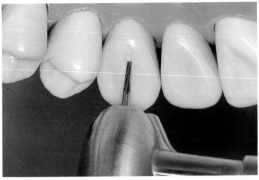

Fig. 11-49 Start the preparation by cutting through the enamel at the incisal end of the cingulum. A lingual dovetail or lock is used to produce resistance to displacement.[20,36,47] It should be 1.0 mm deep.

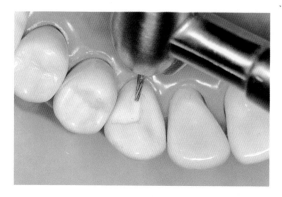

Fig. 11-50 Continue the cut along the midline of the cingulum to within approximately 1.0 mm of the gingiva. A second cut should extend from the incisal end of the roughly formed dovetail to the distal aspect of the lingual surface close to the lesion being restored on the distal surface.

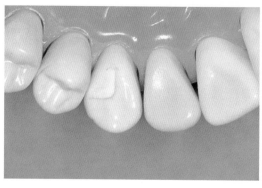

Fig. 11-51 The completed lingual outline consists of an L or reverse L, depending upon whether the preparation is being done on a maxillary right or left canine. It is about 1.0 mm wide.

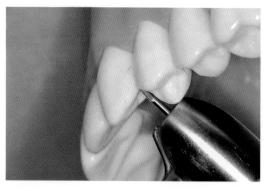

Fig. 11-52 Proximal box: nos. 169L and 170 burs.

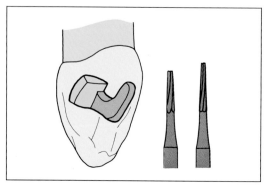

Fig. 11-53 The proximal box is started from the lingual with a no. 170 bur. The lingual approach to a Class III inlay has the best chance of concealing the metal and providing the most esthetic restoration.[65] An incisal approach would lead to unnecessary destruction of tooth structure and create a very unesthetic display of metal as well.

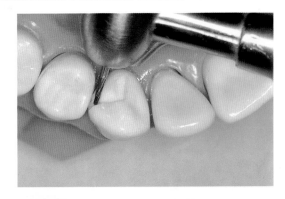

Fig. 11-54 Use the no. 169L bur to accentuate the box corners at the incisal and gingival limits of the preparation. Break contact with the adjacent tooth with the box, being careful not to extend it any farther incisally than is absolutely necessary. If the distal incisal angle is undermined excessively, it may fracture later.

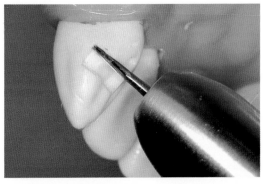

Fig. 11-55 A proximal view of the box form with the adjacent tooth removed shows the incisal and gingival walls of the box formed by the sides of the no. 169L bur. The facial "floor" of the box, which is similar to the gingival floor of the Class I box, extends just slightly to the facial of the proximal contact.

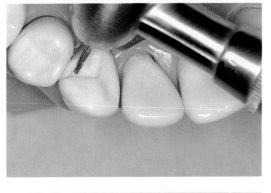

Fig. 11-56 Smooth the axial wall of the box with the no. 169L bur. A no. 170 or 957 bur can be used to smooth the facial wall ("floor") of the box.

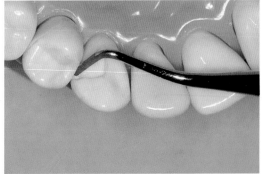

Fig. 11-57 Complete the instrumentation of the box with a 1.0-mm-wide enamel hatchet. The walls of the box, not the angles, are responsible for resistance to displacement.[38]

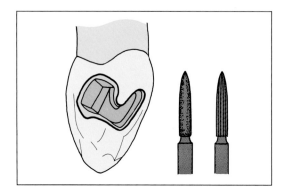

Fig. 11-58 Proximal flares and bevels: flame diamond and bur.

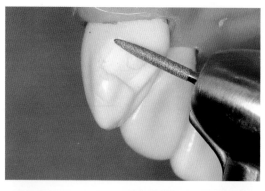

Fig. 11-59 Place a flare on the gingival wall of the proximal box with the flame diamond.

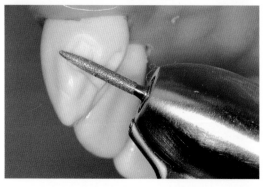

Fig. 11-60 Repeat the process on the incisal wall of the box using the thin tip of the same flame diamond.

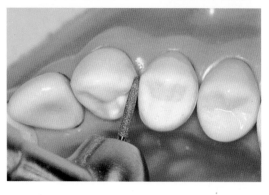

Fig. 11-61 Complete the beveling of the proximal box by placing a facial bevel on the facial "floor" of the box.

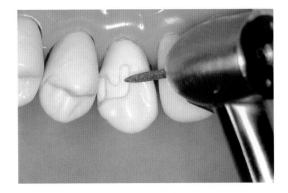

Fig. 11-62 With a flame diamond, place a narrow bevel around the periphery of the lingual dovetail.

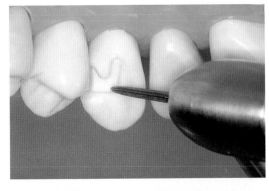

Fig. 11-63 The entire finish line, both proximal and lingual, should be refinished with the flame carbide finishing bur to produce a sharp, smooth finish line.

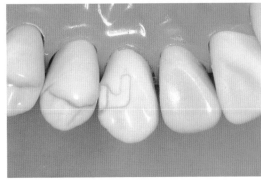

Fig. 11-64 A lingual view of the completed Class III inlay preparation shares many common features with the Class II inlay preparation.

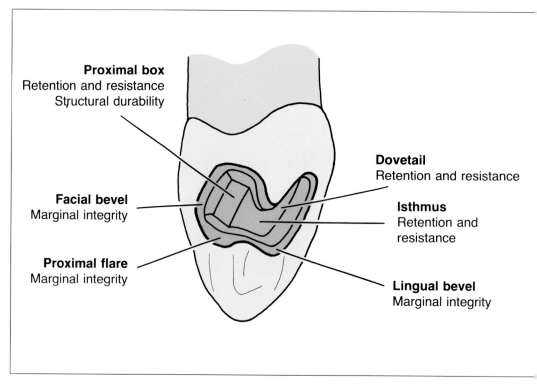

Proximal box
Retention and resistance
Structural durability

Dovetail
Retention and resistance

Facial bevel
Marginal integrity

Isthmus
Retention and
resistance

Proximal flare
Marginal integrity

Lingual bevel
Marginal integrity

Fig. 11-65   The features of a Class III inlay preparation and the function served by each.

Class V inlays

This type of inlay is used less frequently than other types of inlays. It is indicated for severe abrasion[66] or erosion, and large caries. Although it is a long lasting restoration, it is anything but esthetic. It is probably best used on molars.[67] The technique for its preparation is presented in Figs. 11-66 through 11-79.

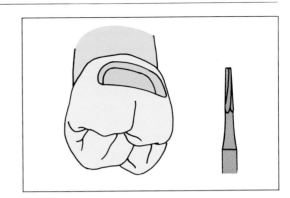

Fig. 11-66 Outline: no. 170 bur.

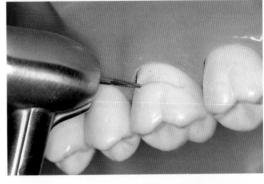

Fig. 11-67 Initial penetration is made in the facial surface with a no. 170 bur, using the edge of the tip of the instrument.

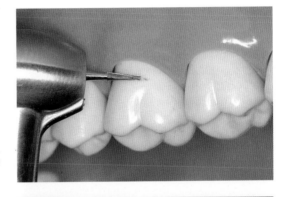

Fig. 11-68 The preparation should be 1.0 mm deep axially. If there is an extensive lesion in the axial wall, create a ledge around the periphery of the preparation extensions.

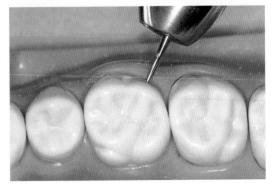

Fig. 11-69 Extend the preparation to the line angle of the tooth. Keep the gingival finish line supragingival, if the damage to tooth structure will permit it.

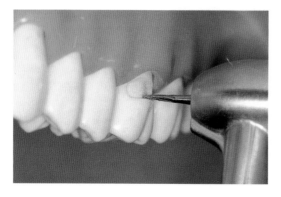

Fig. 11-70 The occlusal finish line should extend no farther occlusally than the height of contour. Curve the axial wall *slightly* to follow the contour of the outer surface of the tooth.

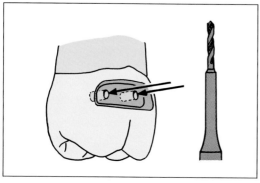

Fig. 11-71 Pinholes: 0.6-mm drill.

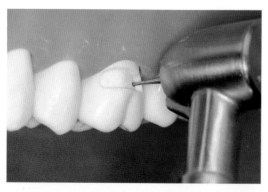

Fig. 11-72 Pinholes are usually placed in this preparation at the mesial and distal edges of the outline form to insure adequate retention and resistance.[67] They should be placed far enough laterally to avoid the pulp chamber, yet far enough in from the edges of the box to avoid interference with the bur and any risk of lateral perforation in any interproximal concavity. Begin the pinholes with a no. 1/2 round bur.

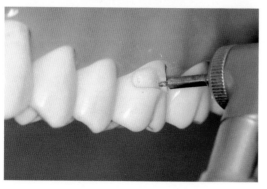

Fig. 11-73 Drill the first pinhole with a 0.6-mm drill held perpendicular to the facial plane of the tooth. Recommended pinhole depths run from 1.5 mm[68] to 3.0 mm[69] for this type of inlay. Experience with cemented pins in other types of restorations would indicate that the longer the pin, the more effective it will be.

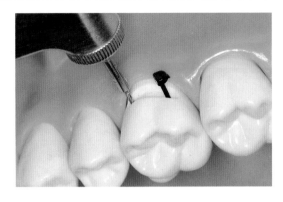

Fig. 11-74 Place the second pinhole on the opposite side of the preparation. A nylon bristle in the first pinhole will assist the parallel alignment of the drill with it.

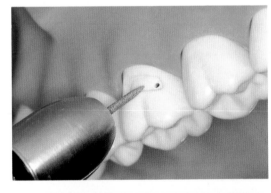

Fig. 11-75 Bevel: flame diamond and bur.

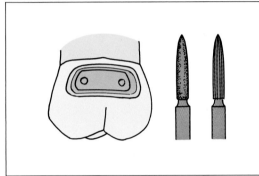

Fig. 11-76 Place a 45-degree bevel around the periphery of the entire outline form of the preparation with a flame diamond. This bevel should be approximately 0.5 mm in width.

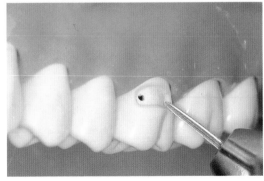

Fig. 11-77 With the flame carbide finishing bur in the handpiece, retrace the entire bevel to make it smooth and to create a definite finish line.

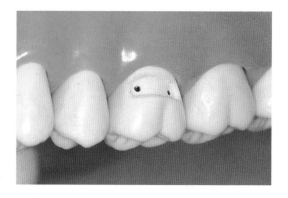

Fig. 11-78 A facial view of the completed Class V inlay preparation.

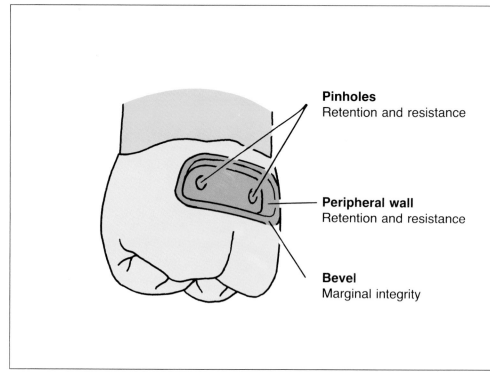

Pinholes
Retention and resistance

Peripheral wall
Retention and resistance

Bevel
Marginal integrity

Fig. 11-79 The features of a Class V inlay preparation and the function served by each.

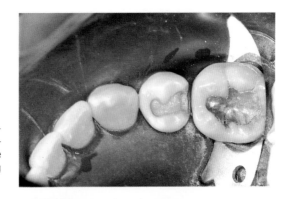

Fig. 11-80 This Class II preparation in a mandibular second premolar exhibits maximum allowable faciolingual isthmus width to prevent the production of dangerous stress in the remaining tooth structure.

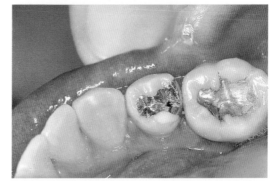

Fig. 11-81 The completed disto-occlusal inlay is shown on the mandibular premolar.

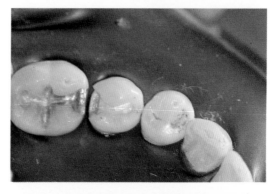

Fig. 11-82 This preparation on a mandibular premolar has an optimum-width isthmus.

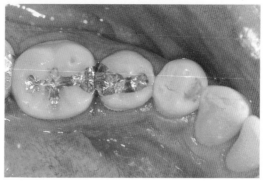

Fig. 11-83 A classic Class II inlay on a mandibular second premolar.

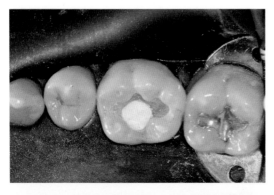

Fig. 11-84 This Class I preparation in a mandibular first molar has a cement base in the vicinity of the central fossa.

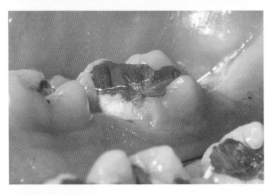

Fig. 11-85 The completed occlusal inlay is as large as it could safely be in a tooth this size without compromising the remaining tooth structure.

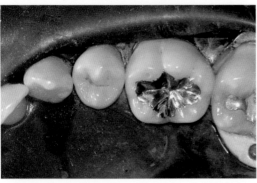

Fig. 11-86 A Class I inlay was used in this situation, which required a restoration with occlusal coverage and greater protection for remaining tooth structure. Undermined tooth structure subsequently fractured, causing the restoration to fail.

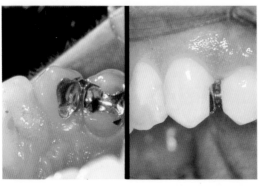

Fig. 11-87 Lingual *(left)* and facial *(right)* views of a Class III inlay show the size of the restoration and its extension on the facial surface. The restoration has been in the mouth for 11 years.

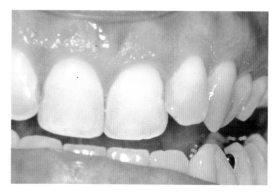

Fig. 11-88 A "conversational" view of the inlay shown in Fig. 11-87 does not reveal any of the "visible" gold.

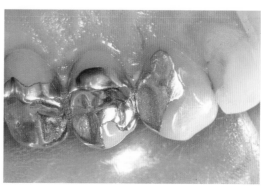

Fig. 11-89 This photograph of a Class III inlay on the distal surface of a maxillary canine was taken 22 years after the restoration was placed. It is highly unlikely that any other restoration, except for a more destructive porcelain-fused-to-metal crown, would be in this serviceable a condition nearly a quarter of a century after being placed.

References

1. McGehee, W. H. O., True, H. A., and Inskipp, E. F. A Textbook of Operative Dentistry. 4th ed. New York: McGraw-Hill Book Co., 1956, 410–443.
2. Vorhees, F. H. History and progress of the cast gold inlay. J. Am. Dent. Assoc 20:2111, 1930.
3. Hinman, T. D. Gold inlays and hoods. Pac. Dent. Gaz. 16:84, 1908.
4. Tucker, R. V. Variation of inlay cavity design. J. Am. Dent. Assoc. 84:616, 1972.
5. Taggart, W. H. A new and accurate method of making gold inlays. Dent. Cosmos 49:1117, 1907.
6. Hollenback, G. M. Science and Technique of the Cast Restoration. St. Louis: The C. V. Mosby Co., 1964, 22–29.
7. Bodecker, H. W. C. The Metallic Inlay. New York: William R. Jenkins Co., 1907, 12.
8. Sigurjons, H. "Extension for prevention": Historical development and current status of G. V. Black's concept. Oper. Dent 8: 57, 1983.
9. Brown, R. K. The present status of the cast gold inlay. J. Am. Dent. Assoc. 20:1841, 1933.
10. Gillett, H. W., and Irving, A. J. Gold inlays by the indirect system: Porcelain and gold inlay cavity preparation compared. Dent. Items Interest 50: 83, 1928.
11. Travis, J. J. The necessity for revising cavity preparation for the cast gold inlay. Dent. Cosmos 67:1141, 1925.
12. Knapp, K. W. Modern conception of proper bridge attachments for vital teeth. J. Am. Dent. Assoc. 14:1027, 1927.
13. Schwartz, J. R. The basic or structural character of abutment preparations. Dent. Items Interest 56:897, 1934.
14. Irving, A. J. A system of cavity preparation which meets the requirements of modern inlay practice. J. Am. Dent. Assoc. 17:1626, 1930.
15. Brown, R. K. Operative procedures incident to the construction of the cast gold inlay. J. Am. Dent. Assoc. 23:99, 1936.
16. Gillett, H. W., and Irving A. J. Gold inlays by the indirect system: Methods to overcome stretching and dislodging thin inlays. Dent. Items Interest 51:493, 1929.
17. Blackwell, R. E. Cavity preparation for inlays to be used as bridge abutments. J. Am. Dent. Assoc. 17:1446, 1930.
18. Doxtater, L. W. Principles underlying the use of the gold inlay as an attachment for bridgework. Dent. Items Interest 51:372, 1929.
19. Gillett, H. W., and Irving, A. J. Gold inlays by the indirect system: Gold inlays as bridge attachments. Dent. Items Interest 51:847, 1929.
20. Thom, L. W. Principles of cavity preparation in crown and bridge prosthesis. III. The inlay abutment. J. Am. Dent. Assoc. 41:541, 1950.
21. Nelson, E. A., and Hinds, F. W. Abutments as applied to fixed as well as removable partial denture prostheses. J. Am. Dent. Assoc. 29:534, 1942.
22. Klaffenbach, A. O. Retention factors in fixed bridge prosthesis. Iowa Dent. Bull. 34:224, 1948.
23. Smith, D. E. Twenty-five years of fixed bridgework J. South. Calif. Dent. Assoc. 7:794, 1936.
24. Bronner, F. J. Is there a common basis for all systems of inlay preparations? Dent. Cosmos 74:1085, 1932.
25. Ingraham, R. The application of sound biomechanical principles in the design of inlay amalgam and gold foil restorations. J. Am. Dent. Assoc. 40:402, 1950.
26. Craig, R. G., El-Ebrashi, M. K., LePeak, P. J., and Peyton, F. A. Experimental stress analysis of dental restorations. I. Two-dimensional photoelastic stress analysis of inlays. J. Prosthet. Dent. 17:277, 1967.
27. Nuckles, D. B., Hembree, J. H., and Beard, J. R. The use of cast alloy restorations by South Carolina dentists. S.C. Dent. J. 38:31, 1980.
28. Clark, N. P., and Smith, G. E. Teaching gold castings in North American dental schools. Oper. Dent. 9:26, 1984.
29. Nuckles, D. B. Inlay vs. amalgam restorations. S.C. Dent. 38:23, 1980.
30. Granath, L. E. Photoelastic studies on certain factors influencing the relation between cavity and restoration. Odont. Rev. 14:278, 1963.
31. Farah, J. W., Dennison, J. B., and Powers, J. M. Effects of design on stress distribution of intracoronal gold restorations. J. Am. Dent. Assoc. 94:1151, 1977.
32. Klaffenbach, A. O. An analytic study of modern abutments. J. Am. Dent. Assoc. 23:2275, 1936.

33. Mahler, D. B., and Terkla, L. G. Relationship of cavity design to restorative materials. Dent. Clin. North Am. 9:149, 1965.

34. Gietzen, C. H. Cavity preparation in relation to inlay fixed bridge construction. J. Am. Dent. Assoc. 18:1117, 1931.

35. Blaser, P. K., Lund, M. R., Cochran, M. A., and Potter, R. H. Effects of designs of Class II preparations on resistance of teeth to fracture. Oper. Dent. 8:6, 1983.

36. Ward, M. L. The American Textbook of Operative Dentistry. 6th ed. New York: Lea & Febiger, 1926, 381–395.

37. Gilmore, H. W. Operative Dentistry. 3rd ed. St. Louis: The C. V. Mosby Co., 1977, 257–263.

38. Smith, G. E., and Grainger, D. A. Biomechanical design of extensive cavity preparations for cast gold. J. Am. Dent. Assoc. 89:1152, 1974.

39. Vale, W. A. Cavity preparation. Ir. Dent. Rev. 2:33, 1956.

40. Mondelli, J., Steagall, L., Ishikiriama, A., Navarro, M. F., and Soares, F. B. Fracture strength of human teeth with cavity preparations. J. Prosthet. Dent. 43:419, 1980.

41. Werrin, S. R., Jubach, T. S., and Johnson, B. W. Inlays and onlays: Making the right decision. Quint. Int. 11:13, 1980.

42. Re, G. J., Norling, B. K., and Draheim, R. N. Fracture resistance of lower molars with varying facio-occlusolingual amalgam restorations. J. Prosthet. Dent. 47:518, 1982.

43. Conzett, J. V. The gold inlay. Dent. Cosmos 52:1339, 1910.

44. Gabel, A. B. Mechanical principles of operative dentistry. J. Am. Dent. Assoc. 43:153, 1951.

45. Gowan, W. C. Cavity preparation for gold inlays. Dominion Dent. J. 24:481, 1912.

46. Brown, R. K. A system of cavity preparation and wax manipulation for the cast gold inlay. J. Am. Dent. Assoc. 25:1974, 1938.

47. Harris, R. The influence of mechanical factors in the design of inlay cavity preparations. Aust. Dent. J. 11:410, 1939.

48. Ferrier, W. I. Cavity preparation for gold foil, gold inlay, and amalgam operations. J. Natl. Dent. Assoc. 4:441, 1917.

49. Sundbe, E. J. Gold inlays. J. Am. Dent. Assoc. 17:2113, 1930.

50. Grundy, J. R. Color Atlas of Conservative Dentistry. Chicago: Year Book Medical Publ., Inc., 1980, 68–75.

51. Gable, A. B. Mechanical principles of operative dentistry. J. Am. Dent. Assoc. 43:153, 1951.

52. Tinker, E. T. Gold inlays. J. Am. Dent. Assoc. 13:317, 1926.

53. McCollum, B. B. Tooth preparation in its relation to oral physiology. J. Am. Dent. Assoc. 27:701, 1940.

54. Frates, F. E. Inlays. Dent. Clin. North Am. 11:163, 1967.

55. McMath, J. F. The gingival groove in gold inlay construction. Dent. Cosmos 67:1162, 1925.

56. Silberhorn, O. W. Fixed bridge retainers—Design and retention features. Ill. Dent. J. 22:641, 1953.

57. Knox, E. L. Slice extension lap preparations and restorations. J. Am. Dent. Assoc. 19:1727, 1932.

58. Metzler, J. C., and Chandler, H. H. An evaluation of techniques for finishing margins of gold inlays. J. Prosthet. Dent. 36:523, 1976.

59. Rosenstiel, E. The marginal fit of inlays and crowns. Br. Dent. J. 117:432, 1964.

60. Rosenstiel, E. To bevel or not to bevel. Br. Dent. J. 138:389, 1975.

61. Ingraham, R., Bassett, R. W., and Koser, J. R. An Atlas of Cast Gold Procedures. 2nd ed. Buena Park, CA: Unitro College Press, 1969, 12.

62. Barnes, I. E. The production of inlay cavity bevels. Br. Dent. J. 137:379, 1974.

63. Christensen, G. J. Clinical and research advancements in cast-gold restorations. J. Prosthet. Dent. 25:62, 1971.

64. Redfern, M. L. The dovetail Class III inlay. Oper. Dent. 8:67, 1983.

65. Gerson, I. V. Invisible gold restorations for anterior teeth. J. Prosthet. Dent. 11:749, 1961.

66. Mack, A. O., and Allan, D. N. Reconstruction of a severe case of attrition and abrasion. Br. Dent. J. 137:379, 1974.

67. Finger, E. M. Restorations for Class V cavities. J. Prosthet. Dent. 10:775, 1960.

68. Lamb, R. T. Varied applications of direct pin inlays. J. Can. Dent. Assoc. 22:282, 1956.

69. Mittleman, G. Use of pins in difficult cases. J. Am. Dent. Assoc. 49:163, 1954.

Chapter 12

MOD Onlays

Although the MOD onlay is a variation of the Class II inlay, there are enough distinct differences between the two restorations that the onlay merits consideration as a separate type of cast restoration. Notwithstanding that the MOD onlay utilizes intracoronal retention almost exclusively, the incorporation of occlusal coverage into this design makes it a partial veneer extracoronal restoration as well.

The retention employed by intracoronal restorations is of the "wedge" variety, which tends to exert pressure outward from the center of the tooth.[1] This force is greatest during try-in and cementation, but it recurs whenever occlusal force is exerted on the tooth. For the restoration to be successful, it must be bolstered by a bulk of sound dentin, or some means must be employed to distribute the force in such a way as to render it nondestructive to the remaining tooth structure.

There is a recent renewed interest in the MOD onlay, based on an occlusion-centered approach to restorative dentistry, rather than one which is solely tooth-oriented. The wedgelike inlay increases the risk of fracture without protecting undermined cusps.[2] The inlay simply replaces missing tooth structure, but it does nothing to reinforce that which remains.[3] If the tooth requires protection from occlusal forces, that protection can be gained by the use of a veneer of casting alloy over the occlusal surface.[4] The use of the more protective restoration is reflected in a recent survey taken in the southeastern United States, in which respondents reported using the MOD onlay about twice as often as the Class II inlay.[5]

Figures 12-1 through 12-61 examine the rationale for the use of MOD onlays and show the technique for preparing a maxillary premolar for this type of restoration.

Photoelastic stress analysis

Craig et al. also used photoelastic stress analysis to show the superiority of the MOD onlay in protecting teeth from stress.[19] Clinicians and researchers alike have linked marginal failures with weakened cusps and preparation walls bending away from the restoration under the kinds of stress demonstrated here.[7,8,20,21] Isthmus width[11,21-23] and depth[10,22] also have been recognized as factors contributing to failure. While some authors have suggested that a preparation whose isthmus width was greater than one-half the intercuspal distance should be restored with an overlay,[6,24] a more conservative one-fourth[25] to one-third[26,27] is probably safer.

237

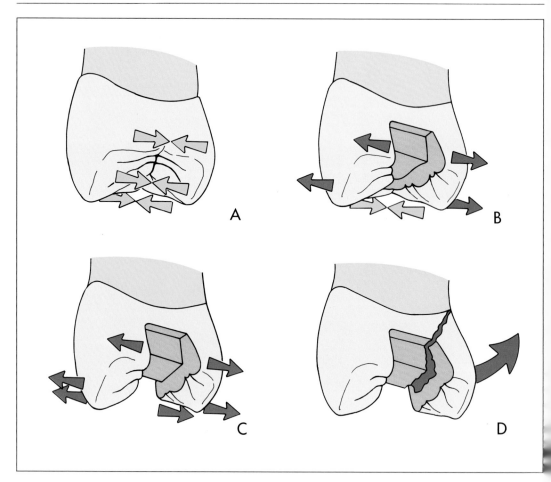

Fig. 12-1 As long as the crown of a tooth is intact, it has structural integrity *(A)*. When an intracoronal preparation is done, the tooth is weakened and made more susceptible to fracture *(B)*. According to Mondelli et al. a premolar has 11% to 52% less fracture resistance (depending on faciolingual width) when a Class I isthmus is cut into the occlusal surface, and 17% to 57% less strength if it has a proximo-occlusal preparation.[6] If both proximal surfaces are weakened by a preparation, the facial and lingual cusps are no longer bound together by tooth structure *(C)*. The tooth is in danger of fracturing if the isthmus has any significant width *(D)*. A premolar has only 36% to 61% of its intact strength (again depending upon faciolingual width of the isthmus) when it has been bisected by an MOD preparation.[6]

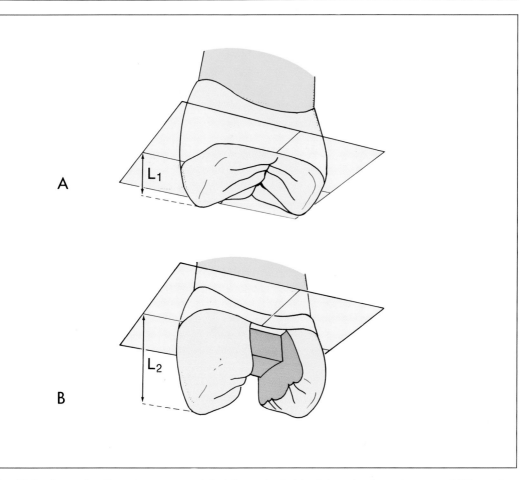

Fig. 12-2 Several authors have appreciated the potential for inlays to elongate cusps. [6-8] Normally cusps have a mechanical cusp height that is equal to the anatomical cusp height, measured from the cusp tip to the level of the central groove (A, L_1). When an MOD preparation is done, the mechanical cusp length is greatly exaggerated, with its effective length becoming the distance from the cusp tip to the gingival extension of the preparation (B, L_2). In a small tooth such as a premolar, this elongation of the lever arm can have disastrous results.

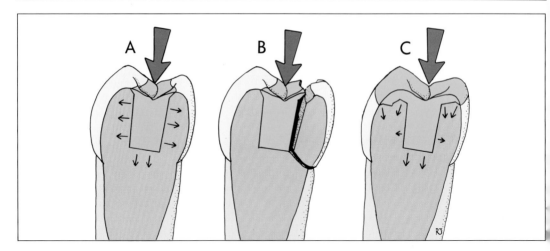

Fig. 12-3 There was also early recognition by clinicians that the inlay had a tendency to wedge the cusps apart,[9,10] particularly when there was a wide isthmus. [11] Occlusal force applied to an inlay produces stress along the sides of the restoration and at its base, as the restoration pushes against the tooth structure surrounding it *(A)*. The situation in *A* could lead to fracture of the tooth, [12] with cracks caused by MOD restorations typically occurring at a 40- to 50-degree angle from the corner of the cavity preparation apically *(B)*. [13] An onlay will distribute the force over a wide area, thus drastically reducing the potential for breakage *(C)*. For this reason the MOD onlay is well suited for restoring endodontically treated teeth with sound facial and lingual surfaces. [14–17]

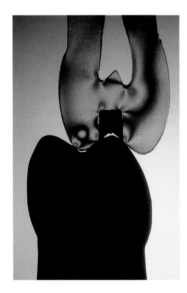

Fig. 12-4a The wedging stresses produced by inlays were shown by photoelastic stress analysis by Fisher et al.[18] The inlay produced very high stress concentrations at the walls of the isthmus and at the line angles. (Courtesy of Dr. D. W. Fisher, Los Angeles.)

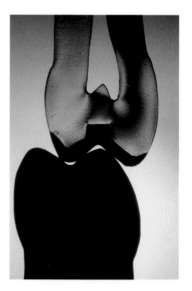

Fig. 12-4b The onlay, on the other hand demonstrated very little stress. (Courtesy of Dr D. W. Fisher, Los Angeles.)

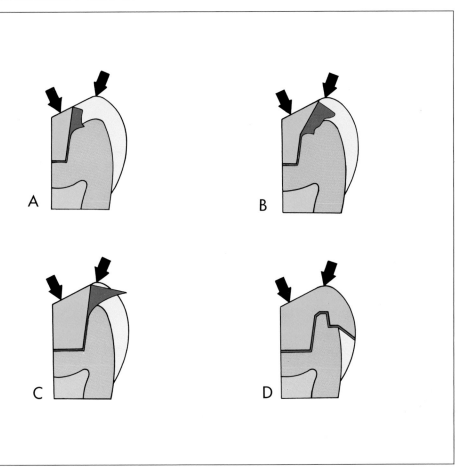

Fig. 12-5 In a stress analysis study utilizing the finite element technique with computer-generated models, Farah et al. clearly demonstrated the stress-producing potential of the ordinary inlay *(A)* and some common variations in the standard design.[28] Stress is designated in these illustrations by red. An overextended bevel increases the stress to a dangerous level *(B)*. An inlay that is too wide could result in the catastrophic failure of tooth structure because of the extent of the stress generated *(C)*. The use of an onlay, on the other hand, keeps stress at a low level, which creates no hazard for the remaining tooth structure *(D)*. (Adapted from Farah et al.[28])

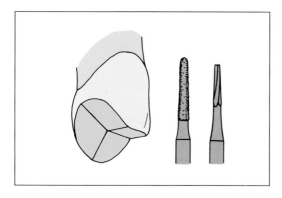

Fig. 12-6 Planar occlusal reduction: round-end tapered diamond and no. 171 bur.

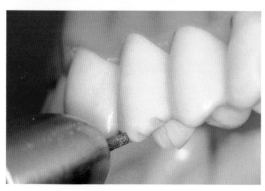

Fig. 12-7 The occlusal reduction is started by placing depth-orientation grooves on the occlusal surface with the round-end tapered diamond. There should be one along the crest of each triangular ridge and one in each major developmental groove.

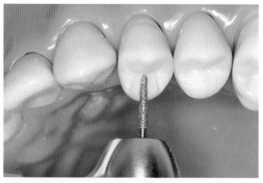

Fig. 12-8 The occlusal reduction and, therefore, the depth-orientation grooves, should be 1.5 mm deep on the functional cusp and 1.0 mm deep over most of the nonfunctional cusp. On a maxillary tooth where the nonfunctional facial cusp will be highly visible, care should be taken not to overcut the facio-occlusal extension, which would produce an unnecessary display of metal. The depth of the orientation grooves and the occlusal reduction itself, should be approximately 0.5 mm in depth at the facio-occlusal line angle.

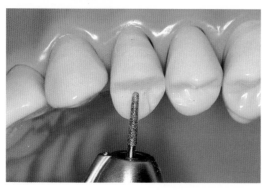

Fig. 12-9 Occlusal reduction is accomplished by removing the tooth structure remaining between the depth-orientation grooves with the round-end tapered diamond. The reduction should follow the original contours of the cusp,[1] reproducing the basic geometric inclined planes of the occlusal surface in the process.[1] In addition to creating space for a uniform bulk of metal, it has been hypothesized that this corrugated multiplanar design will add even more strength to the restoration.[29]

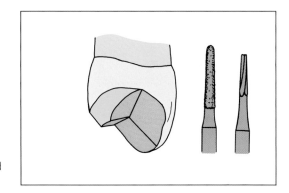

Fig. 12-10 Functional cusp bevel: round-end tapered diamond and no. 171 bur.

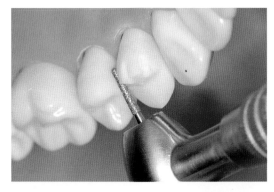

Fig. 12-11 Make depth-orientation cuts on the outward facing inclines of the functional cusp. These grooves should be 1.5 mm deep at the cusp tip and fade out along the line that will later mark the location of the occlusal shoulder.

Fig. 12-12 Complete the reduction for the functional cusp bevel by removing the tooth structure remaining between the orientation grooves. The functional cusp bevel will approximate the angle of the cuspal inclines in the opposing arch. This bevel will extend around to the central groove on the mesial and distal surfaces of the tooth. However, because the proximal boxes have not yet been prepared, it may be difficult to extend the functional cusp bevel as far as it should be extended at this time. If it creates a difficult situation, the final extension of the bevel can be delayed until the boxes have been instrumented.

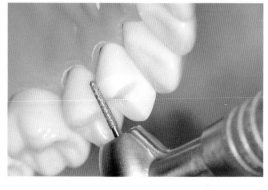

Fig. 12-13 Smooth the planes of the occlusal reduction and the funtional cusp bevel with the no. 171 tapered fissure carbide bur. Although the inclined planes are well defined, there should be no sharp line or point angles where these planes meet. A smooth surface on the occlusal reduction will remove the kinds of defects that might later interfere with the complete seating of the cast restoration.

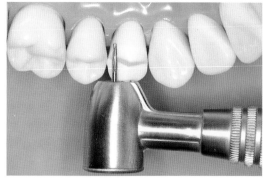

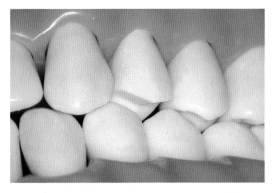

Fig. 12-14 Check the occlusal reduction Visual inspection is an important and frequently overlooked means of assessing the adequacy of the occlusal reduction. It is limited to those segments of the reduction in the facial half of the occlusal surface. The reduction on the lingual cusp can be verified with red utility wax, or with a thickness gauge.*

*Flexible Clearance Guide, Belle de St. Claire, Van Nuys, Calif.

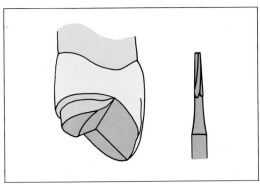

Fig. 12-15 Occlusal shoulder: no. 171 bur.

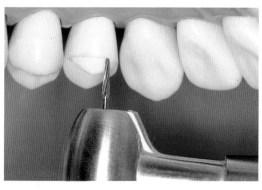

Fig. 12-16 Cut the occlusal shoulder with a no. 171 bur, following the termination line of the functional cusp bevel on the axial surface of the functional cusp. The shoulder is 1.0 mm wide and it extends from the central groove on one proximal surface to the central groove on the other proximal surface. This feature provides space for a bulk of metal to reinforce the occlusal margin on the funtional cusp.

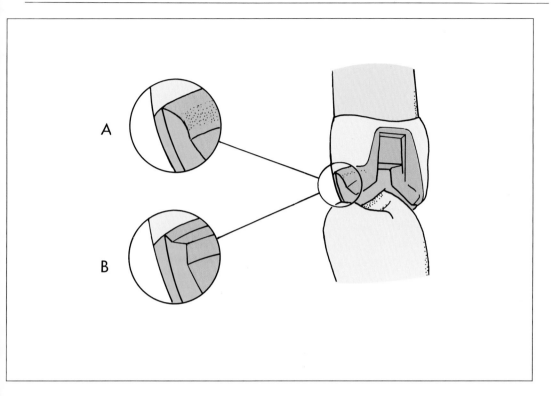

Fig. 12-17 Either a chamfer *(A)* or an occlusal shoulder *(B)* can be used for the occlusal finish line on the functional cusp bevel, since they both meet the requirement of accommodating an acute edge in the restoration margin, with a nearby bulk of metal for reinforcement. However, the shoulder with a bevel is easier to prepare properly and should be used by the novice operator.

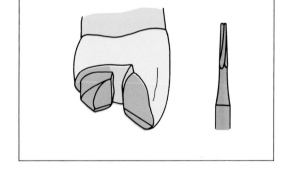

Fig. 12-18 Isthmus: no. 170 bur.

Fig. 12-19 Make the isthmus at this time, if it was not created earlier when existing restorations were removed. Because the occlusal surface has been reduced already, the isthmus on an onlay is 1.0 mm shallower than the isthmus on an inlay. The opposing facial and lingual walls of this feature should be smooth, with a minimum taper. This feature can provide about one-fifth of the retention of an MOD onlay, and a great deal more of the resistance.[30]

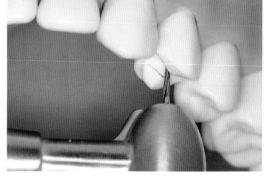

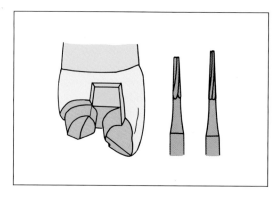

Fig. 12-20 Proximal box: nos. 169L and 170 burs.

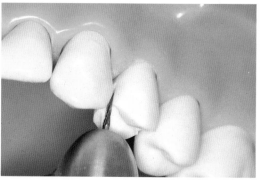

Fig. 12-21 Begin the proximal box with a no. 170 bur. If the surface is relatively intact, it may be easier to start the box with the no. 169L bur, which is smaller in diameter and easier to keep away from the proximal surface of the adjacent tooth. The box should barely break contact with the adjacent tooth on the mesial surface. The gingival floor should be approximately 1.0 mm wide. Use the no. 169L bur to accentuate the facioaxial and linguoaxial line angles.

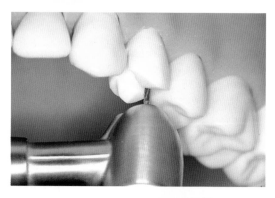

Fig. 12-22 After completing the mesial box, repeat the process with the distal box. It is not necessary to be quite as conservative with the facial extensions of the distal box.

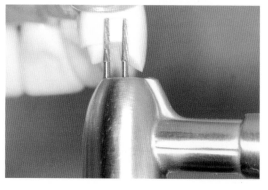

Fig. 12-23 The no. 169L bur is used for forming the facial and lingual walls and the line angles of the proximal boxes. If this bur is used to accentuate the angles of the box, the preparation will need very little hand instrumentation.

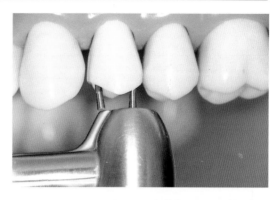

Fig. 12-24 The bur is leaned slightly to the center of the tooth and to the facial or lingual side in forming the facial and lingual walls of the boxes respectively. This will insure facial and lingual walls that will diverge occlusally, and axial walls that will converge occlusally.

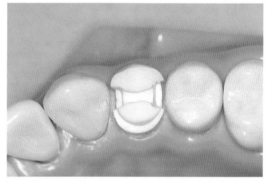

Fig. 12-25 This occlusal view of the completed boxes shows that they are the width of the proximal contact areas with the adjacent teeth. At this point in the preparation of the tooth, no part of the proximal flares has been started. The flares are added *after* the boxes have been finished.

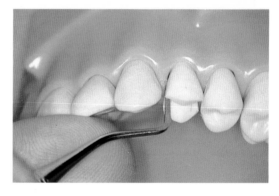

Fig. 12-26 A 1.0-mm-wide enamel chisel, such as a binangle chisel or the hatchet shown here, can be used to plane the facial and lingual walls of the preparation. It is these flat walls perpendicular to the direction of oblique or rotating forces that will provide resistance to the restoration, and not the angle between the axial and the facial or lingual surfaces.

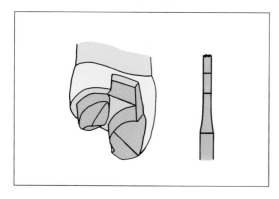

Fig. 12-27 Planing horizontal surfaces: no. 957 bur.

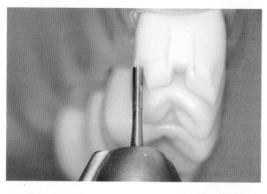

Fig. 12-28 The no. 957 end-cutting bur is used to smooth the pulpal floor of the isthmus that joins the proximal boxes.

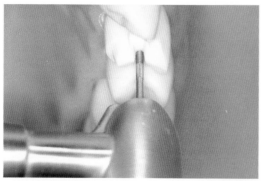

Fig. 12-29 The same instrument is needed to smooth the occlusal shoulder on the functional cusp bevel. This feature should be 1.0 mm wide.

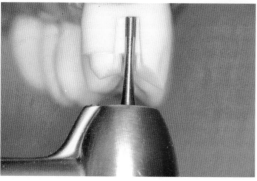

Fig. 12-30 The last of the horizontal surfaces to be planed smooth are the gingival floors of the proximal boxes. This aspect of the proximal box will help to improve the resistance of the finished onlay to displacement when compressive occlusal forces occur on the restoration.

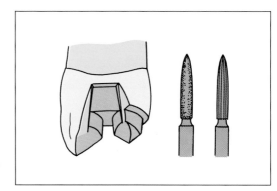

Fig. 12-31 Proximal flares: flame diamond and flame bur.

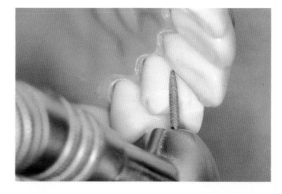

Fig. 12-32 Place the flares on the proximal box from within, starting with the tip of the flame diamond, which is small enough to allow the instrument to be inserted into the restricted embrasure space next to the tooth without scarring the adjacent tooth.

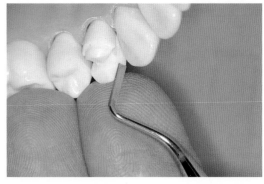

Fig. 12-33 A wide enamel hatchet (1.5 to 2.0 mm) can be used to shape the mesiofacial flare where esthetic considerations are important. The instrument must be sharp in order to achieve the planing action needed to produce a smooth, unmarred flare and finish line.

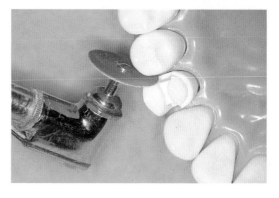

Fig. 12-34 A sandpaper disk can also be used for forming the flares. Be careful not to cut the soft tissues surrounding the tooth. It is best to reserve this technique for use with a rubber dam, which will retract the cheeks and lips, and keep the tongue out of harm's way.

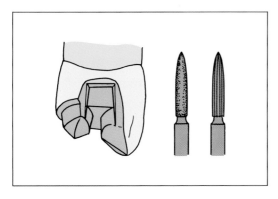

Fig. 12-35   Gingival bevel: flame diamond and flame bur.

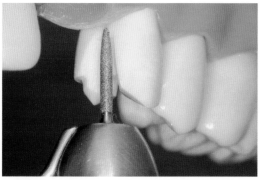

Fig. 12-36   Use a flame diamond to produce a narrow bevel (0.5 to 0.7mm wide) along the entire gingival floor of the box. The bevel should blend into the flares on the facial and lingual walls of the box, without forming an undercut.

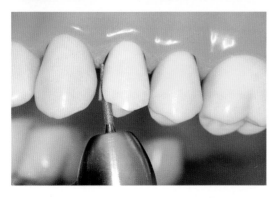

Fig. 12-37   It is very likely that it will be necessary to lean the flame diamond over into the proximal box to produce a bevel that is not excessively long or obtuse. This will probably round over the proximo-occlusal line angle which is acceptable.

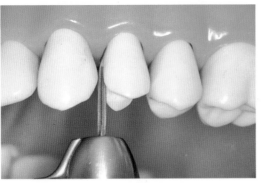

Fig. 12-38   Reinstrument the flares and the gingival bevel with a flame-shaped carbide finishing bur.* This will smooth the flares and bevels and produce a sharp, distinct finish line. The definite line will facilitate the fabrication of a well-fitting restoration.

*No. H48L-010, Brasseler USA Inc., Savannah, Ga.

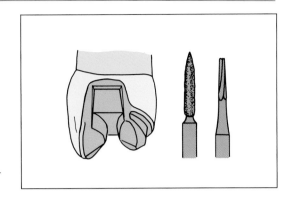

Fig. 12-39 Facial and lingual bevels: flame diamond and no. 170 bur.

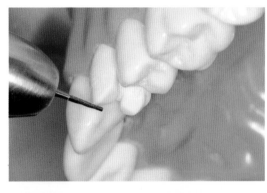

Fig. 12-40 The occlusal finishing bevel is placed on the facial cusp with a no. 170 carbide bur held perpendicular to the long axis of the tooth. The bevel is approximately 0.5 mm in width. If the bur is leaned over to the faciogingival, the bevel will be wider and more obtrusive esthetically.

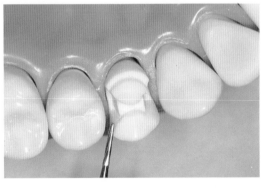

Fig. 12-41 Round the bevel over onto the facial flares. To insure a smooth, unbroken finish line in this transitional area, take care to make the outer edge of the occlusal bevel (the actual finish line) continuous with the outer edge of the facial flare. A sharp angle in the finish line in this area would result in a negative angle in the wax pattern, which could easily produce an unfinishable gap in the casting margin.

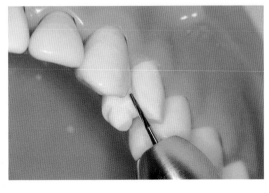

Fig.12-42 You should also round over the line angle between the occlusal reduction and the flare to remove any other sharp projections that might interfere with the complete seating of the final cast restoration.

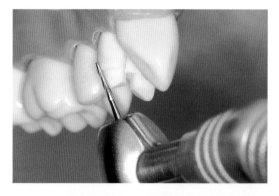

Fig. 12-43 Place a narrow (0.5 mm) bevel on the occlusal shoulder, making sure that it also will blend smoothly with the lingual flares where it joins them. Be careful not to extend this bevel too far gingivally. If it does, the resulting bevel on the wax pattern will be wide and thin, which can result in an incomplete casting.

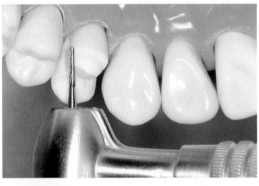

Fig. 12-44 Use the same bur to round over the angle between the funtional cusp bevel and the flares.

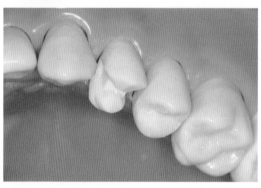

Fig. 12-45 Occlusofacial view of the completed MOD onlay preparation on a maxillary premolar.

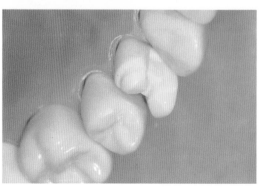

Fig. 12-46 An occlusolingual view of the same preparation.

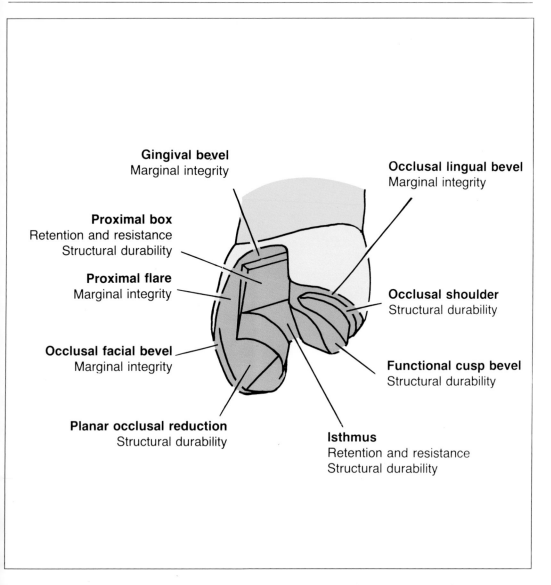

Gingival bevel
Marginal integrity

Occlusal lingual bevel
Marginal integrity

Proximal box
Retention and resistance
Structural durability

Proximal flare
Marginal integrity

Occlusal shoulder
Structural durability

Occlusal facial bevel
Marginal integrity

Functional cusp bevel
Structural durability

Planar occlusal reduction
Structural durability

Isthmus
Retention and resistance
Structural durability

Fig. 12-47   The features of an MOD onlay preparation, and the function served by each.

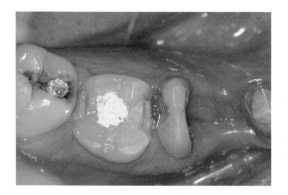

Fig. 12-48 This mandibular second molar has been prepared for an MOD onlay. The distal root of the first molar has been retained after endodontic treatment and surgery to be used as an abutment for a short-span fixed bridge replacing the mesial root of the first molar, which was extracted for periodontal reasons.

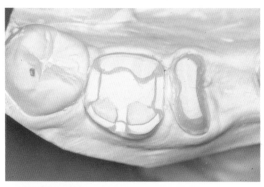

Fig. 12-49 An occlusal view of the stone cast shows more details of the MOD onlay preparation.

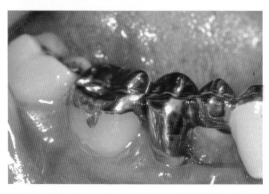

Fig. 12-50 The completed MOD onlay is shown in place on the mandibular second molar. The bridge restoring the first molar has also been inserted.

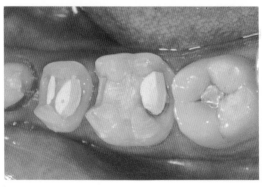

Fig. 12-51 MOD onlay preparations are shown on a mandibular premolar and molar. Extensive destruction of tooth structure has required the placement of large bases in both axial walls of the second premolar preparation and in the distal axial wall of the first molar preparation. These bases were placed for insulating purposes and to aid the operator in visualizing the retention and resistance features needed for the preparations. The bases add *nothing* to the retention and resistance of the preparations themselves.

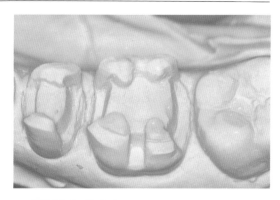

Fig. 12-52 The detail of the preparations is more easily seen on the stone casts. The distal boxes of both preparations, especially that of the premolar, are larger than normal because of caries and previous restorations.

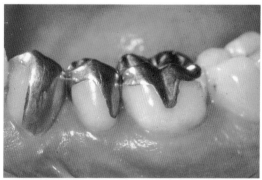

Fig. 12-53 A facial view of the completed restorations shows the distal facial extension of the premolar. The first premolar has been restored with a seven-eighths crown. Notice the gingival extension of the facial occlusal margin of the molar to include a carious facial groove.

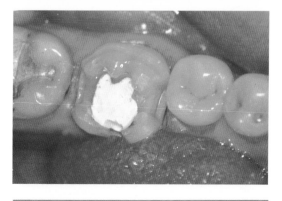

Fig. 12-54 An MOD restoration was selected for this tooth because of the extensive defect in the center of the tooth that had structurally weakened the tooth. There were several small fracture lines in the proximal surfaces.

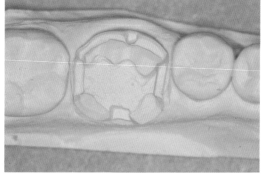

Fig. 12-55 Occlusal view of the stone cast of this prepared tooth showing the extreme width of the isthmus of the preparation.

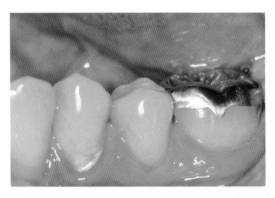

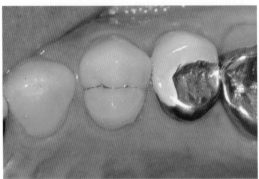

Fig. 12-56 Facial view of the completed restoration.

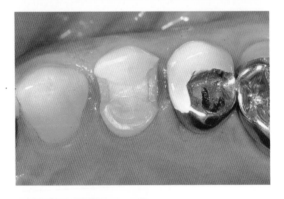

Fig. 12-57 Occlusal view of an unrestored maxillary premolar with minimal distal caries. There was a fracture line on the mesial marginal ridge, however, and the tooth was sensitive to thermal changes and occlusal pressure (but not to percussion).

Fig. 12-58 Occlusal view of a classic MOD onlay preparation. This is not frequently seen because teeth requiring MOD onlays usually have been previously restored and extensively damaged to make this restoration necessary.

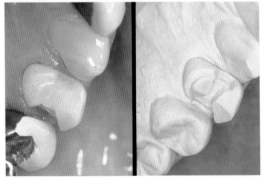

Fig. 12-59 Mesio-occlusal views of the completed preparation on the tooth *(left)* and on the stone cast *(right.)*

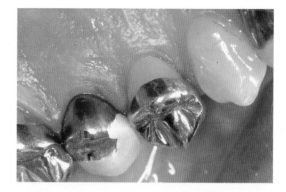

Fig. 12-60 Lingual view of the finished MOD onlay, showing the extent of coverage on the lingual cusp.

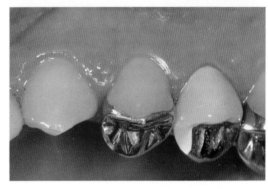

Fig. 12-61 A facial view of the completed restoration.

References

1. Shillingburg, H. T. Conservative preparations for cast restorations. Dent. Clin. North Am. 20:259, 1976.
2. Kayser, A. F., Battistuzzi, P. G., Snoek, P. A., and Spanauf, A. J. The rationale for the indication and design of the MOD inlay. Aust. Dent. J. 27:22, 1982.
3. Shillingburg, H. T., and Fisher, D. W. The MOD onlay—A rational approach to a restorative problem. N.M. Dent. J. 21:12, 1970.
4. Tanner, H. Ideal and modified inlay and veneer crown preparations. Ill. Dent. J. 26:240, 1957.
5. Nuckles, D. B., Hembree, J. H., and Beard, J. R. The use of cast alloy restorations by South Carolina dentists. S.C. Dent. J. 38:31, 1980.
6. Mondelli, J., Steagall, L., Ishikiriama, A., Navarro, M. F., and Soares, F. B. Fracture strength of human teeth with cavity preparations. J. Prosthet. Dent. 43:419, 1980.
7. Smith, D. E. Fixed bridgework in the various phases of dental practice. J. South. Calif. Dent. Assoc. 13:13, 1942.
8. Ingraham, R. The application of sound biomechanical principles in the design of inlay, amalgam and gold foil restorations. J. Am. Dent. Assoc. 40:402, 1950.
9. Smith, D. E. Twenty-five years of fixed bridgework. J. South. Calif. Dent. Assoc. 7:794, 1936.
10. Meyer, F. S. Inlays, crowns and full cast bridges. Am. Dent. Surg. 52:33, 1932.
11. Gietzen, C. H. Cavity preparation in relation to inlay fixed bridge construction. J. Am. Dent. Assoc. 18:1117, 1931.
12. Maxwell, E. H., and Braly, B. V. Incomplete tooth fracture: Prediction and prevention. J. Calif. Dent. Assoc. 5:51, 1977.
13. Bell, J. G., Smith, M. C., and de Pont, J. J. Cuspal failures of MOD restored teeth. Aust. Dent. J. 27:283, 1982.
14. Potter, H. R., and Smith, D. E. Practical bridgework. III. Non-vital teeth in bridgework. Pac. Dent. Gaz. 40:519, 1932.
15. Werrin, S. R., Jubach, T. S., and Johnson, B. W. Inlays and onlays: Making the right decision. Quint. Int. 11:13, 1980.
16. Perel, M. L. Crown and bridge and partial coverage castings. R.I. Dent. J. 14:19, 1981.
17. Draheim, R. N. Current concepts in intracoronal casting preparations: A new look at the gold casting preparation. Comp. Cont. Educ. Dent. 6:373, 1985.
18. Fisher, D. W., Caputo, A. A., Shillingburg, H. T., and Duncanson, M. G. Photoelastic analysis of inlay and onlay preparations. J. Prosthet. Dent. 33:47, 1975.
19. Craig, R. G., El-Ebrashi, M. K., LePeak, P. J. and Peyton, F. A. Experimental stress analysis of dental restorations. I. Two-dimensional photoelastic stress analysis of inlays. J. Prosthet. Dent. 17:277, 1967.
20. Klaffenbach, A. O. An analytic study of modern abutments. J. Am. Dent. Assoc. 23:2275, 1936.
21. Mahler, D. B., and Terkla, L. G. Relationship of cavity design to restorative materials. Dent. Clin. North Am. 9:149, 1965.
22. Blaser, P. K., Lund, M. R., Cochran, M. A., and Potter, R. H. Effects of designs of Class II preparations on resistance of teeth to fracture. Oper. Dent. 8:6, 1983.
23. Larson, T. D., Douglas, W. H., and Gustfeld, R. E. Effect of prepared cavities on the strength of teeth. Oper. Dent. 6:2, 1981.
24. Ward, M. L. The American Textbook of Operative Dentistry. 6th ed. New York: Lea & Febiger, 1926, 381–395.
25. Smith, G. E., and Grainger, D. A. Biomechanical design of extensive cavity preparations for cast gold. J. Am. Dent. Assoc. 89:1152, 1974.
26. Christensen, G. J. Clinical and research advancements in cast-gold restorations. J. Prosthet. Dent. 25:62, 1971.
27. Gilmore, H. W. Operative Dentistry. 3rd ed. St Louis: The C. V. Mosby Co., 1977, 257–263.
28. Farah, J. W., Dennison, J. B., and Powers, J. M. Effects of design on stress distribution of intracoronal gold restorations. J. Am. Dent. Assoc. 94:1151, 1977.
29. Racowsky, L. P., and Wolinsky, L. E. Restoring the badly broken-down tooth with esthetic partial coverage restorations. Comp. Cont. Educ. Dent. 2:322, 1981.
30. Kishimoto, M., Shillingburg, H. T., and Duncanson, M. G. Influence of preparation features on retention and resistance. I. MOD onlays. J. Prosthet. Dent. 49:35, 1983.

Chapter 13

Anterior Porcelain-Fused-to-Metal Crowns

The norm for what constitutes an esthetically acceptable restoration varies from culture to culture, country to country, and time to time. Usually it is influenced by the capabilities of available technology. Today it is possible to fabricate crowns from a material which, under ideal circumstances, can be almost indistinguishable from natural enamel.

The healthy untreated look is the ideal in the *appearance zone.* This zone varies from patient to patient. For most people it includes all the anterior teeth, the maxillary premolars and first molars, and the mandibular first premolars. The dentist should observe the patient speaking and smiling to determine its extent *objectively,* and talk with the patient to establish its extent *subjectively.* If the patient's perception of the appearance zone extends past that which is readily apparent, the dentist must accommodate the patient's self-concept. To do otherwise invites patient dissatisfaction.

When preparing teeth in the appearance zone for crowns, the dentist has two general types from which to choose: partial veneer metal restorations that leave the facial surfaces uncovered, or full crowns with a veneer of tooth-colored material covering the facial surface.

Partial veneer restorations such as onlays, three-quarter crowns, and seven-eighths crowns require less removal of peripheral tooth structure. They should be selected if enough of the facial surface is sound. If facial and incisal extensions are kept to a minimum, gold restorations that are almost invisible can be fabricated. If the mesial surface of an anterior tooth is intact, it need not be covered at all. Carefully placed pinholes and grooves can substitute for that wall.

When a substantial part of the facial surface of a tooth has been destroyed or undermined, an alternative restoration must be selected. The use of acrylic resin veneers was the first way of restoring teeth that allowed the use of full veneer retainers for fixed bridges in situations demanding maximum esthetics. It was seriously limited, however, by the lack of color stability and abrasion resistance.

The porcelain-fused-to-metal restoration is a combination of an esthetic porcelain veneering material and a metal substructure. By fusing porcelain to metal, it became possible to produce a full-coverage restoration with a stable, esthetic veneer and adequate strength to be used for replacing missing teeth.

While a porcelain-fused-to-metal crown can serve as a strong and esthetic restoration, patients too often receive this type of restoration for minor irregularities that could have been better handled by conservative treatment or none at all.

The use of porcelain-fused-to-metal restorations has grown from the development of the first commercially successful porcelain/gold alloy restoration by Weinstein et al. in the 1950s.[1] Unless the preparations for porcelain-fused-to-metal restorations are meticulously done, however, the restorations will not be as esthetic as sound natural tooth structure. They can often be identified by their opacity, bulkiness, exposed gingival metal collar, or by a cuff of inflamed tissue at the gingival margin. All of these problems have their roots in faulty crown preparation.

The proper preparation for this restoration is a reflection of the materials used in its fabrication and the space required to provide an adequate bulk for both durability and an esthetic result.

Creation of a lifelike porcelain veneer requires a thin layer of opaque porcelain to mask the underlying metal and a thicker layer of translucent porcelain to produce the illusion of natural enamel.[2] The metal itself should be 0.3 to 0.5 mm thick if it is a noble metal alloy,[3] while a coping made of the more rigid base metal alloys can be thinned to 0.2 mm.[4] Some simple arithmetic shows that an absolute minimum of 1.2 mm of facial reduction is needed for a porcelain-fused-to-metal crown with a base metal alloy coping, while at least 1.4 mm is recommended for a restoration fabricated of a noble metal alloy.[5] Inadequate reduction will lead to overcontouring of the restoration in the laboratory, which in turn will produce gingival inflammation.[5–10]

Figures 13-1 through 13-39 show the steps in the preparation of a maxillary central incisor for a porcelain-fused-to-metal crown. Figures 13-40 through 13-53 are clinical examples of porcelain-fused-to-metal crowns and their tooth preparations on anterior teeth.

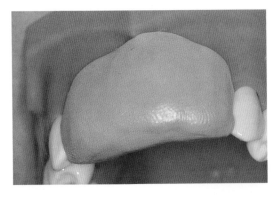

Anterior porcelain-fused-to-metal crown preparation (Figs. 13-1 through 13-39)

Fig. 13-1 Before beginning the preparation, make an index by adapting one-half scoop of condensation reaction silicone putty to the facial and lingual surfaces of the tooth to be prepared and to at least one tooth on each side of it.

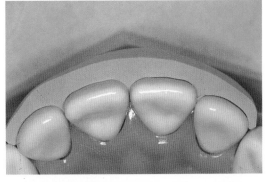

Fig. 13-2 A facial index can be made by cutting the adapted putty into facial and lingual halves, and then splitting the facial half. The gingivofacial segment formed in this manner is placed against the teeth to check for adaptation. If the contour of the facial surface of the tooth will be significantly altered by the restoration, the index should be made from a diagnostic wax-up of the proposed changes.

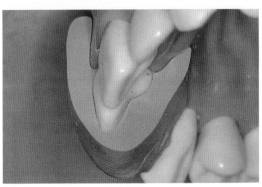

Fig. 13-3 A midsagittal index can be created by sectioning the silicone putty from gingivofacial to gingivolingual along the midline of the tooth to be prepared. This index gives a better indication of overall reduction, including the incisal and lingual aspects, but it does not provide any information about the facial reduction mesiodistally. Each operator must decide which index provides the most useful information for him or her. Two indices can be made from two separate mixes of putty, if the dentist has the time to spend doing it.

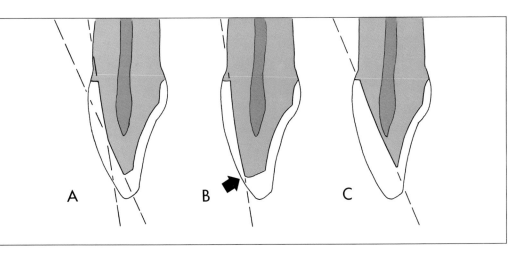

Fig. 13-4 When a tooth is being prepared to receive a crown with an esthetic veneer, the facial surface should be reduced in two planes:[5,8] one nearly parallel with the path of insertion, and one parallel with the incisal two-thirds of the facial surface of the tooth (A). Reduction only in the plane parallel with the path of insertion may result in insufficient space for porcelain in the incisal one-third, which is a common error (B).[11] One-plane reduction, which creates adequate space for the restoration in both the shoulder and incisal areas, will come dangerously close to the pulp in the midfacial area and may also produce an overtapered preparation (C).

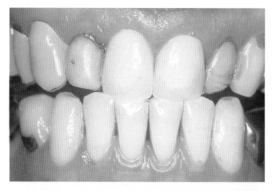

Fig. 13-5 Failure to use biplanar facial reduction can result in a facial veneer of porcelain that is too thin. This will produce an ugly display of opaque porcelain corresponding to the incisofacial angle of the preparation, as seen in the crown on this maxillary left central incisor. (Photograph courtesy of Dr. Royce A. Hatch of Denver.)

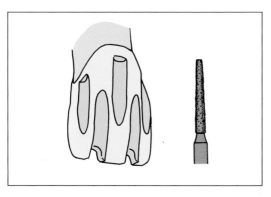

Fig. 13-6 The preparation on this incisor also was done with only one plane of reduction on the facial surface. In an effort to reduce enough bulk to avoid the esthetic problem just seen, this tooth was overreduced facially. The resulting exposure of the pulp horns required endodontic treatment.

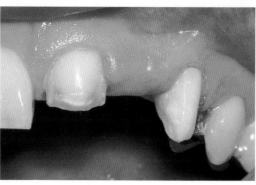

Fig. 13-7 Depth-orientation grooves: flat-end tapered diamond.

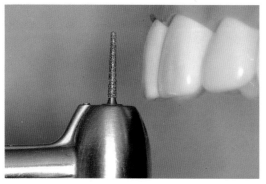

Fig. 13-8 Placement of gauging or orientation cuts is recommended by Preston[5] and Miller.[1] The key to their proper application is use of instruments of known diameters and use of remaining tooth structure as a benchmark against which the reduction can be measured.[1] Align the flat-end tapered diamond with the incisal portion of the facial surface.

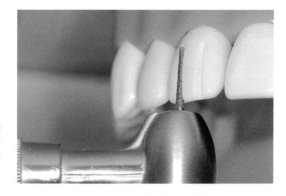

Fig. 13-9 Make at least two vertical cuts in the incisal portion of the facial surface. These will be made to the full diameter of the diamond, fading out at the "break" where the curvature of the facial surface is greatest.

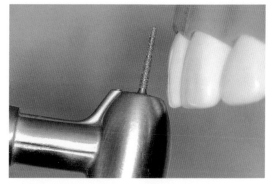

Fig. 13-10 Next align the flat-end tapered diamond with the gingival portion of the facial surface.

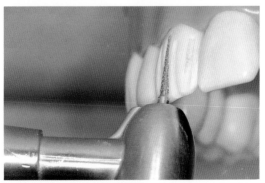

Fig. 13-11 Sink the side of the diamond into the mesiodistal center of the facial surface, maintaining the same instrument alignment parallel to the gingival segment of the facial surface. Make sure the diamond is inserted into the tooth to its full diameter, or slightly deeper. Keep the tip of the diamond slightly supragingival at this point, even if it is ultimately to be flush with the gingival crest, or slightly subgingival. Repeat the process at least twice, placing these orientation grooves closer to the line angles of the tooth.

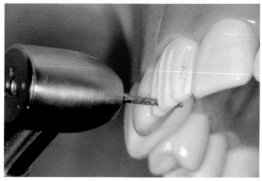

Fig. 13-12 Make two incisal orientation grooves that are 2.0 mm deep. The diamond should parallel the angle of the uncut incisal edge faciolingually.

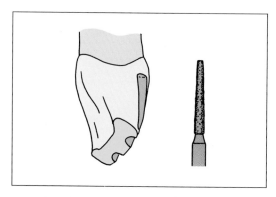

Fig. 13-13 Incisal reduction: flat-end tapered diamond.

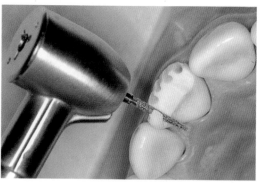

Fig. 13-14 Reduce the incisal edge by 2.0 mm, to the level of the depth-orientation grooves. Keep the plane of the reduced surface parallel to the former incisal edge.

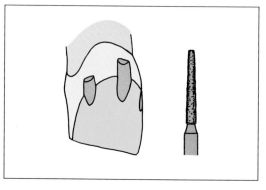

Fig. 13-15 Facial reduction, incisal half: flat-end tapered diamond.

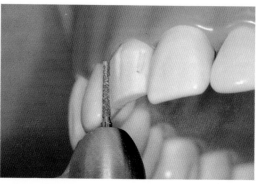

Fig. 13-16 The incisal portion of the facial surface is reduced with the flat-end tapered diamond, removing the tooth structure remaining between the orientation grooves.

Fig. 13-17 Facial reduction, gingival half: flat-end tapered diamond.

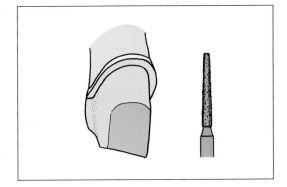

Fig. 13-18 Be sure that the gingival segment of the reduction extends well into the proximal surface. Recommendations for the depth of facial axial reduction have included 1.0 mm,[12,13] 1.2 mm,[14] 1.25 mm,[15] and 1.5 mm.[13,16,17] These are reasonable amounts if 1.2 to 1.4 mm is accepted as a desirable thickness for the veneer of porcelain and alloy. If reduction of less than 1.2 mm is done for a porcelain-fused-to-base-metal or 1.4 mm for a porcelain-fused-to-noble-metal restoration, the dentist must be willing to accept either a slightly opaque restoration or an overcontoured one. The reduction interproximally is wider than the diameter of the diamond, so it is safe to favor the proximal contacts by keeping some tooth structure between the adjacent teeth and the instrument.

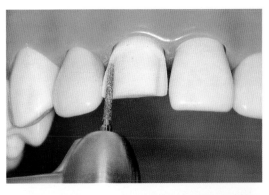

Fig. 13-19 The "lip" or undermined edge of tooth structure thus formed can be easily removed with a sharp enamel chisel, such as a hatchet or binangle chisel.

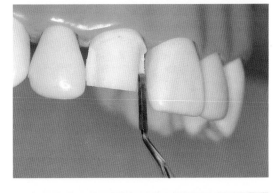

Fig. 13-20 If there is sound tooth structure interproximally, a vertical wall, or "wing" of it, is left standing in each interproximal area, lingual to the proximal contact. Besides preserving tooth structure, it also adds some torque resistance to the preparation. The shoulder must be extended lingual to the contact to permit an adequate bulk of interproximal porcelain for good esthetics.[5] If the termination of the shoulder and wings occurs at or facial to the proximal contact, the interproximal area of the restoration will have an opaque, "dead" appearance. If, as so often happens to teeth requiring porcelain-fused-to-metal crowns, the proximal surfaces have been damaged by caries or have been previously restored, the wing is deleted.

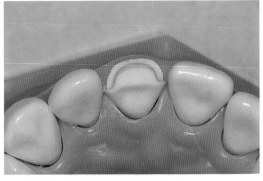

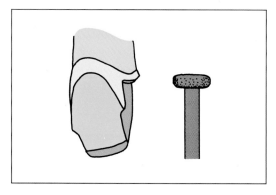

Fig. 13-21 Lingual reduction: small wheel diamond.

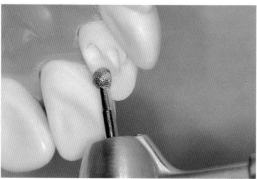

Fig. 13-22 Begin the reduction of the lingual surface by using a small round diamond with a diameter 1.4 mm larger than the shaft. By sinking this instrument into lingual tooth structure until the shaft touches enamel, it is possible to produce index marks that are 0.7 mm deep. Distribute several of these "potholes" over the lingual surface of the tooth.

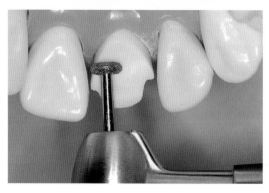

Fig. 13-23 Reduce the cingulum portion of the lingual surface with the small wheel diamond. Be careful not to extend the lingual reduction so far gingivally over the cingulum that the vertical lingual wall is overshortened. Overreduction at this point will produce a retention deficiency that will be hard to compensate for later.

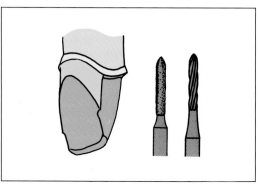

Fig. 13-24 Lingual axial reduction: torpedo diamond and carbide finishing bur.

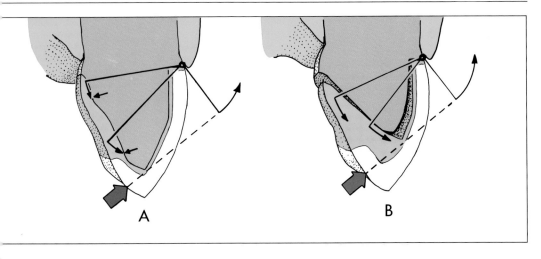

Fig. 13-25 It is necessary to form the lingual surface of an anterior tooth so that there is a vertical wall on the lingual surface of the cingulum and a separate concave surface incisal to it *(A)*. This provides steplike resisting areas to counteract the tipping effect of forces from the lingual. The lingual concavity also creates space for a crown with proper contours and occlusion with minimum removal of tooth structure. If the lingual surface is formed into a single sloping plane *(B)*, the arcs of rotation of all points in the crown will be either parallel with or directed away from the tooth, and the crown, lacking resistance form, will fail.

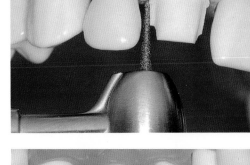

Fig. 13-26 If there is limited space between the facioproximal angle of the wing and the proximal surface of the adjacent tooth, use a long-needle diamond to reduce the axial wall lingual to the wing.

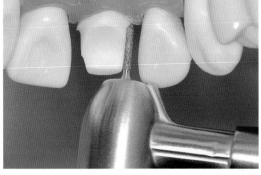

Fig. 13-27 In this portion of the tooth preparation where the coping will not be veneered by porcelain, the torpedo diamond is used to reduce the lingual axial surface, simultaneously forming a chamfer finish line. If the lingual axial wall is too short, it may be possible to lengthen it by using a shoulder with a bevel to move the lingual wall farther toward the center of the tooth. The lingual axial wall should be parallel with the cervical one-third of the facial surface.[8]

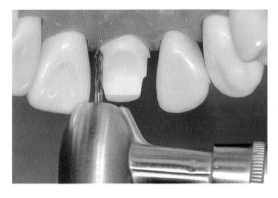

Fig. 13-28 Redefine and smooth the lingual chamfer with a torpedo carbide finishing bur.

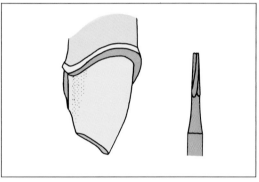

Fig. 13-29 Facial axial finishing: no. 171 bur.

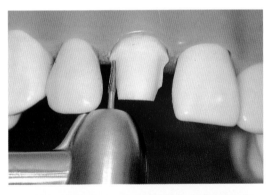

Fig. 13-30 Smooth the entire facial surface with a no. 171 bur. As you do, eliminate any undercuts. Pay particular attention to the facial aspect of the proximal wings, if they are present. Make sure that they are parallel with or slightly lingually inclined to the path of insertion of the preparation.

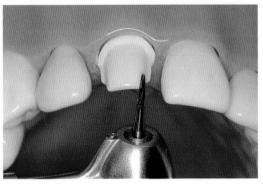

Fig. 13-31 Round over any sharp angles on the incisal angle or along the edges of the incisal notches with the no. 171 bur. The incisal notches themselves were automatically created by placing the wings lingual to the proximal contacts. The heavier facial reduction cut through the lingual surface, creating the notches on the proximal ends of the incisal angle as it did.

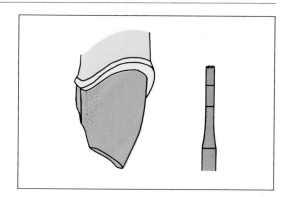

Fig. 13-32 Shoulder finishing: no. 957 bur.

Finishing the shoulder

It is possible to gouge the shoulder (Fig. 13-33) with the bur edges when instrumenting a shoulder that is not level. The operator must be careful *not* to drop the shoulder at the facioproximal line angles to the same level as the facial surface midpoint while trying to eliminate nicks in the shoulder. The result will be serious damage to the interdental papilla and a vertical finish line where the facial shoulder meets the proximal finish line.

Some form of the shoulder has been widely used for the facial finish line of the preparation for the porcelain-fused-to-metal crown for many years. Some clinicians have recommended it alone[8,12,18–21] or with a narrow finishing bevel.[5,6,22–24] McLean and Wilson have refuted the argument that the facial finish line should be a bevel, stating that the bevel on the shoulder would have to form an angle of 160 to 170 degrees to produce a significant effect.[25] Because a bevel on the shoulder requires a metal collar at the margin of the restoration,[26] a 135-degree shoulder has also been proposed[5,27] to allow an acute margin while minimizing the edge of metal at the actual margin.

A highly skilled technician can meticulously trim a facial metal margin under a stereomicroscope to produce an extremely thin edge, but metal will still be present, nonetheless. It is fragile and susceptible to distortion, and the metal line at the margin, albeit a very fine one, will eventually become visible when there is a gingival recession.

The interest in an all-porcelain margin is occasioned not only by the ugly display of metal when a collar is bared by gingival recession, but also by the gingival inflammation that often accompanies the subgingival placement of restoration margins. This can best be avoided by keeping the crown margin as shallow as possible. The solution to both problems would seem to be the elimination of metal in the facial margin of porcelain veneered crowns in esthetically critical areas.

Many techniques have been described for fabricating porcelain-fused-to-metal crowns with porcelain shoulders. The use of a platinum foil matrix was a logical extension of a technique used in fabricating porcelain jacket crowns.[6,28] Refractory casts have been employed for adding and firing the porcelain for the shoulder on the die.[29] Others have used a direct-lift

269

technique, forming the porcelain shoulder against a treated die and then lifting it off for firing. Opaque porcelain[30] or special shoulder porcelain[31] can be used, or the porcelain used for forming the shoulder can be mixed with wax.[32]

Quantitative evaluations of the marginal fit in vivo[33,34] and in vitro[35] have indicated satisfactory adaptation of the porcelain to the preparation finish line. The clinician's decision to use porcelain-fused-to-metal crowns with all-porcelain margins will depend on whether he or she has access to a technician who is able to produce restorations with accurate porcelain margins.

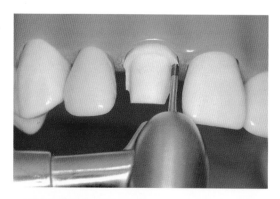

Fig. 13-33 The shoulder, roughed out with the flat-end tapered diamond, is completed at this stage with an endcutting bur and hand instruments. The finish line should follow the undulating contours of the gingival tissues, rising incisally in the interproximal region.

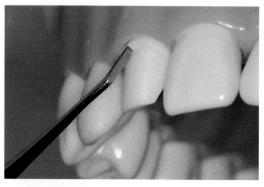

Fig. 13-34 The shoulder is instrumented with a sharp 1.0-mm-wide chisel to produce a smooth finish line. It is not necessary to accentuate the internal angle. In fact, a rounded internal angle has been proposed by some authors because it reduced stress.[36,37] It is important to make sure that there is no "lip" or reverse bevel of enamel at the finish line. Otherwise, this edge may fail to reproduce when the impression is poured, or it may fracture off the cast, resulting in an ill-fitting casting. It is also susceptible to fracture on the tooth, which would cause an open margin. The shoulder should be no less than 1.0 mm in width. The enamel chisel helps to verify this dimension.

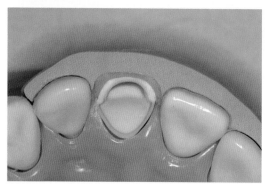

Fig. 13-35 Use the horizontal gingivofacial silicone index to check the reduction across the entire facial surface. If there is any question, use the width of the blade of a 1.5-mm-wide enamel chisel for a comparative measurement.

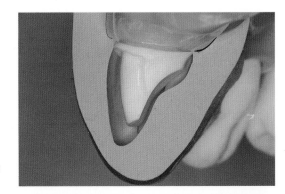

Fig. 13-36 A vertical midsagittal index can also be used for checking the amount of reduction.

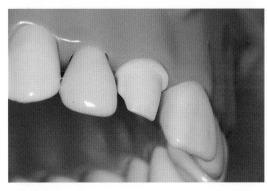

Fig. 13-37 This is an incisofacial view of a preparation for a porcelain-fused-to-metal crown on a maxillary central incisor.

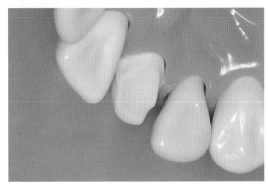

Fig. 13-38 A linguo-incisal view of the same preparation on a maxillary central incisor.

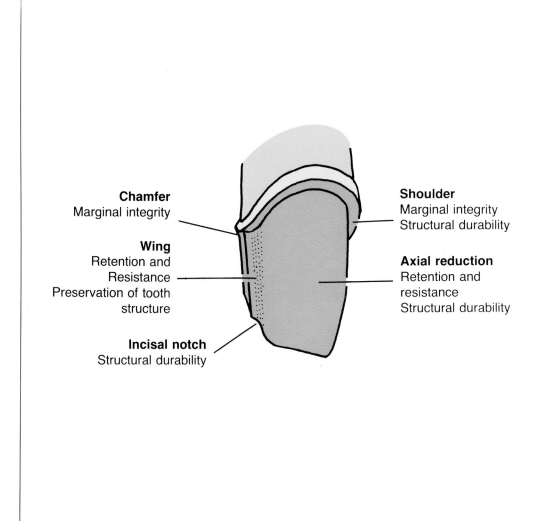

Fig. 13-39 The features of a preparation for a porcelain-fused-to-metal crown on an anterior tooth and the function served by each.

Clinical examples: Porcelain-fused-to-metal (Figs. 13-40 through 13-53)

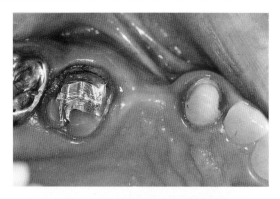

Fig. 13-40 Incisal view of a preparation for a porcelain-fused-to-metal bridge retainer on a maxillary canine. The patient is a 19-year old male who lost these and several other teeth in an automobile accident.

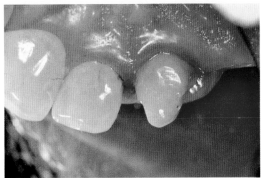

Fig. 13-41 A lingual view of the same preparation.

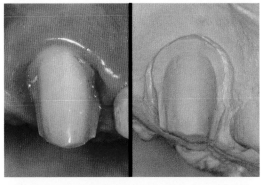
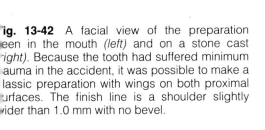

Fig. 13-42 A facial view of the preparation seen in the mouth *(left)* and on a stone cast *(right)*. Because the tooth had suffered minimum trauma in the accident, it was possible to make a classic preparation with wings on both proximal surfaces. The finish line is a shoulder slightly wider than 1.0 mm with no bevel.

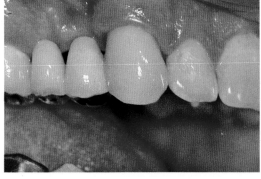
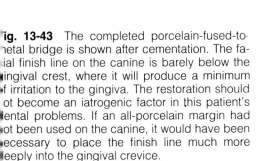

Fig. 13-43 The completed porcelain-fused-to-metal bridge is shown after cementation. The facial finish line on the canine is barely below the gingival crest, where it will produce a minimum of irritation to the gingiva. The restoration should not become an iatrogenic factor in this patient's dental problems. If an all-porcelain margin had not been used on the canine, it would have been necessary to place the finish line much more deeply into the gingival crevice.

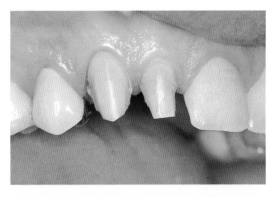

Fig. 13-44 A facial view of porcelain-fused-to metal preparations on a maxillary right lateral incisor and canine.

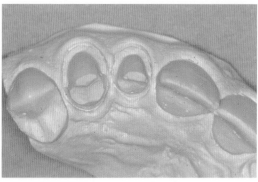

Fig. 13-45 An incisal view of the stone casts of the same preparations shows smooth facial shoulders of uniform width. All-porcelain margins were used, so there are no bevels.

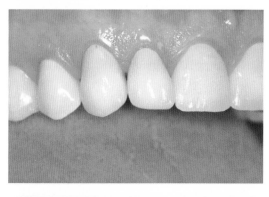

Fig. 13-46 These porcelain-fused-to-metal crowns were placed on the preparations seen in the preceding photographs.

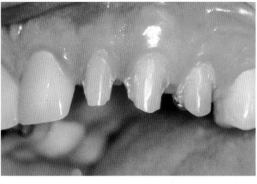

Fig. 13-47 Preparations for porcelain-fused-to metal crowns are shown on the lateral incisor, canine, and first premolar on the contralateral side of the same arch.

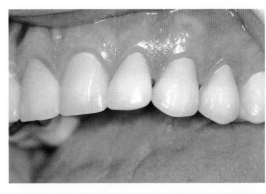

Fig. 13-48 The stone casts of the same three preparations.

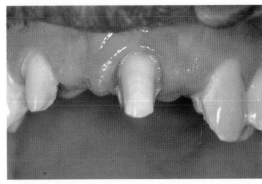

Fig. 13-49 A close-up view of the cemented crowns shows that all-porcelain shoulders just barely beneath the gingival crest can produce a good cosmetic result.

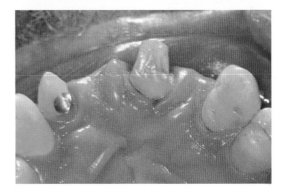

Fig. 13-50 A facial view of a preparation for a porcelain-fused-to-metal retainer on a central incisor pier abutment.

Fig. 13-51 A linguo-incisal view of the same preparation. It has been modified with a box form on the distal surface to accommodate a nonrigid connector. The other retainer preparations are for a porcelain-fused-to-metal crown on the lateral incisor, and an acid-etch resin-bonded retainer on the canine.

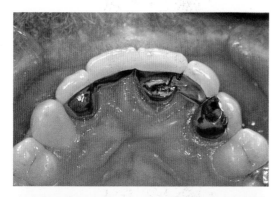

Fig. 13-52 A linguo-incisal view of the completed prosthesis.

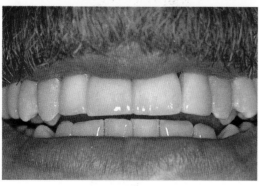

Fig. 13-53 A conversational view of the facial aspect of the cemented restoration.

References

1. Tuccillo, J.J., and Cascone, P. J. The evolution of porcelain-fused-to-metal (PFM) alloy systems. pp. 347–370 In J. W. McLean (ed.) Dental Ceramics: Proceedings of the 1st International Symposium on Ceramics. Chicago: Quintessence Publishing Co., 1983.
2. McLean, J. W. The Science and Art of Dental Ceramics. Vol. I. Chicago: Quintessence Publishing Co., 1979, 138.
3. Mumford, G. The porcelain fused to metal restoration. Dent. Clin. North Am. 9:241, 1965.
4. Weiss, P. A. New design parameters: Utilizing the properties of nickel chromium superalloys. Dent. Clin. North Am. 21:769, 1977.
5. Preston, J. D. Rational approach to tooth preparation for ceramo-metal restorations. Dent. Clin. North Am. 21:683, 1977.
6. Brecker, S. C. Porcelain baked to gold. A new medium in prosthodontics. J. Prosthet. Dent. 6:801, 1956.
7. Stein, R. S., and Kuwata, M. A dentist and a dental technologist analyze current ceramo-metal procedures. Dent. Clin. North Am. 21:729, 1977.
8. Romanelli, J. H. Periodontal considerations in tooth preparation for crown and bridge. Dent. Clin. North Am. 21:683, 1977.
9. Wilson, R. D. Intracrevicular restorative dentistry. Int. J. Periodont. Rest. Dent. 1:(4):35,1981.
10. Miller, L. A clinician's interpretation of tooth preparations and the design of metal substructures for metal-ceramic restorations. pp. 173–206 In J. W. McLean (ed.) Dental Ceramics: Proceedings of the 1st International Symposium on Ceramics. Chicago: Quintessence Publishing Co., 1983.
11. Tjan, A. H. Common errors in tooth preparation. Gen. Dent. 28:20, 1980.
12. Johnston, J. F., Mumford, G., and Dykema, R. W. The porcelain veneered gold crown. Dent. Clin. North Am. 7:853, 1963.
13. Sozio, R. B. The marginal aspects of the ceramo-metal restoration: The collarless ceramo-metal restoration. Dent. Clin. North Am. 21:787, 1977.
14. Schöler, A. Überlegungen, analysen, und praktische erkentnisse zur Kronenstumpfpräparation (I). Die Quint. 31:71, 1980.
15. Engleman, M. A. Simplified esthetic ceramo-metal restorations. N.Y. J. Dent. 49:252, 1971.
16. Silver, M., Klein, G., and Howard, M. C. Platinum-porcelain restorations. J. Prosthet. Dent. 6:695, 1956.
17. Hoffman, E. J. How to utilize porcelain fused to gold as a crown and bridge material. Dent. Clin. North Am. 9:57, 1965.
18. Shelby, D. S. Practical considerations and design of porcelain fused to metal. J. Prosthet. Dent. 12:542, 1962.
19. Behrand, D. ·A. Ceramometal restorations with supragingival margins. J. Prosthet. Dent. 47:625, 1982.
20. Grundy, J. R. Color Atlas of Conservative Dentistry. Chicago: Year Book Medical Publ., Inc., 1980, 68.
21. Johnston, J. F., Dykema, R. W., Mumford, G., and Phillips, R. W. Construction and assembly of porcelain veneer gold crowns and pontics. J. Prosthet. Dent. 12:1125, 1962.
22. Hobo, S., and Shillingburg, H. T. Porcelain fused to metal: Tooth preparation and coping design. J. Prosthet. Dent. 30:28, 1973.
23. Goldstein, R. E. Esthetic principles for ceramo-metal restorations. Dent. Clin. North Am. 21:803, 1977.
24. Silver, M., Howard, M. C., and Klein, G. Porcelain bonded to a cast metal understructure. J. Prosthet. Dent. 11:132, 1961.
25. McLean, J. W., and Wilson, A. D. Butt joint vs. bevelled gold margins in metal ceramic crowns. J. Biomed. Materials Res. 14:239, 1980.
26. Strating, H., Pameijer, C. H., and Gildenhuys, R. R. Evaluation of the marginal integrity of ceramo-metal restorations. Part I. J. Prosthet. Dent. 46:59, 1981.
27. McAdam, D. B. Preparation of a 135-degree shoulder for a ceramometal margin using an end-cutting bur. J. Prosthet. Dent. 54:473, 1985.
28. Goodacre, C. J., Van Rockel, N. B., Dykema, R. W., and Ullman, R. B. The collarless metal-ceramic crown. J. Prosthet. Dent. 38:615, 1977.

29. Sozio, R. B. The marginal aspect of the ceramo-metal restoration: The collarless ceramo-metal restoration. Dent. Clin. North Am. 21:787, 1977.

30. Vryonis, P. A simplified approach to the complete porcelain margin. J. Prosthet. Dent. 42:592, 1979.

31. Kessler, J. C., Brooks, T.D., and Keenan, M. P. The direct lift technique for constructing porcelain margins. Quint. Dent. Technol. 10:150, 1986.

32. Prince, J., and Donovan, T. The esthetic metal-ceramic margin: A comparison of techniques. J. Prosthet. Dent. 50:185, 1983.

33. Belser, U. C., MacEntee, M. I., and Richter, W. A. Fit of three porcelain-fused-to-metal marginal designs in vivo: A scanning electron microscope study. J. Prosthet. Dent. 53:24, 1985.

34. Hunt, J. L., Cruickshanks-Boyd, D. W., and Davies, E. H. The marginal characteristics of collarless bonded porcelain crowns produced using a separating medium technique. Quint. Dent. Technol. 2:21, 1978.

35. West, A. J., Goodacre, C. J., Moore, B. K., and Dykema, R. W. A comparison of four techniques for fabricating collarless metal-ceramic crowns. J. Prosthet. Dent. 54:636, 1985.

36. El-Ebrashi, M. K., Craig, R. G., and Peyton, F. A. Experimental stress analysis of dental restorations. III. The concept of the geometry of proximal margins. J. Prosthet. Dent. 22:333, 1969.

37. Nally, J. N., Farah, J. W., and Craig, R. G.: Experimental stress analysis of dental restorations. IX. Two-dimensional photoelastic stress analysis of porcelain bonded to metal crowns. J. Prosthet. Dent. 25:307, 1971.

Chapter 14

Posterior Porcelain-Fused-To-Metal Crowns

The use of porcelain-fused-to-metal crowns allows an esthetic restoration on a posterior tooth in the appearance zone, which requires placement of a full crown. As discussed in the previous chapter, the *objective* limits of this zone (as viewed by others in conversation) and the *subjective* limits (as perceived by the patient) may differ.

The maxillary premolars and first molars and the mandibular first premolars are almost always in the appearance zone. The mandibular second premolars can also fall into this category. Maxillary second molars and mandibular molars may also have to be included if the patient is bothered by the presence of metal on those teeth. Routinely placing porcelain-fused-to-metal crowns on all posterior teeth, regardless of objective or subjective criteria, represents overtreatment because of the additional tooth structure that must be removed to accommodate the combination of porcelain and metal. There is also an increased risk of failure due to fracture of the porcelain veneer.

The routine use of porcelain occlusal surfaces is not without its critics.[1] It offers maximum cosmetic effect when indicated for a highly visible area or because of patient preference. However, it again requires the removal of greater quantities of tooth structure which can pose a real threat to the structural integrity of the opposing occlusal sur-faces. Although, theoretically, abrasion should not occur if attention is paid to the occlusion when the restorations are fabricated and inserted, inspection of mouths restored in this manner all too frequently exhibits heavy facets opposing these types of restorations. Patients who demand porcelain occlusal surfaces should be informed of these potential problems.

Preparations for porcelain-fused-to-metal crowns should be done with a plan in mind for the extension of the porcelain coverage, since areas to be veneered with porcelain will require greater depth of reduction than those which will simply be overlaid with metal alone.

Figures 14-1 through 14-39 show the detailed steps for the preparation of a maxillary premolar for a porcelain-fused-to-metal crown. Figures 14-40 through 14-50 demonstrate the use of porcelain-fused-to-metal crowns to restore actual premolars and molars.

Enhanced distortion resistance

Crowns made over shoulder finish lines have been shown by some investigators to be less likely to distort during porcelain firing. Shillingburg et al. found porcelain-fused-to-noble-metal crown margins fabricated on shoulders exhibited less marginal gap opening than those made on some form of chamfer.[23] Faucher and Nicholls found a similar distortion resistance of shoulders over chamfers, demonstrating that the changes actually occurred as increases in the mesiodistal dimension and decreases in the faciolingual dimension of the coping.[24] It has been hypothesized that the shoulder configuration provides space for an internal bulk of metal to buttress the margin.[5,11] Other investigators have not found these differences in marginal fit and believe that marginal gaps following porcelain firing may be caused either by technical difficulties in forming a knife-edge of metal and porcelain[25] or by differences in metal-porcelain combinations.[26]

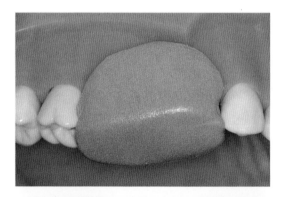

Posterior porcelain-fused-to-metal crown preparation (Figs. 14-1 through 14-39)

Fig. 14-1 Before beginning the preparation on the tooth or teeth to receive a porcelain-fused-to-metal crown, adapt condensation-reaction silicone to the facial, lingual, and occlusal surfaces of the tooth or teeth to be prepared and one tooth on either side.

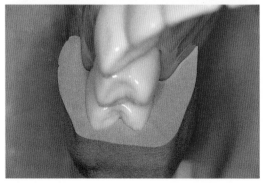

Fig. 14-2 After polymerization, a midsaggital index can be formed from the silicone by cutting it in half along the faciolingual midline of the tooth to be prepared. Try it back on the tooth to be sure it is still well adapted. If the tooth being restored is badly broken down, make an index from the diagnostic waxup.

Fig. 14-3 The more conventional facial index is fabricated by cutting through the silicone along the facial cusps of the teeth. The facial piece thus formed is further divided along a line midway between the cervical lines of the teeth and the facial cusp tips. Discard the occlusal portion and use the gingival portion as an index. It is shown here after it has been placed back onto the facial surfaces of the maxillary right premolars and first molar.

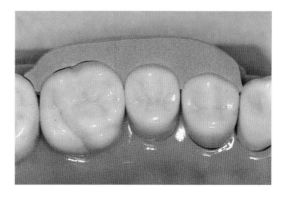

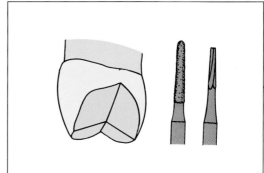

Fig. 14-4 Planar occlusal reduction: round-end tapered diamond and no. 171 bur.

Fig. 14-5 Begin the occlusal reduction by making depth-orientation grooves with a round-end tapered diamond. In those areas where there is to be occlusal coverage with porcelain, reduction should be 1.5 mm^2 to 2.0 mm.[3–5] Therefore, the 1.6-mm-diameter diamond should be sunk into enamel to its full diameter, and frequently farther.

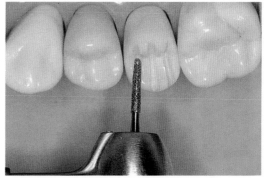

Fig. 14-6 The occlusal reduction is then accomplished by using the same diamond to remove the strips of intact enamel left between the depth-orientation grooves. The reduction should take the form of definite planes reproducing the general occlusal morphology,[6] or basic geometric shape, of the occlusal surface.

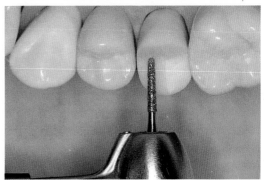

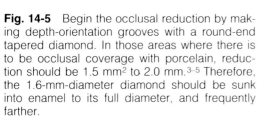

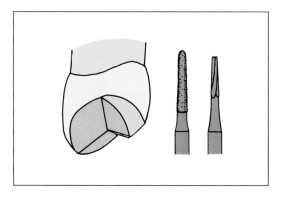

Fig. 14-7 Functional cusp bevel: round-end tapered diamond and no. 171 bur.

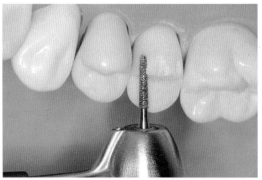

Fig. 14-8 The functional cusp bevel, to provide a uniform bulk of restorative material on the lingual incline of maxillary lingual cusps and the facial incline of mandibular facial cusps, is begun by placing depth-orientation grooves with the 1.4-mm-diameter diamond used for the occlusal reduction. The depth required will be 1.5 mm if the cusp is to be covered by metal only and 2.0 mm if it will be veneered with porcelain.

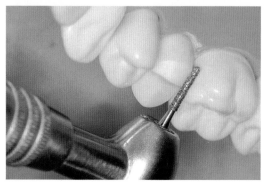

Fig. 14-9 Complete the functional cusp bevel by removing the tooth structure between the depth-orientation grooves. The angle of the bevel should approximate the inclination of the opposing cusps, which in this case would mean paralleling the facial inclines of the mandibular lingual cusps.

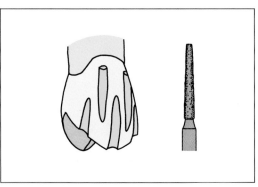

Fig. 14-10 Depth-orientation grooves: flat-end tapered diamond.

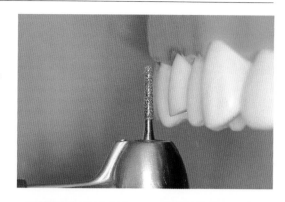

Fig. 14-11 Depth-orientation cuts, recommended by Preston[5] and Miller,[7] provide a means of judging the amount of tooth structure to be removed. An instrument of known diameter is cut into the tooth, and the surface of the remaining tooth structure is used as a reference point against which the depth of reduction can be measured.[7] Align the flat-end tapered diamond (1.6 mm in diameter at the shank) with the occlusal segment of the facial surface.

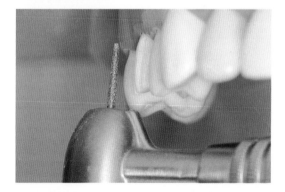

Fig. 14-12 Cut three vertical grooves in the occlusal portion of the facial surface. These are placed to the full diameter of the instrument, fading out in the area where the facial surface is most curved.

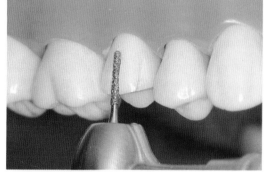

Fig. 14-13 Now align the flat-end tapered diamond with the gingival component of the facial surface.

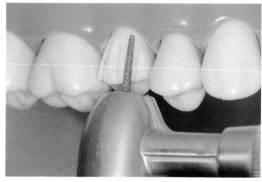

Fig. 14-14 Use the side of the instrument to cut into the facial surface, keeping the diamond aligned parallel with the uncut gingival portion of the facial surface. At the very least, the full diameter of the instrument must cut into the tooth. The tip of the diamond should be slightly supragingival at this point, even if the final intended position of the finish line is to be flush with or slightly beneath the gingival crest. Place at least two more orientation grooves, positioning them near the line angles of the tooth.

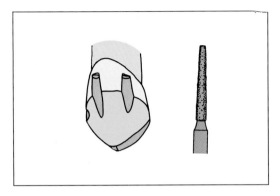

Fig. 14-15 Facial reduction, occlusal half: flat-end tapered diamond.

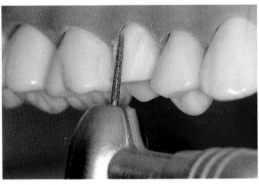

Fig. 14-16 Reduce the occlusal segment of the facial surface with the flat-end tapered diamond, removing all of the tooth structure remaining between the depth-orientation grooves.

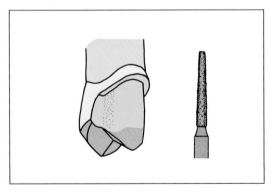

Fig. 14-17 Facial reduction, gingival half: flat-end tapered diamond.

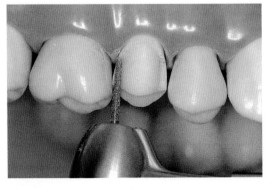

Fig. 14-18 Extend the gingival portion of the reduction well into the proximal surface. The depth of facial axial reduction has been recommended to be 1.0,[8,9] 1.2,[10] 1.25,[11] and 1.5 mm.[9,12,13] These are reasonable depths for restorations whose combined thicknesses of porcelain and alloy will be 1.2 to 1.4 mm. If reduction of less than 1.2 mm is done for a porcelain-fused-to-base-metal or 1.4 mm for a porcelain-fused-to-noble-metal crown, the restoration will be either slightly opaque or slightly overcontoured.

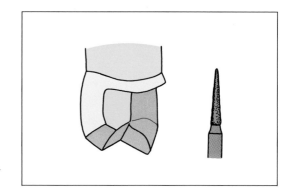

Fig. 14-19 Proximal axial reduction: short-needle diamond.

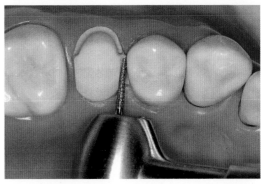

Fig. 14-20 The proximal axial reduction is begun with a short-needle diamond, whose narrow diameter will facilitate interproximal reduction without nicking the adjacent tooth.

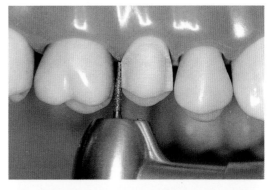

Fig. 14-21 Use the same thin diamond on the other proximal surface. The instrument can be used in either an up-and-down motion on the facial or lingual aspect of the interproximal tooth structure, or it can be held horizontally and used on the occlusal portion with a faciolingual movement. At this stage the only objective is to achieve separation between the teeth without overtapering the wall being prepared, or mutilating the adjacent tooth surface.

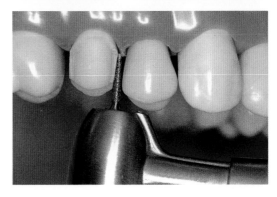

Fig. 14-22 The final step in the initial reduction of the proximal surface is the use of the needle diamond to plane the axial wall smooth.

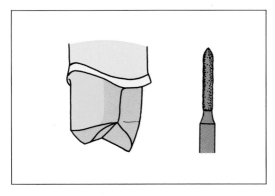

Fig. 14-23 Lingual axial reduction: torpedo diamond.

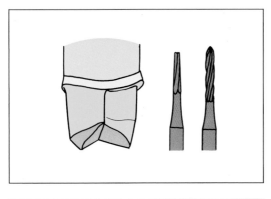

Fig. 14-24 Reduce the lingual axial wall with a torpedo diamond. Produce adequate reduction on both the lingual and proximal axial walls to have a distinct chamfer finish line in all areas of the tooth where there will not be a porcelain veneer. Take care to round over the corner created at the line angles with the proximal surfaces. Inadequate reduction of transitional line angles is a common error that causes overcontouring of the restoration and inflammation of the interdental papilla.[6]

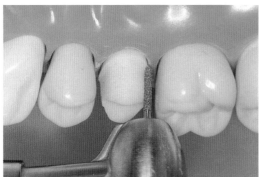

Fig. 14-25 Axial finishing: Torpedo finishing bur and no. 171 bur.

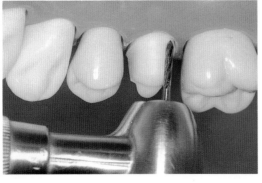

Fig. 14-26 The chamfer finish line and the axial surfaces adjacent to it are smoothed with the torpedo carbide finishing bur. All axial surfaces of the preparation to be veneered with metal only are finished in this way.

Fig. 14-27 The facial surface and those areas of the proximal surfaces to be veneered with porcelain are smoothed with the no. 171 bur. At the lingualmost extension of the facial reduction, lingual to the proximal contact, the transition from the deeper facial reduction to the relatively shallower lingual axial reduction results in a vertical wall or "wing" of tooth structure. Be sure that the wings are not undercut with the lingual axial wall of the preparation or with the preparation path of insertion. If the shoulder and wings terminate at the proximal contact or facial to it, the interproximal region of the facial porcelain will have a lifeless appearance. If there was an amalgam restoration in the tooth prior to preparing it for a porcelain-fused-to-metal crown, the wing will usually coincide with the lingual wall of the amalgam's proximal box form. Besides conserving tooth structure, the wing adds torque resistance to the preparation. If the entire proximal surface is to be veneered with porcelain, the shoulder should be extended across the entire proximal surface without a wing.

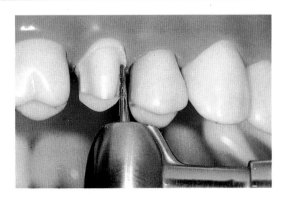

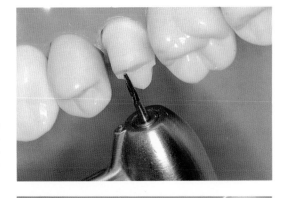

Fig. 14-28 At this time, use the no. 170 bur to smooth the planes of the occlusal reduction to remove any roughness or pits that might interfere with the complete seating of the finished restoration.

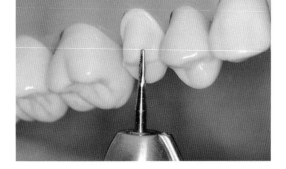

Fig. 14-29 Also round over any sharp corners or edges on the preparation that might present problems in impression pouring, investing, casting, and, ultimately, in the seating of the completed crown.

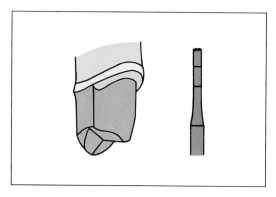

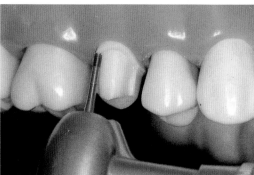

Fig. 14-30 Shoulder finishing: no. 957 bur.

Fig. 14-31 The shoulder, which was begun with the flat-end tapered diamond at the time the facial reduction was accomplished, is finished at this point with an end-cutting bur. A form of shoulder has been advocated for the facial finish line of porcelain-fused-to-metal preparations either alone,[2,8,14–17] or with a narrow finishing bevel.[3,5,18-20] The metal collar demanded by a shoulder with a bevel[21] often requires that the finish line be placed deep into the gingival sulcus to hide the metal.[22] In a posterior area of the mouth that is particularly visible, such as the maxillary premolar region, an all-porcelain margin may have to be used to achieve a good esthetic result without intruding into the gingival sulcus. There will be occasions, nonetheless, when a shoulder with a bevel will be the finish line of choice: in those areas where the esthetic needs are not so critical, or when the dental technician is unable to consistently produce a well fitting all-porcelain margin.

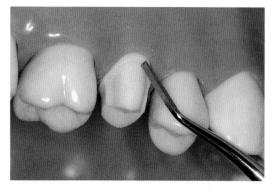

Fig. 14-32 To produce a smooth finish line, the shoulder is planed with a sharp 1.0-mm-wide chisel. No special effort is made to accentuate the internal angle. Remove any "lip" or reverse bevel of enamel at the cavosurface line. Small, sharp edges in this area may not be reproduced when the impression is poured, and they are susceptible to fracture on the cast or on the tooth in the mouth. The shoulder should be at least 1.0 mm wide. An instrument of that dimension is very helpful in checking the width.

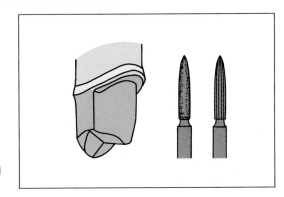

Fig. 14-33 Gingival bevel: Flame diamond and finishing bur.

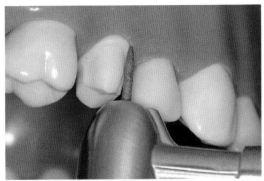

Fig. 14-34 A narrow bevel, no wider than 0.3 mm, is placed on the shoulder with the tip of a flame-shaped diamond. Keep the bevel narrow, since the metal collar on the resulting crown will have to be as wide as the bevel is. A more distinct bevel with an angle conducive to waxing and casting is formed by leaning the diamond and the head of the handpiece toward the center of the tooth as much as possible.

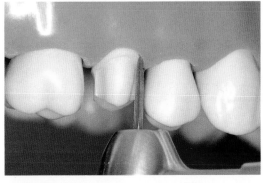

Fig. 14-35 Finish the bevel with the flame-shaped carbide finishing bur to create as smooth a surface and as clear a finish line as possible.

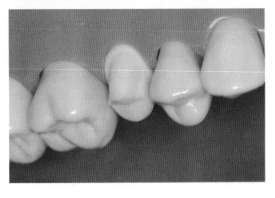

Fig. 14-36 The completed preparation for a porcelain-fused-to-metal crown is shown on a maxillary second premolar. The presence of wings midway through the proximal surfaces indicate that the crown made for this tooth would have an occlusal surface whose lingual two-thirds would be unveneered polished metal.

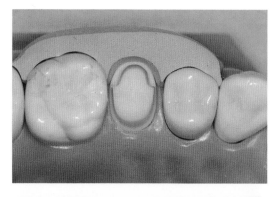

Fig. 14-37 The facial silicone putty index is positioned to demonstrate adequate and uniform axial reduction across the facial surface from the mesial to distal aspects.

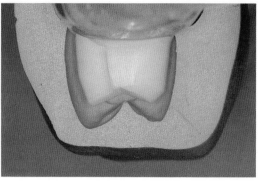

Fig. 14-38 A midsagittal index shows uniform reduction occlusogingivally on the facial surface. Occlusal reduction on the facial cusp, which is to be veneered with porcelain, is slightly greater than that on the lingual cusp, which will be covered with metal only. The axial reduction and chamfer finish line on the lingual surface also reflect the need for less reduction where metal only will be placed in the completed restoration.

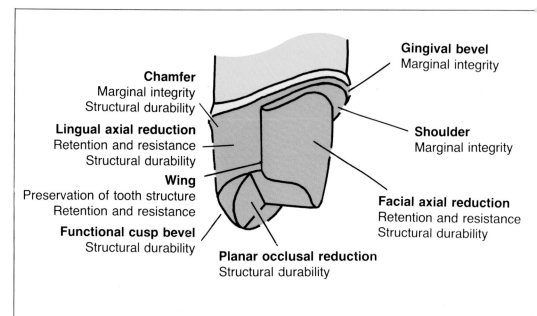

Gingival bevel
Marginal integrity

Chamfer
Marginal integrity
Structural durability

Lingual axial reduction
Retention and resistance
Structural durability

Wing
Preservation of tooth structure
Retention and resistance

Functional cusp bevel
Structural durability

Shoulder
Marginal integrity

Facial axial reduction
Retention and resistance
Structural durability

Planar occlusal reduction
Structural durability

Fig. 14-39 The features of a preparation for a porcelain-fused-to-metal-crown on a posterior tooth and the function served by each.

Clinical examples: Porcelain-fused-to-metal (Figs. 14-40 through 14-50)

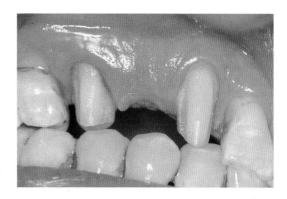

Fig. 14-40 This is a facial view of preparations for porcelain-fused-to-metal bridge retainers on a maxillary second premolar and canine. The combination of length and minimal taper made these preparations very retentive.

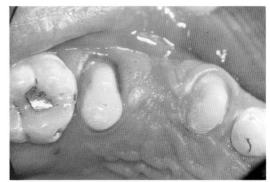

Fig. 14-41 An occlusal view of the same two preparations. Notice the wings on both preparations.

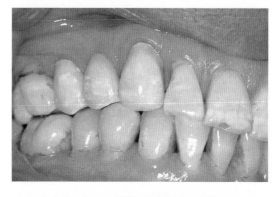

Fig. 14-42 This is the completed bridge fabricated for the preparations seen in Figs. 14-40 and 14-41.

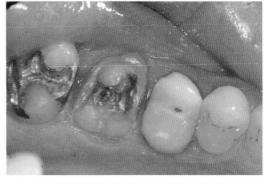

Fig. 14-43 An occlusal view of a porcelain-fused-to-metal preparation on a maxillary first molar that had been previously restored with a large four-surface amalgam.

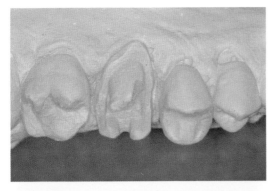

Fig. 14-44 The stone cast of this preparation shows the uniform width of the shoulder. The shoulder was not placed in or near the gingival sulcus, although erosion dictated that the crown margin extend that far. If the shoulder had been extended apically to the cervical constriction of the tooth, a normal-width shoulder would have required that the axial wall be placed so far into the center of the tooth that it would have endangered the pulp.

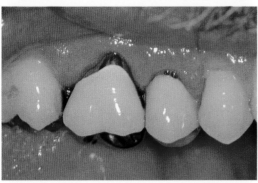

Fig. 14-45 A facial view of the completed restoration with the cheek retracted shows a wide metal collar along the gingival margin. This collar allows the restoration contours to be minimal near the gingival sulcus, thereby presenting less a risk of gingival inflammation than if the technician tried to overlay it with porcelain. It is not visible when the patient speaks or smiles.

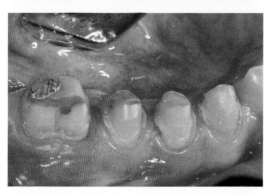

Fig. 14-46 These four teeth have been prepared for porcelain-fused-to-metal crowns on the canine and premolars and a full veneer crown on the molar.

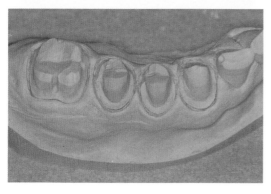

Fig. 14-47 A facial view of the stone cast shows the uniform-width shoulders on the canine and premolar preparations. There are no wings on the premolar preparations because of the planned extension of the porcelain.

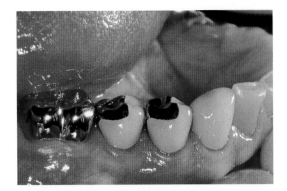

Fig. 14-48 The completed full veneer crown and porcelain-fused-to-metal crowns are shown cemented on the prepared teeth.

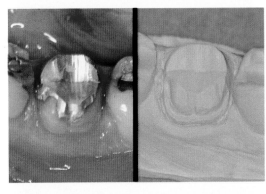

Fig. 14-49 An occlusal view of a preparation for a porcelain-fused-to-metal crown on a mandibular first molar in the mouth *(left)* and on the stone cast *(right)*.

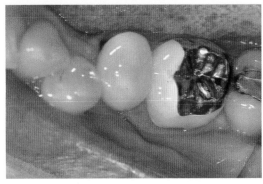

Fig. 14-50 The completed porcelain-fused-to-metal crown on the mandibular molar.

References

1. Nabers, C. L., Christensen, G. J., Markely, M. R., Miller, E. F., Pankey, L. D., Potts, J. W., and Pugh, C. E. Porcelain occlusions—To cover or not to cover? Texas Dent. J. 100:6, 1983.
2. Johnston, J. F., Dykema, R. W., Mumford, G., and Phillips, R. W. Construction and assembly of porcelain veneer gold crowns and pontics. J. Prosthet. Dent. 12:1125, 1962.
3. Brecker, S. C. Porcelain baked to gold—A new medium in prosthodontics. J. Prosthet. Dent. 6:801, 1956.
4. Goldstein, R. E. Esthetics in Dentistry. Philadelphia: J. B. Lippencott Co., 1976, 65, 332–341.
5. Preston, J. D. Rational approach to tooth preparation for ceramo-metal restorations. Dent. Clin. North Am. 21:683, 1977.
6. Tjan, A. H. Common errors in tooth preparation. Gen. Dent. 28:20, 1980.
7. Miller, L. A clinician's interpretation of tooth preparations and the design of metal substructures for metal-ceramic restorations. pp. 173–206 In J. W. McLean (ed.) Dental Ceramics: Proceedings of the 1st International Symposium on Ceramics. Chicago: Quintessence Publishing Co., 1983.
8. Johnston, J. F., Mumford, G., and Dykema, R. W. The porcelain veneered gold crown. Dent. Clin. North Am. 7:853, 1963.
9. Sozio, R. B. The marginal aspects of the ceramo-metal restoration: The collarless ceramo-metal restoration. Dent. Clin. North Am. 21:787, 1977.
10. Schöler, A. Überlegungen, analysen, und praktische erkentinisse zur Kronenstumpfpräparation (I). Die Quint. 31:71, 1980.
11. Engleman, M. A. Simplified esthetic ceramo-metal restorations. N.Y. J. Dent. 49:252, 1971.
12. Silver, M., Klein, G., and Howard, M. C. Platinum-porcelain restorations. J. Prosthet. Dent. 6:695, 1956.
13. Hoffman, E. J. How to utilize porcelain-fused-to-gold as a crown and bridge material. Dent. Clin. North Am. 9:57, 1965.
14. Shelby, D. S. Practical considerations and design of porcelain-fused-to-metal. J. Prosthet. Dent. 12:542, 1962.
15. Romanelli, J. H. Periodontal considerations in tooth preparation for crown and bridge. Dent. Clin. North Am. 21:683, 1977.
16. Grundy, J. R. Color Atlas of Conservative Dentistry. Chicago: Year Book Medical Publ., Inc., 1980, 68.
17. Behrand, D. A. Ceramometal restorations with supragingival margins. J. Prosthet. Dent. 47:625, 1982.
18. Silver, M., Howard, M. C., and Klein, G. Porcelain bonded to a cast metal understructure. J. Prosthet. Dent. 11:132, 1961.
19. Hobo, S., and Shillingburg, H. T. Porcelain fused to metal: Tooth preparation and coping design. J. Prosthet. Dent. 30:28, 1973.
20. Goldstein, R. E. Esthetic principles for ceramo metal restorations. Dent. Clin. North Am. 21:803, 1977.
21. Strating, H., Pameijer, C. H., and Gildenhuys, R. R. Evaluation of the marginal integrity of ceramo-metal restorations: Part I. J. Prosthet. Dent. 46:59, 1981.
22. Wilson, R. D. Intracrevicular restorative dentistry. Int. J. Periodont. Rest. Dent. 1(4): 35, 1981.
23. Shillingburg, H. T., Hobo, S., and Fisher, D. W. Preparation design and margin distortion in porcelain-fused-to-metal restorations. J. Prosthet. Dent. 29:276, 1973.
24. Faucher, R. R., and Nicholls, J. I. Distortion related to margin design in porcelain-fused-to-metal restorations. J. Prosthet. Dent. 43:149, 1980.
25. Hamaguchi, H., Cacciatore, A., and Tueller, V. M. Marginal distortion of the porcelain-bonded-to metal complete crown: An SEM study. J. Prosthet. Dent. 47:146, 1982.
26. DeHoff, P. H., and Anusavice, K. J. Effect of metal design on marginal distortion of metal-ceramic crowns. J. Dent. Res. 63:1327, 1984.

Chapter 15

All-Ceramic Crowns

For many years, the only type of all-ceramic crown was the porcelain jacket crown, which was built up in increments over a matrix or shell formed by thin platinum foil adapted to a cast or die of the prepared tooth. From a technological standpoint, this was analogous to early inlays[1] and three-quarter crowns[2] formed by flowing solder over a foil matrix that had been adapted to the cavity preparation or prepared tooth in the mouth.

In recent years, there have been other forms of all-ceramic crowns developed that use some form of casting. A substrate or coping of aluminous porcelain is formed in one process. Upon it the full-contour restoration of conventional dental porcelains will be built.[3] In two other systems, the actual full contour restoration is cast in molten glass, using the lost wax technique.[4,5]

Porcelain jacket crowns

The original porcelain jacket crown, made of feldspathic porcelain, possessed excellent esthetics but was very prone to fracture. With the development of aluminous reinforcement the restoration again generated interest amongst dentists.[6] It is still an inherently weak restoration, however; its use should be restricted to incisors, where a maximum cosmetic result is necessary.

More than any other restoration, the porcelain jacket crown depends for its very survival on the tooth preparation beneath. Tooth support is more critical for the fracture resistance of the restoration than is the bulk of porcelain.[7] The "crescent moon fracture" often seen in this type of restoration is a direct result of inadequate preparation length.[7–10]

The technique followed for preparing an incisor for a porcelain jacket crown is shown in Figs. 15-1 through 15-40. Preparations for cast ceramic crowns are shown in Figs. 15-41 through 15-71.

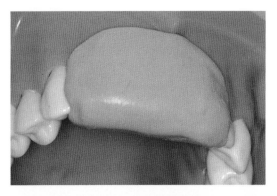

Porcelain jacket crowns (Figs. 15-1 through 15-40)

Fig. 15-1 Before the preparation is begun, start a depth-reduction index by adapting some condensation reaction silicone putty to the facial and lingual surfaces of the tooth or teeth to be prepared. The putty should extend to at least one tooth on either side of the tooth to be prepared.

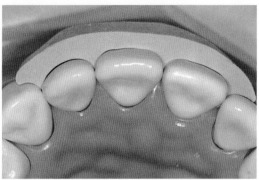

Fig. 15-2 A facial index is made by sectioning the adapted putty along the incisal edges of the tooth imprints. The facial segment is then cut into incisal and gingival halves. The gingivofacial portion thus formed is replaced against the teeth to insure that it is well adapted. If the facial contour of the tooth is to be significantly altered by the crown, make the index from a diagnostic wax-up of the proposed contour.

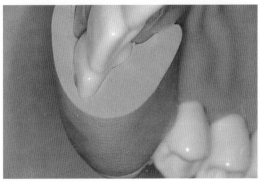

Fig. 15-3 It is also possible to make an index by sectioning the putty along the midsagittal line of the tooth from the gingivofacial to the gingivolingual aspects. This type of index provides more information about reduction all along the midline of the preparation, including the incisal and lingual aspects. On the other hand, it provides no information about the facial reduction mesiodistally. If desired, both indices can be made by using two separate mixes of putty.

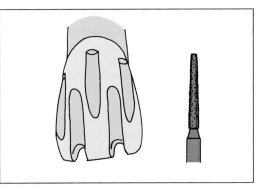

Fig. 15-4 Depth-orientation grooves: flat-end tapered diamond.

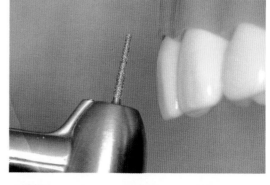

Fig. 15-5 Depth-orientation grooves have been used for the porcelain jacket crown preparation for many years.[11,12] A rotary instrument of known diameter is used so that the depth of reduction can be measured against the surface of the untouched enamel. Position the flat-end tapered diamond so it will be parallel with the gingival portion of the facial surface.

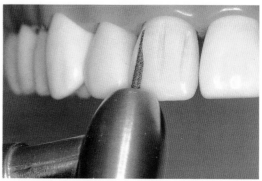

Fig. 15-6 Cut into the mesiodistal center of the facial surface with the side of the diamond, keeping the instrument parallel with the gingival portion of the facial surface. The diamond must be inserted into the tooth to its full diameter, or slightly deeper. The tip of the diamond should be slightly supragingival at this point, even if the finish line will eventually be even with the gingival crest, or slightly below it. Repeat the process twice, placing an orientation groove halfway between the midsagittal groove and each proximal line angle.

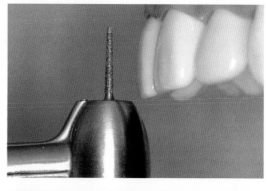

Fig. 15-7 Now orient the flat-end tapered diamond with the incisal aspect of the facial surface.

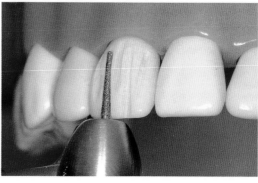

Fig. 15-8 Make two or more vertical cuts in the incisal portion of the facial surface. These must be sunk into the enamel to the full diameter of the diamond. They will disappear near the middle of the facial surface along the horizontal, where the curvature of the surface is greatest.

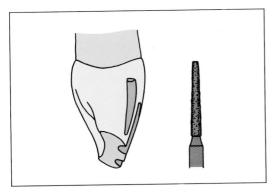

Fig. 15-9 Incisal reduction: flat-end tapered diamond.

Fig. 15-10 Make at least two faciolingual incisal orientation grooves 2.0 mm deep. The diamond should parallel the angle of the uncut incisal edge faciolingually.

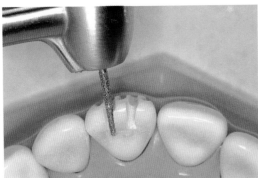

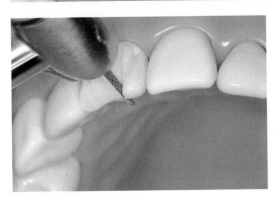

Fig. 15-11 Recommendations for incisal reduction range from 1.0[13,14] to 1.5,[14,15] to 2.0 mm.[13,16] To produce an adequate esthetic result, it is best to reduce the incisal edge by 2.0 mm, to the level of the depth-orientation grooves. Any greater reduction will increase the stress on the facial surface,[17–19] which can result in the facial half-moon fracture mentioned previously.[7–10] The plane of the reduced incisal surface should be parallel with the former incisal edge and, more importantly, perpendicular to the forces of mastication.[11,15,20] Failure to create this near-45-degree incisolingual bevel will produce excessive stress at the shoulder.[21]

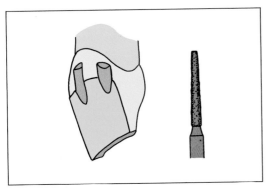

Fig. 15-12 Facial reduction, incisal half: flat end tapered diamond.

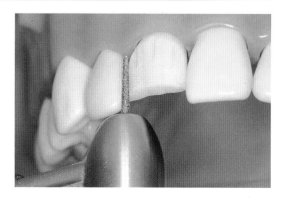

Fig. 15-13   The facial reduction should be done in two planes.[22] This permits the facio-incisal angle to be moved far enough lingually to permit enough porcelain for an esthetically satisfactory result, without endangering the pulp or over-tapering the preparation. The flat-end tapered diamond is employed for this purpose, removing all of the tooth structure remaining between the depth-orientation grooves incisal to the horizontal "break" across the facial surface of the tooth.

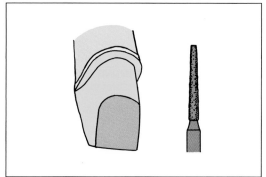

Fig. 15-14   Facial reduction, gingival half: flat-end tapered diamond.

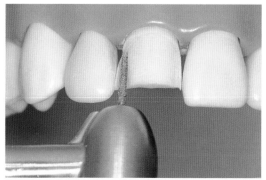

Fig. 15-15   The gingival half of the facial reduction is done with the same diamond, roughly cutting a shoulder finish line at the same time. This portion of the facial reduction is done so that it will exhibit a minimum amount of taper with the vertical lingual wall. There is general agreement that the axial reduction should be about 1.0 mm deep.[7,8,14,22]

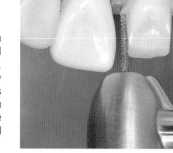

Fig. 15-16   Extend the facial reduction through the proximal surfaces with the flat-end tapered diamond, producing a shoulder in the process. The shoulder can be extended all the way around the lingual surface at this time, but in this sequence it is delayed until after the cingulum has been reduced. This helps to emphasize the distinction between the vertical lingual wall and the concave cingulum reduction.

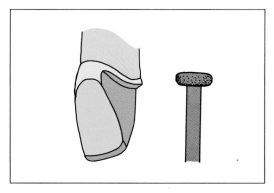

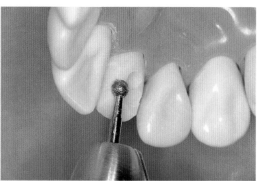

Fig. 15-17 Lingual reduction: small wheel diamond.

Fig. 15-18 To insure adequate reduction of the cingulum portion of the lingual reduction, make depth-orientation marks with a small ball diamond whose diameter is 1.4 mm larger than its shank. When the side of the diamond is sunk into the lingual surface to the shaft of the instrument, the cut will be 0.7 mm deep. Most teeth will require three of these benchmark cuts. Recommendations for reduction of the lingual surface range from 0.5 to 1.0 mm.[16,23–25]

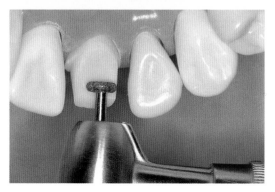

Fig. 15-19 Use the small round-edge wheel diamond to produce the concave cingulum reduction. By producing this concave shape, it is possible to achieve the greatest possible reduction in the middle of the lingual surface, where maximum clearance is needed on the majority of teeth. A distinct curve in the cingulum reduction also breaks the lingual surface into a horizontal component and an upright vertical segment, which can add to the retention and resistance of the preparation. Finally, the curved surface in this area will reduce stress,[17] while reduction done in a tapered plane or incline will produce greater tensile stress.[19] On a canine, the cingulum is reduced with a slight lingual ridge to divide the surface into two concavities, which increases rotational resistance.[11]

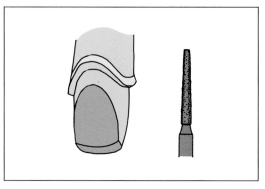

Fig. 15-20 Lingual axial reduction: flat-end tapered diamond.

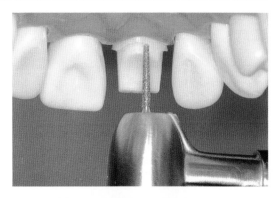

Fig. 15-21 Use the flat-end tapered diamond employed for the other axial reduction to prepare the vertical lingual wall. It should extend 1.0 mm into the tooth, and should exhibit very little taper in relation to the gingival portion of the facial surface. Minimal taper is highly recommended,[26–29] since an overtapered preparation lacks resistance[28] and can exert wedgelike forces on a restoration,[27] increasing stress[18] and even causing the crown to fracture.[9]

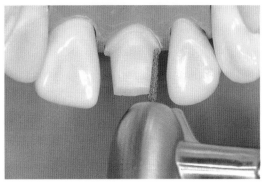

Fig. 15-22 Carefully blend the reduction of each axial surface with that on the adjacent axial surface (in this case the lingual and distal surfaces). If these junctions are not rounded over, the crown will be thin and prone to fracture in these transitional areas. A rectangular preparation with corners might create better stability, but a rounded preparation produces greater strength.[30]

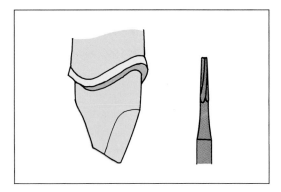

Fig. 15-23 Axial finishing: no. 171 bur.

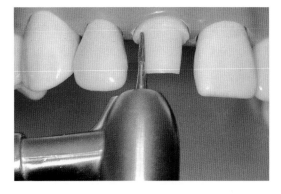

Fig. 15-24 Smooth the axial surfaces with a nondentate tapered fissure bur. Special burs of large diameter and extra length are less likely to nick and gouge the surface of the tooth, but a no. 171 will work well if used carefully.

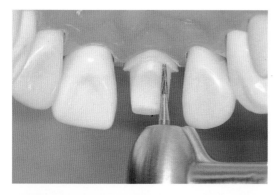

Fig. 15-25 Finish all of the axial surfaces of the preparation, again taking care to remove any residual angles at the corners of the tooth. Be especially careful to avoid creating any undercuts near the gingival shoulder of the preparation.

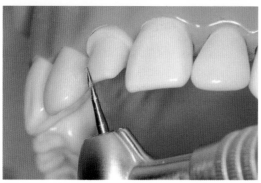

Fig. 15-26 Use the tapered fissure bur to round over all distinct positive angles on the preparation. If allowed to remain, sharp line angles will cause the crown to fracture.[9,27,31]

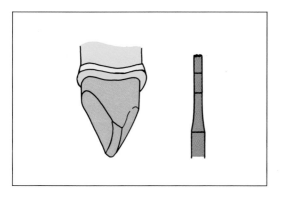

Fig. 15-27 Shoulder finishing: no. 957 bur.

Finishing the shoulder

A shoulder with a rounded internal angle is a different matter from that shown in Fig. 15-28. A sharp internal angle will not be reproduced by the porcelain[32] and is ineffective in supporting the porcelain.[16] A shoulderless crown, on the other hand, is likely to result in poor marginal fit and overcontouring.[33] The absence of interproximal shoulders will increase the strain on the mesial and distal aspects of the crown.[21]

A shoulder 1.0 mm wide is generally preferred.[8,13,16,22,23,25,31,34] Although widths of 0.5 to 1.0 mm have been mentioned,[11,13,15,22,23,25,26,29,31,35] shoulders narrower than 1.0 mm should be re-

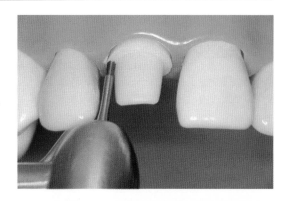

Fig. 15-28 A smoothly cut shoulder is generally accepted as the finish line of choice for this restoration. It should be perpendicular to the line of force,[8,20,24] or to the long axis of the tooth.[13,16,24] It will form a near right angle with the outer surface of tooth structure.[26] Although chamfers have occasionally been recommended for this purpose, a true chamfer forms an obtuse angle with the outer surface of the tooth, increasing stress as the shoulder angle is increased.[17]

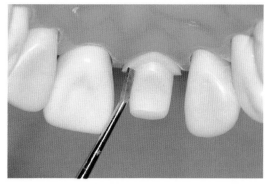

Fig. 15-29 To insure as even a shoulder as possible, a 1.0-mm-wide enamel hatchet is used to plane the surface of the shoulder and to check its width. It is neither necessary nor desirable to produce a sharp internal angle at the junction of the axial wall and the shoulder. A smoothly cut shoulder is essential to a well-fitting margin for the porcelain jacket crown.[24,32]

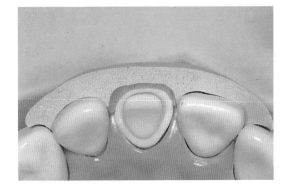

Fig. 15-30 The horizontal facial index is shown in place to verify the amount of facial reduction done incisogingivally at midpreparation.

served for those teeth too small to safely permit more than minimal destruction of tooth structure.

The shoulder is instrumented first with a flat-end diamond. An end-cutting diamond with a beveled edge, as recommended by Goldstein,[23] can produce less soft-tissue trauma. It also permits following the "up-and-down" incisogingival contours traced by the shoulder from the facial to the interproximal to the lingual aspects, without gouging nicks in the shoulder. The shoulder may be further smoothed with an end-cutting bur whose edge has been slightly beveled to prevent its digging in where the shoulder rises incisally.

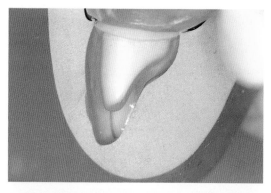

Fig. 15-31 Overall reduction can be checked with a midsaggital index. It can be seen here that the quality of reduction is essentially uniform.

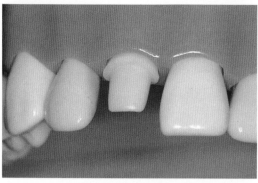

Fig. 15-32 This is an incisofacial view of the completed porcelain jacket crown preparation on a maxillary central incisor.

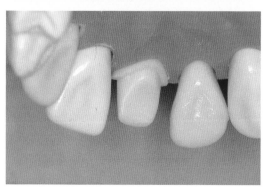

Fig. 15-33 A lingual view of the same preparation. Notice the absence of sharp line angles on the lingual and incisal aspects of the tooth preparation.

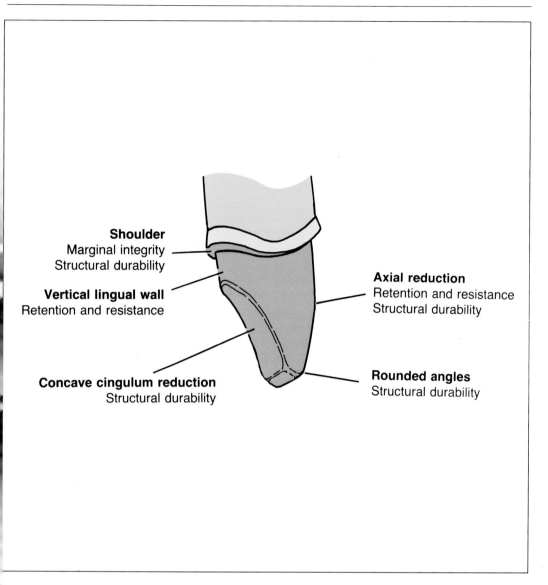

Shoulder
Marginal integrity
Structural durability

Vertical lingual wall
Retention and resistance

Concave cingulum reduction
Structural durability

Axial reduction
Retention and resistance
Structural durability

Rounded angles
Structural durability

Fig. 15-34 The features of a preparation for a porcelain jacket crown on an anterior tooth and the function served by each.

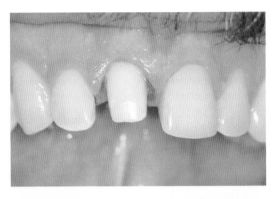

Fig. 15-35 Facial view of a porcelain jacket crown preparation on a maxillary central incisor.

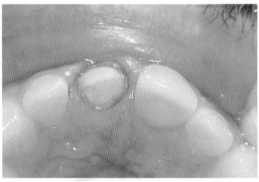

Fig. 15-36 Incisal view of the porcelain jacket crown preparation shown in Fig. 15-35.

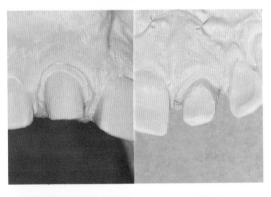

Fig. 15-37 Facial *(left)* and lingual *(right)* views of a stone cast of the porcelain jacket crown preparation.

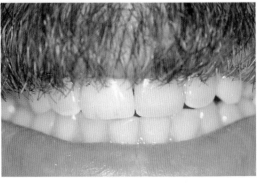

Fig. 15-38 The completed porcelain jacket crown.

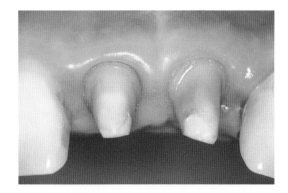

Fig. 15-39 Porcelain jacket crown preparations on both maxillary central incisors. (Photograph courtesy of Dr. Sumiya Hobo of Tokyo.)

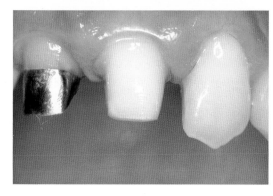

Fig. 15-40 A porcelain jacket crown preparation can be done on natural tooth structure or on a cast dowel-core if the tooth has been endodontically treated. (Photograph courtesy of Dr. Sumiya Hobo of Tokyo.)

There are several types of all-porcelain restorations whose fabrication processes involve some form of casting to produce part or all of the restoration.

Cast core

The Cerestore crown,* introduced in 1982,[3] utilizes a cast core. A coping wax pattern is fabricated on a heat-stable epoxy resin die. The die and wax pattern are invested in plaster, and the wax is removed with boiling water.

A thermoplastic pellet of compacted aluminous ceramic is heated to 160°C and is forced into the preheated mold cavity under pressure, forming a transfer-molded coping directly against the die. After cooling, the "green" ceramic coping is sufficiently strong to permit refinement with stones or burs. It is then removed from the die and fired at 1,295°C. Veneering layers of porcelain are added over the coping to complete the restoration.

Because the first layer of ceramic in this technique is molded directly against a die of the preparation, an excellent marginal fit is possible. Its compressive strength does not differ significantly from that of conventional aluminous porcelain crowns.[36] At the present time, this system is limited to single-unit restorations.

Ceramco Inc., East Windsor, N.J.

Cast crown

The second new way of fabricating all-ceramic crowns is by constructing a full-contour anatomic wax pattern and imbedding it in a special phosphate-bonded investment. Once the wax has been eliminated in a burnout furnace, a castable ceramic material is heated to a molten state and cast into the mold on a motor-driven centrifugal casting machine.

After cooling to room temperature, the casting of transparent amorphous glass is removed from the investment and imbedded in a refractory material for heat treatment to convert it into a semicrystalline translucent restoration. The first system using this technique was the Dicor,* whose "cerammed" restoration contains tetrasilicic fluormica crystals $(K_2Mg_5Si_8O_{20}F_4)$.[4] The other system is the Cerapearl,† whose end product is an artificial hydroxyapatite $Ca_{10}(PO_4)_6O$.[37] The specific shades for both systems are accomplished by applications of a surface colorant.

Each of these methods, whether using an injection cast ceramic coping or an entire cast crown, requires generous reduction of tooth structure to permit an adequate bulk of ceramic materials to give the restoration the strength needs. The following sequence show the preparation being done on a mandibular premolar (Figs. 15-41 to 15-71) and a clinical example is shown on a maxillary premolar (Figs. 15-72 to 15-78).

*Dentsply International, York, Pa.
†Bioceram Division, Kyocera International, Inc., San Diego, Calif.

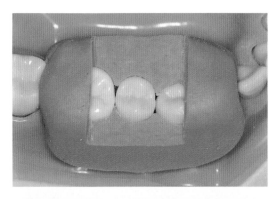

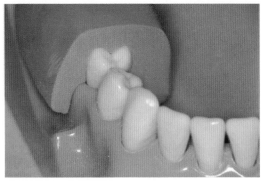

Cast ceramic crowns (Figs. 15-41 through 15-78)

Fig. 15-41 A combination facial and lingual index is made by adapting condensation-reaction silicone putty to the facial, lingual, and occlusal surfaces of a posterior tooth. After the material has polymerized it is removed from the mouth. The segment is removed by first making cuts along the midlines of the cusps mesial and distal to the tooth being prepared. These cuts are joined by a horizontal slice made on each of the facial and lingual surfaces. By virtue of its orientation on the occlusal surfaces of the adjacent teeth, this index will provide an accurate reference for both facial and lingual reduction.

Fig. 15-42 A midsagittal index, cut along the vertical midline of a single-rooted tooth or the midline of the mesial cusp of a molar, can also be used to check reduction. It can be used instead of, or in addition to, the facial/lingual index. It will, of course, require a second mix of silicone putty.

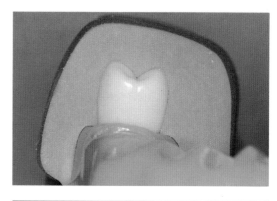

Fig. 15-43 This closeup of the midsaggital index with the adjacent teeth removed demonstrates the close adaptation of the silicone putty to the midline of the unprepared tooth.

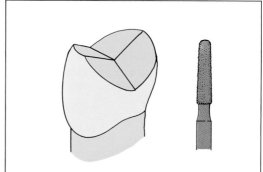

Fig. 15-44 Occlusal reduction: large round-end tapered diamond.

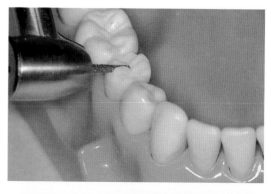

Fig. 15-45 Use a large round-end tapered diamond to place depth-orientation grooves on the occlusal surface. There should be one on each triangular ridge, and one in each major groove to the mesial or distal of the triangular ridge.

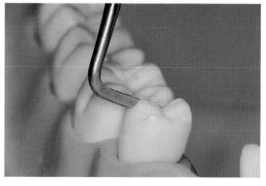

Fig. 15-46 Use a 1.5- or 2.0-mm-wide enamel hatchet to measure the depth of the orientation grooves. The final occlusal reduction should be 1.5[4,38–40] to 2.0 mm deep.[4,38–41]

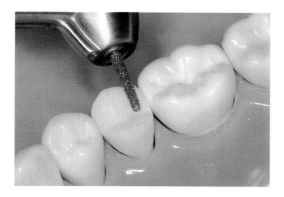

Fig. 15-47 Remove the tooth structure remaining between the depth-orientation grooves with the large round-end tapered diamond. The reduction will follow the geometric inclined planes of the occlusal surface to insure sufficient bulk of material, support for porcelain, and preparation length.

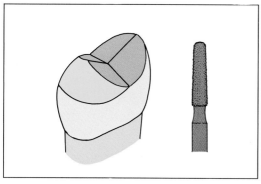

Fig. 15-48 Functional cusp bevel: large round-end tapered diamond.

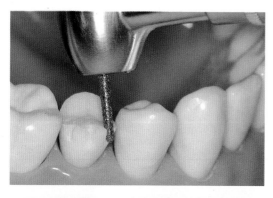

Fig. 15-49 Use the same round-end tapered diamond to produce depth-orientation grooves for the functional cusp bevel, which in this case is the facial incline of the facial cusp.

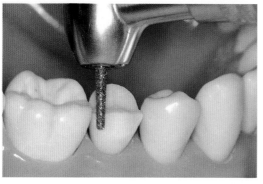

Fig. 15-50 Create the functional cusp bevel to insure that the facial incline of the facial cusp will have the same porcelain thickness as the lingual incline. On a maxillary tooth, the reduction would be on the lingual incline of the lingual cusp. The functional cusp bevel roughly parallels the inclines of the cusps of the opposing teeth.

Fig. 15-51 Check the occlusal reduction by having the patient bite on a 1.5-mm leaf of a thickness gauge.* If the guide can be pulled through the reduced area from the facial, it indicates that a minimum of 1.5 mm of clearance has been achieved. If the guide cannot be drawn through, more reduction will be required. Have the patient bite on a piece of red utility wax to determine where the extra reduction is needed.

*Flexible Clearance Guide, Belle de St. Claire, Van Nuys, Calif.

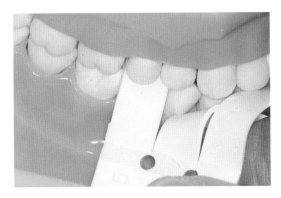

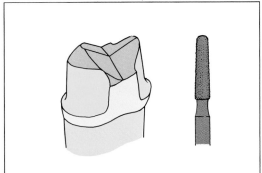

Fig. 15-52 Facial and lingual axial reduction: large round-end tapered diamond.

Fig. 15-53 Make depth-orientation grooves on the facial and lingual surfaces to insure that adequate reduction will be achieved. Axial reduction amounts of 1.0, 1.2, and 1.5 mm have been recommended.[4,38,40,41] In order to achieve a minimum thickness of 1.0 mm of porcelain at the gingival finish line, it is necessary to have 1.5 mm or slightly less of axial reduction at mid-crown. Because more tooth structure is removed for the occlusal reduction and the functional cusp bevel of this preparation than for most preparations, the functional cusp bevel will probably serve the function of making the facial reduction in two planes.

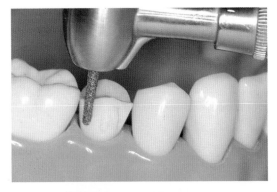

Fig. 15-54 Remove the tooth structure remaining between the depth-orientation grooves, carrying the axial reduction as far into the facial embrasures as possible without nicking the adjacent teeth. A large round-end tapered diamond is used for the axial reduction so that a shoulder with a rounded internal angle can be formed at the same time as the axial reduction. Although either a 135-degree chamfer or a shoulder can be used to prepare this type of crown,[38,40,41] a shoulder is preferred because it insures enough material in the axial walls and marginal area of the restoration.

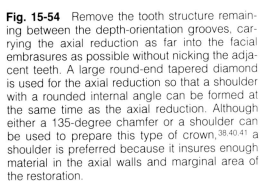

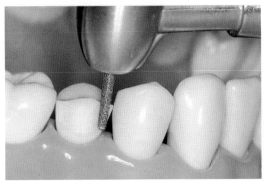

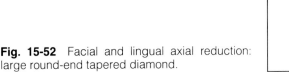

311

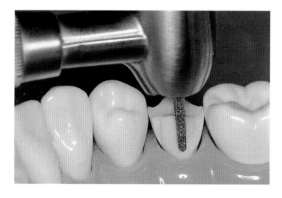

Fig. 15-55 Repeat the process on the lingual surface, making sure to achieve the same amount of reduction produced on the facial surface. A shoulder finish line, with a rounded internal angle, will result from this reduction.

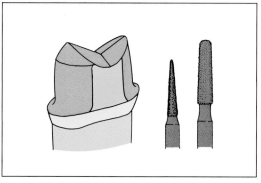

Fig. 15-56 Complete axial reduction: short-needle and large round-end tapered diamonds.

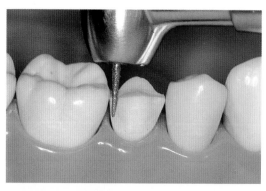

Fig. 15-57 Use the short-needle diamond to begin the proximal axial reduction. Avoid touching the adjacent tooth with the instrument, but do not overtaper the wall in the process.

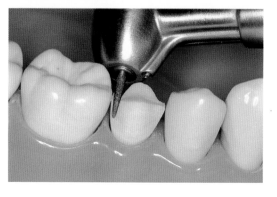

Fig. 15-58 It may be necessary to lay the diamond over in a horizontal attitude along the marginal ridge to begin the cut into the interproximal area.

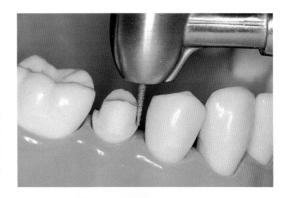

Fig. 15-59 Repeat the process on the other proximal surface. As more space is created, the needle diamond can be brushed across the entire proximal surface to produce more reduction and a smoother surface. The finish line may still be a bit irregular at this point, but that will be remedied shortly.

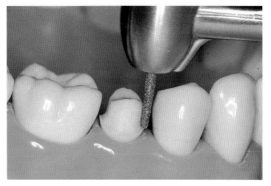

Fig. 15-60 Complete the axial reduction interproximally by running the round-end tapered diamond, which will now fit, across the mesial and distal surfaces. Carefully blend the proximal axial reduction and shoulder with those of the facial and lingual surfaces. Sharp angles at the junctions of the proximal and facial or lingual surfaces will produce unacceptable irregularities or notches in the shoulder and stress points in the axial surfaces of the ceramic crown.

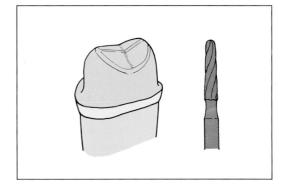

Fig. 15-61 Preparation finishing: round-end tapered carbide bur.

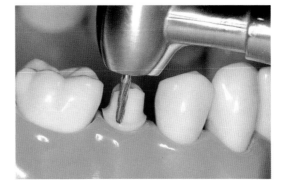

Fig. 15-62 The axial surfaces should be planed smooth at this time, using a carbide finishing bur. A large torpedo-shaped bur, such as an H282-016* whose tip has been blunted to facilitate its use on a shoulder, or an 1157L long rounded fissure bur* can be used.

*Brasseler USA Inc., Savannah, Ga.

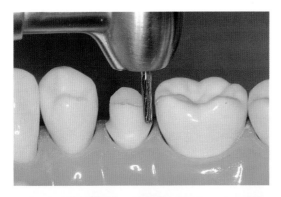

Fig. 15-63 Continue the smoothing process into the interproximal areas, taking care to blend in any corners that might still be present in the line angle regions of the tooth. Smooth the shoulder itself at this time.

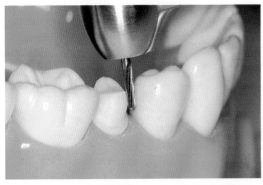

Fig. 15-64 Use the carbide finishing bur to finish the functional cusp bevel, removing all sharp angles in the process.

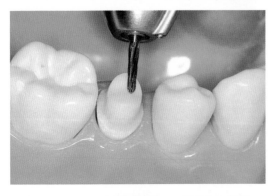

Fig. 15-65 Go over the occlusal reduction in the same manner. While the inclined planes should be distinct, any sharp angles where they intersect should be removed.

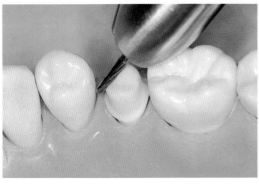

Fig. 15-66 Because of their stress-generating potential in the final restoration, no sharp angles can be permitted on this type of preparation.[38,40,41]

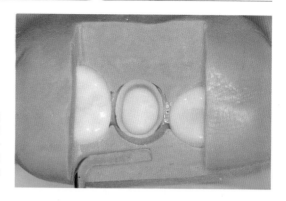

Fig. 15-67 The horizontal index, when viewed from the occlusal aspect, shows the amount of axial reduction on both the facial and lingual surfaces. A 1.5-mm-wide enamel hatchet has been placed on the index to allow comparison of the axial reduction with it.

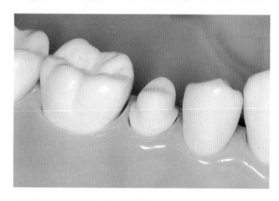

Fig. 15-68 The 1.5-mm-wide enamel hatchet is shown superimposed over a midsaggital index to reveal the amount of occlusal and axial reduction.

Fig. 15-69 Facial view of the preparation for an all-ceramic crown on a mandibular premolar.

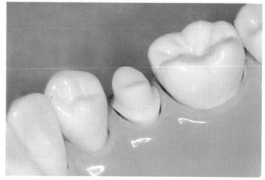

Fig. 15-70 Lingual view of the preparation for an all-ceramic crown.

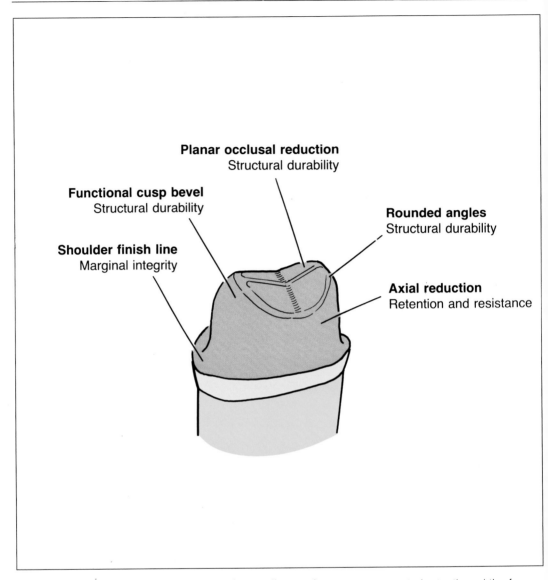

Planar occlusal reduction
Structural durability

Functional cusp bevel
Structural durability

Rounded angles
Structural durability

Shoulder finish line
Marginal integrity

Axial reduction
Retention and resistance

Fig. 15-71 The features of a preparation for an all-ceramic crown on a posterior tooth and the function served by each.

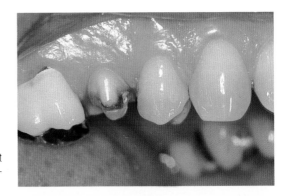

Fig. 15-72 Facial view of preparation for a cast ceramic crown on maxillary right second premolar. Notice the ample occlusal reduction.

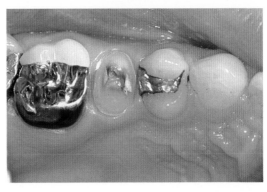

Fig. 15-73 Occlusal view of the preparation seen in Fig. 15-72. In this view, the shoulder of uniform width can be seen completely encompassing the tooth.

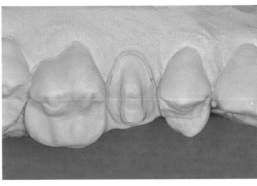

Fig. 15-74 An occlusofacial view of a stone cast of the same preparation.

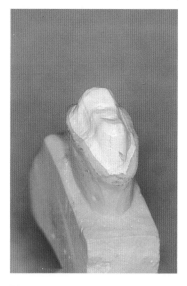

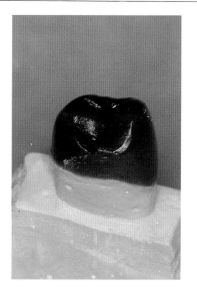

Fig. 15-75a The die has been painted with a cement spacer whose color is keyed to the desired shade of the restoration, matching the color of the final cement.

Fig. 15-75b The completed wax pattern for the cast ceramic crown.

Fig. 15-76 The cast ceramic crown* is shown on the die. After casting and removal of investment *(left)*. After ceramming *(middle)*. After shading and glazing*(right)*.

*Dicor, Dentsply International, York, Pa.

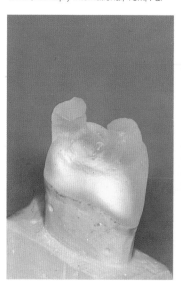

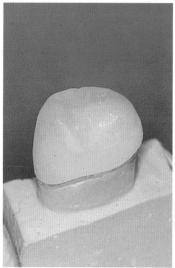

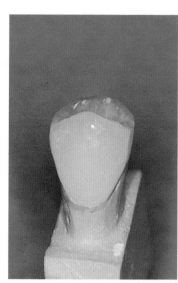

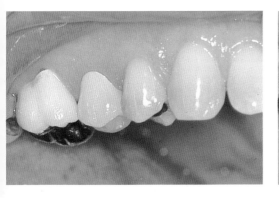

Fig. 15-77 Facial view of the completed crown in the mouth.

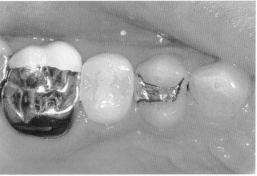

Fig. 15-78 Occlusal view of the cemented cast ceramic crown.

References

1. Vorhees, F. H. History and progress of the cast gold inlay. J. Am. Dent. Assoc. 17:2111, 1930.
2. Carmichael, J. P. Attachment for inlay and bridgework. Dent. Rev. 15:82, 1901.
3. Sozio, R. B., and Riley, E. J. The shrink-free ceramic crown. J. Prosthet. Dent. 49:182, 1983.
4. Grossman, D. G. Processing a dental ceramic by casting methods. Presented at Conference on Recent Developments in Ceramic and Ceramic-Metal Systems for Crown and Bridge. Ann Arbor: W. K. Kellogg Foundation Institute, Oct. 10–12, 1983. Available from Dentsply, York, Pa.
5. Hobo, S., and Iwata, T. Castable apatite ceramics as a new biocompatible restorative material. II. Fabrication of the restoration. Quint. Int. 16:207, 1985.
6. McLean, J. W., and Hughes, T.H. The reinforcement of dental porcelain with ceramic oxides. Br. Dent. J. 119:251, 1965.
7. Bartels, J. C. Preparation of the anterior teeth for porcelain jacket crowns. J. South. Calif. Dent. Assoc. 30:199, 1962.
8. Klaffenbach, A. O. Science, art and ceramic fundamentals involved in porcelain jacket prosthesis. Aust. Dent. J. 55:88, 1951.
9. Ewing, J. E. Beautiful but glum: Porcelain jacket crowns. J. Prosthet. Dent. 4:94, 1954.
10. Saklad, M. J. The disclosure of cleavage and fracture lines in porcelain restorations. J. Prosthet. Dent. 8:115, 1958.
11. LeGro, A. L. Ceramics in Dentistry. Brooklyn: Dental Items of Interest Publishing Co., 1925, 12.
12. Walton, C. B. Methodical jacket crown preparation. J. Am. Dent. Assoc. 47:1, 1953.
13. Avary, H. Classification of teeth as a guiding factor in the correct preparation for porcelain jacket crowns. J. Natl. Dent. Assoc. 63:233, 1921.
14. Bartels, J. C. Full porcelain veneer crowns. J. Prosthet. Dent. 7:533, 1957.
15. Doxtater, L. W. The porcelain jacket crown. Dent. Items Interest 50:886, 1928.

16. Southan, D. E. The porcelain jacket crown. pp. 207–230 In J. W. McLean (ed.) Dental Ceramics: Proceedings of the 1st International Symposium on Ceramics. Chicago: Quintessence Publishing Co., 1983.

17. Derand, T. Studies of porcelain jacket crowns by means of two-dimensional photoelastic experiments. Odont. Rev. 24:373, 1973.

18. Derand, T. Effect of variation of the shape of the core on stresses in a loaded model of a porcelain crown. Odont. Rev. 25:11, 1974.

19. Derand, T. Analysis of stresses in loaded models of porcelain crowns. Odont. Rev. 25:189, 1974.

20. Oppice, H. W. A resume of ideas on porcelain jacket crown preparations. J. Am. Dent. Assoc. 21:1030, 1934.

21. Lehman, M. L., and Hampson, E. L. A study of strain patterns in jacket crowns on anterior teeth resulting from different tooth preparations. Br. Dent. J. 113:337, 1962.

22. Fairley, J. M., and Deubert, L. W. Preparation of a maxillary central incisor for a porcelain jacket restoration. Br. Dent. J. 104:208, 1958.

23. Goldstein, R. E. Esthetics in Dentistry. Philadelphia: J. B. Lippencott Co., 1976, 333.

24. Bastian, C. C. The all porcelain jacket crown by the indirect method. Dent. Cosmos 65:1285, 1923.

25. McLean, J. W. The alumina reinforced porcelain jacket crown. J. Am. Dent. Assoc. 75:621, 1967.

26. Vehe, W. D. Some basic principles underlying porcelain veneer crown technic. J. Am. Dent. Assoc. 17:2167, 1930.

27. Pettrow, J. N. Practical factors in building and firing characteristics of dental porcelain. J. Prosthet. Dent. 11:334, 1961.

28. Nuttall, E. B. Factors influencing success of porcelain jacket restorations. J. Prosthet. Dent. 11:743, 1961.

29. Minker, J. S. Simplified full coverage preparations. Dent. Clin. North Am. 9:355, 1965.

30. Walton, C. B., and Levin, M. M. A preliminary report of photoelastic tests of strain patterns within jacket crowns. J. Am. Dent. Assoc. 50:44, 1955.

31. Argue, J. E. The preparation of teeth for porcelain jacket crowns. J. Am. Dent. Assoc. 17:1259, 1930.

32. Derand, T. The importance of an even shoulder preparation in porcelain crowns. Odont. Rev. 23:305, 1972.

33. Bastian, C. C. The porcelain jacket crown: Its usefulness in removable bridgework. J. Am. Dent. Assoc. 13:226, 1926.

34. Sharp, T. B. Preparations for and construction of baked porcelain crowns and inlays. J. Prosthet. Dent. 9:113, 1959.

35. Iwansson, R. Porcelain jacket crown construction: Some frequent causes of failure and how to avoid them. Dent. Cosmos 73:329, 1931.

36. Philip, G. K., and Brukl, C. E. Compressive strengths of conventional, twin foil, and all-ceramic crowns. J. Prosthet. Dent. 52:215, 1984.

37. Hobo, S., and Iwata, T. Castable apatite ceramics as a new biocompatible restorative material. I. Theroretical considerations. Quint. Int. 16:135, 1985.

38. Adair, P. J., and Grossman, D. G. The castable ceramic crown. Int. J. Periodont. Rest. Dent. 4:(2):33, 1984.

39. Malament, K. The castable ceramic crown: A new evolution in the science and art of fixed prosthodontics. In J. Preston (ed.) Proceedings of the 4th International Symposium on Ceramics. Chicago: Quintessence Publishing Co., 1987 (in press).

40. Cerestore System: Clinical Procedures. East Windsor, NJ: Ceramco, Inc., 1983, 5.

41. Hobo, S., and Iwata, T. Castable apatite ceramics as a new biocompatible restorative material. II. Fabrication of the restoration. Quint. Int. 16:207, 1985.

Chapter 16

Preparation Modifications for Damaged Teeth

The preparations described in the preceding chapters are designed to provide the maximum retention and resistance consistent with the principles of tooth preparation: preservation of tooth structure, structural durability, periodontal health, and marginal integrity. However, classic preparation designs can be employed without modification only on bridge abutments that are virtually intact, and on severely damaged teeth following the restoration of coronal bulk with amalgam, composite resin, or cast dowel-cores.

Most individual teeth requiring cemented restorations and a large percentage of bridge abutments will have suffered enough damage from caries or trauma to necessitate deviation from the classic preparation form. Although unmodified classic tooth preparations can be used in relatively few clinical situations, they should be firmly fixed in the operator's mind. Every feature has a definite purpose, and when conditions preclude placement of a feature in a classic pattern, some other geometric feature must be improvised to fill its role.

Because every damaged tooth is different, it would be impossible to describe a "correct" preparation for each individual circumstance. Following are general rules and examples of typical situations to guide the operator in selecting and executing a suitable restoration and preparation design.

It should be noted that for many teeth, the objectives of tooth restoration are best met with direct filling materials such as amalgam and composite resin. The greatest advantage of cast metal over direct filling materials is its greater tensile strength. For small restorations which are held in place and protected by surrounding tooth structure, that greater tensile strength is not needed. A gold inlay might be selected for restoration of a small lesion where above normal abrasion is expected, such as under the clasp of a partial denture, or where amalgam in contact with an existing gold restoration might cause objectionable galvanism.

If the restoration is to extend outside the dimensions of the original tooth in order to restore contact with adjacent or opposing teeth, cast metal would be in-

Fig. 16-1 Treatment planning for vital and endodontically treated anterior teeth.

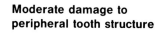

Vital Teeth

Minimal damage to peripheral tooth structure	**Moderate damage to peripheral tooth structure**	**Moderate to severe damage to peripheral tooth structure**

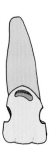 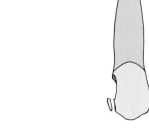 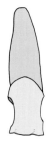

Proximal caries or small Class V lesion.

One incisal angle involved.

Both incisal angles involved.

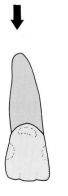 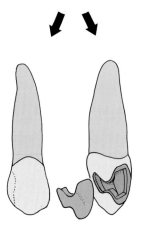 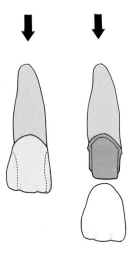

Composite resin.

Composite resin.
Class III inlay on distal of canine only.

Composite resin can be used, but prognosis is guarded.
Porcelain jacket crown or porcelain-fused-to-metal crown.

| **Severe damage to peripheral tooth structure** | **Moderate damage to central tooth structure** | **Severe damage to central tooth structure** | **Minimal damage** | **Moderate damage** |

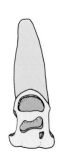 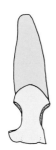 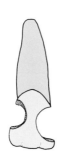 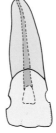 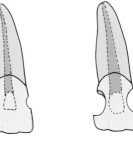

| More than 50% of tooth surface (peripheral) involved. | Deep proximal lesions impinging on "vital core" (central). | More than 50% of "vital core" destroyed (central). | Endodontic access and small proximal lesions (combined). | Endodontic access; large proximal lesions; possible loss of incisal angle(s) (combined). |

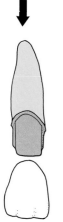 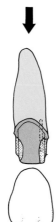 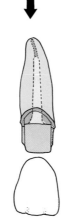 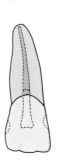 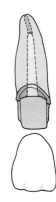

| Porcelain jacket crown or porcelain-fused-to-metal crown. | Porcelain jacket crown or porcelain-fused-to-metal crown with cement base and/or pin-composite resin core. | Devitalization, dowel-core and porcelain jacket crown or porcelain-fused-to-metal crown. | Composite resin restorations on lingual as well as proximal surfaces. | Dowel-core and porcelain jacket crown or porcelain-fused-to-metal crown. |

Fig. 16-2 Treatment planning for vital posterior teeth.

Minimal damage

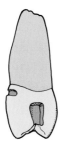 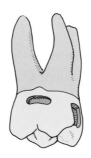

Small occlusal (central) lesion, proximal and/or facial lesions (peripheral), occlusal and proximal (combined).

Moderate damage

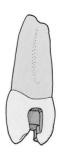 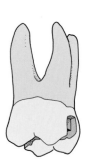

Occlusal lesion 1.0 mm past DEJ (central), proximal or facial lesion 1.0 mm past DEJ (peripheral), occlusal and proximal (combined).

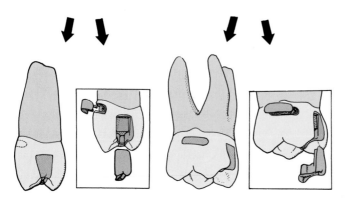

Occlusal and Class II restorations done in amalgam except in esthetically critical areas where composite resin is used. Inlays can be used. Composite resin used on facial surface in esthetic zone.

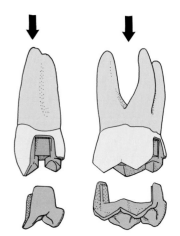

Amalgam over cement base for occlusal and Class II lesions in molars. Combined lesions may require MOD onlays. Composite resin over base used on facial surface in esthetic zone.

Moderate to severe damage

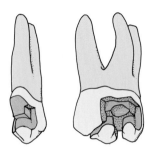

Severe damage

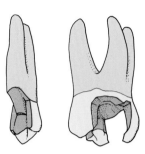

Total coronal destruction

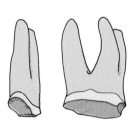

Central destruction extends into core of tooth. Peripheral destruction may cover up to 50% of tooth surface. One missing cusp (combined).

Central destruction extends into core of tooth and much of supporting dentin. Peripheral damage greater than 50% of tooth surface.

Central destruction includes most of core. Any remaining enamel is undermined.

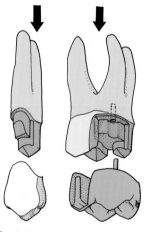

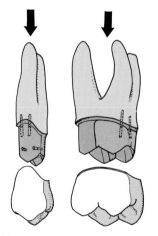

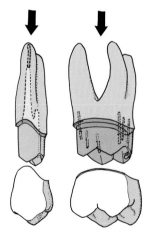

Peripheral damage alone restored with crown. Core (central) involvement alone may be restored with onlay.

Extensive peripheral damage without core (central) involvement restored with crown only. Pin-amalgam core needed before crown placement with extensive central destruction.

Pin-amalgam core needed before fabrication of crown on molar. Elective devitalization and dowel-core usually required on premolars before crown is constructed.

Fig. 16-3 Treatment planning for endodontically treated posterior teeth.

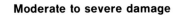

| **Minimal damage** | **Moderate to severe damage** |

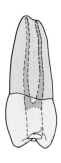 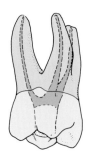 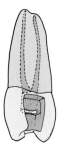 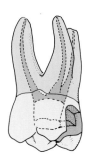

Minimal core destruction (central) from endodontic access with slight proximal (peripheral) involvement. No facial or lingual damage.

Loss of supporting dentin, wider proximal boxes, or more extensive surface (peripheral) involvement.

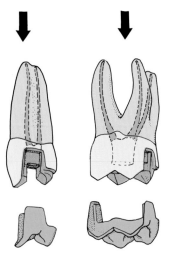 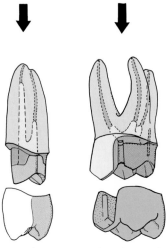

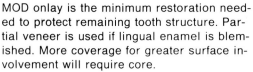

MOD onlay is the minimum restoration needed to protect remaining tooth structure. Partial veneer is used if lingual enamel is blemished. More coverage for greater surface involvement will require core.

Dowel-core (cast or made with prefabricated dowels and amalgam or composite resin) and crown for premolars. Amalgam core (with or without pins) for molar.

Total coronal destruction

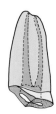
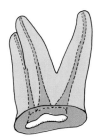

Loss of all supragingival tooth structure.

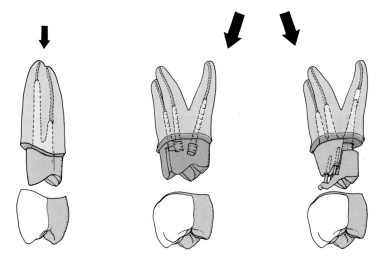

Dowel-core and crown for premolar may need to be preceded by crown lengthening surgery. Molar should have dowels to give lateral resistance to amalgam core, or two-piece dowel-core under crown.

dicated because of the greater restoration extension required to distribute the contour change over a wide area, and because of the greater stress to which the material would be subjected.

The amount of tooth structure destroyed is not the only factor to be considered in selecting a restorative material and designing a preparation. Of equal importance is the location of the destruction and the amount of the tooth surface involved. Location can be classified as *peripheral,* or occurring on the axial surfaces of the tooth; *central,* occurring in the center of the tooth; and *combined,* which includes destruction in both sites.[1]

Treatment planning guides are presented for anterior teeth (Fig. 16-1), vital posterior teeth (Fig. 16-2), and endodontically treated posterior teeth (Fig. 16-3).

Modifications for damaged vital teeth

Most modifications consist of squaring the walls of cavities left by removal of caries and old restorations, and adding features to enhance retention and resistance. Because this requires cutting into an already weakened tooth, two rules must be observed to avoid excessive tooth destruction for the sake of retention:

1. When treating vital teeth, the central or "vital core," consisting of the pulp and the surrounding layer of protective dentin approximately 1.0 mm thick, must not be invaded.[2] No retentive features should be cut deeper into the tooth than 1.5 mm at the

cervical line or down 1.5 mm from the central fossa (Fig. 16-4). If caries removal results in a deeper cavity, any part lying within the vital core should be filled with an insulating cement. Any tooth preparation done for mechanical retention is kept in the safe area of the tooth that is peripheral to the vital core.

2. No remaining wall of dentin should ever be reduced for the sake of retention to a thickness less than its height. Sometimes this may preclude the use of a full veneer crown, or if one must be used, it might first require the placement of a core.

The restoration of damaged teeth should be approached in an organized manner. For vital teeth, the steps are as follows:

1. Evaluate the condition of the pulp and periodontal tissues and make a preliminary decision on the design of the restoration.
2. Remove all caries and old restorations.
3. Reevaluate the strength of the remaining walls and decide on the final preparation design.
4. Execute the chosen design.

Pulpal considerations

The condition of the pulp is an important factor in determining the design of the preparation. If the tooth has not suffered a pulp exposure, is asymptomatic, displays no radiographic evidence of periapical pathology, responds normally to an electric pulp tester, and has adequate coronal tooth structure for retention and resistance, every effort should be made to maintain the vitality

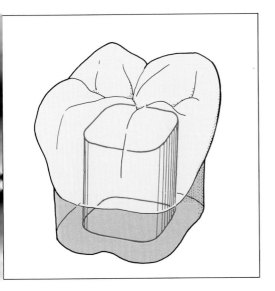

Fig. 16-4 No retentive features should be cut into the "vital core" of the tooth (shaded area) if its vitality is to be preserved.

of the pulp. While skillfully performed endodontic treatment is usually successful, there is always some risk of failure. Even when successful, it weakens the tooth and increases the expense for the patient.

However, if the condition of the pulp is doubtful, or if an exposure, however small, should occur during tooth preparation, the pulp should be removed and the canals obturated before a cast restoration is placed.[3] Otherwise there is too great a risk that the restoration will subsequently need to be perforated to perform endodontic treatment. If there is any likelihood that the pulp will become involved, the patient should be warned before the preparation is started that endodontic treatment may become necessary. A statement that is accepted as a reasonable explanation before the fact will sound like a feeble alibi when proffered after the fact.

Periodontal condition

Carefully evaluate the periodontal tissue surrounding the tooth to be restored, with special emphasis on deep subgingival extensions of caries, fractures, or previous restorations. Deep placement of the finish line which violates the "biologic width" of 2.0 mm of epithelial and connective tissue attachment, may require periodontal surgery before an adequate restoration can be made.[4,5] To do otherwise could result in a compromised restoration surrounded by chronically inflamed tissue.

Removal of caries and previous restorations

Before the final design of the restoration can be selected, all caries and old restorations must be removed. Even though an existing restoration appears sound on the surface, it may conceal caries or a pulp exposure. A calcium-hydroxide–containing cavity liner should be placed in deep cavities as soon as practicable to protect the pulp from the effects of drying and temperature changes while the preparation is being completed.

Reevaluation

The decision must now be made whether to incorporate the defects left in the tooth by removal of caries and old restorations into the preparation, or to fill them in. If more than 50% of the coronal tooth structure of a posterior tooth is sound, and the tooth will not be a bridge abutment, sufficient retention can be achieved by adding supplemen-

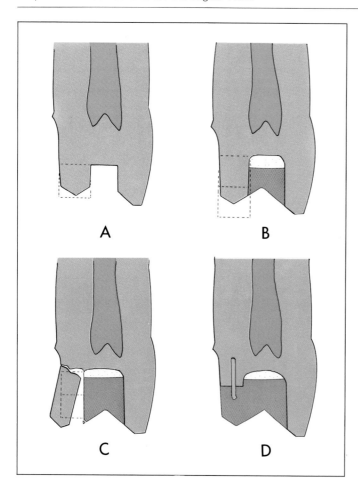

A   B

C   D

Fig. 16-5 A cavity can be used as an internal retention feature if the surrounding walls are at least as thick as they are long *(A)*. If a cusp's thickness is less than its height, an amalgam core should be placed *(B)*. If the thickness is less than half the height, there is danger of fracture even with an amalgam core *(C)*. Tall thin cusps should be shortened and built up with pin-retained amalgam *(D)*.

tal features to the tooth. For an internal feature such as an isthmus or a box form to be effective, the surrounding walls of dentin should be at least as wide as they are tall (Fig. 16-5, *A*). If the thickness/height ratio of the remaining walls lies between 1:1 and 1:2, the cavity should be filled with amalgam to support the weakened walls (Fig. 16-5, *B*). Any walls with thickness/height ratios of less than 1:2 are subject to fracture (Fig. 16-5, *C*) and should be shortened (Fig. 16-5, *D*).

The choices for anterior teeth are more limited because of esthetic requirements and the smaller bulk of dentin in which supplemental features can be placed. Modifications of the classic anterior preparations are limited to substitution of a box for a groove to encompass a carious lesion, or addition of extra grooves or pinholes. If more than one-third of the coronal structure is lost, placement of a pin-retained core followed by a porcelain-fused-to-metal crown is usually indicated.

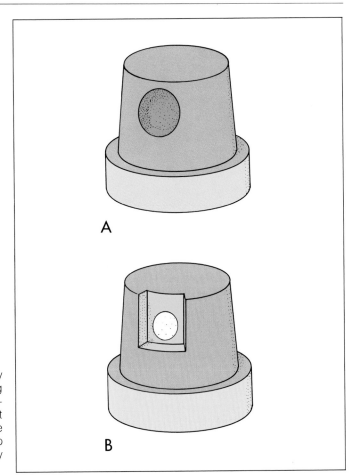

A

B

Fig. 16-6 A cavity was formed by removal of caries *(A)*. Converting the cavity into a box increases retention *(B)*. The part of a cavity that extends into the vital core of the tooth must be filled with cement to protect the pulp and eliminate any remaining undercut.

Protection of remaining tooth structure

An important aspect of restoring damaged teeth is the protection of remaining tooth structure. Teeth already weakened by the loss of large amounts of tooth structure are ill equipped to withstand unassisted the forces of occlusion. Protection can be provided by capping the cusps with the occlusal surface of the cast restoration.[6,7] The occlusal thickness should be 1.0 mm over the nonfunctional cusps and 1.5 mm over the functional cusps.

Conversion of defects into retentive features

Defects can be incorporated into the preparation if they are not too extensive. Any carious lesion or previous restoration that extends deeper than 1.5 mm into a vital tooth should be filled to that level with an insulating cement. The walls of the remaining defect should be shaped to remove undercuts and provide vertical walls nearly parallel with the path of insertion (Fig. 16-6).

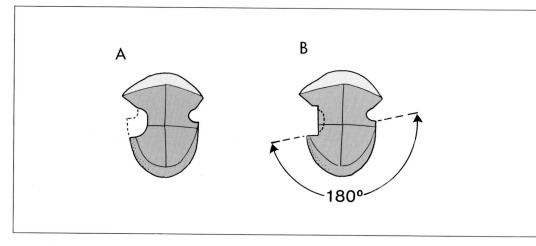

Fig. 16-7 In this occlusal view of a premolar being prepared for a three-quarter crown, destruction has occurred beyond the outline of a standard mesial groove *(A)*. The defect is converted into a box to substitute for the groove of the classic design *(B)*. Ideally, there should be no less than 180 degrees of sound tooth structure remaining between the box and the opposite groove.

Fig. 16-8 If less than 180 degrees of the tooth's circumference remains between the box and the groove, the lingual cusp may fracture during function *(A)*. Moving the distal groove onto the facial surface compensates for the overextended mesial box *(B)*.

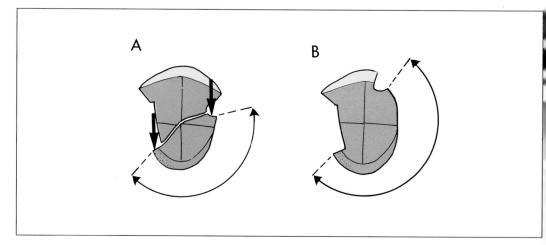

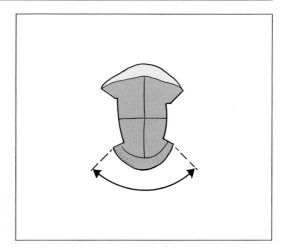

Fig. 16-9 Not enough of the lingual cusp remains to support a three-quarter crown. Supplemental pin retention or full coverage must be employed.

Box forms

By using a box form, it is possible to take advantage of well defined opposing upright surfaces of tooth structure at the periphery of a damaged area. It is the walls of the box, and not the line angles, that will resist displacement.[8] Because it does require removal of large quantities of tooth structure, the box is not usually used on an intact surface.

If there is a small interproximal carious lesion or prior restoration, a box usually can be substituted for the classic grooves to serve the dual purpose of caries removal and retention form (Fig. 16-7, A).[9-15] Boxes provide excellent retention and resistance for three-quarter crown preparations, if at least half the circumference (180 degrees) remains in the area between the lingual walls of the boxes or grooves (Fig. 16-7, B). If the preparation encircles less than 180 degrees, the lingual cusp may be overstressed and could fracture under lingually directed forces (Fig. 16-8, A). If esthetics permit, the distal groove can be placed farther than normal onto the facial surface to compensate for a large mesial box (Fig. 16-8, B).

If both mesial and distal surfaces are involved too extensively, another means must be found to compensate for the diminished lingual tooth structure (Fig. 16-9). Possible solutions include changing the design to a full-coverage restoration, or placing a pin-retained amalgam core followed by a classic three-quarter crown preparation.

Orientation of sloping surfaces

On broad sloping surfaces left after cusp fracture or excavation of large carious lesions, it is better to form multiple small steps than to excessively weaken the remaining dentin or risk pulpal encroachment by attempting to form one long vertical wall (Fig. 16-10). The incline is broken into vertical and horizontal components. Horizontal surfaces are perpendicular to the path of insertion and increase resistance to compression, while the vertical surfaces are aligned with the path of insertion to assist retention and resistance to tipping.

If the sloping surface does not cover too much of the tooth, there will be only

333

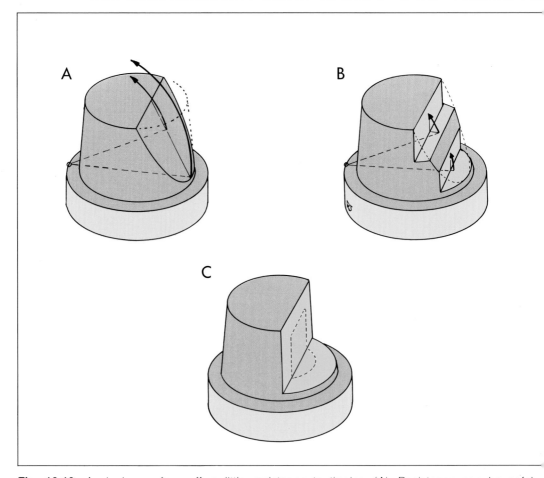

Fig. 16-10 A sloping surface offers little resistance to tipping *(A)*. Resistance can be safely enhanced by breaking the slope into steps with vertical walls and horizontal surfaces *(B)*. Conversion of the inclined surface into one long vertical wall is contraindicated. This would unnecessarily weaken the tooth and endanger the vitality of the pulp *(C)*.

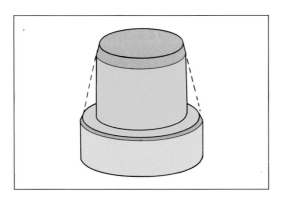

Fig. 16-11 An overtapered axial wall (broken outline) has been made more retentive by creating a gingival shoulder. This allows the vertical walls to be more nearly parallel.

one horizontal component, which will take the form of a peripheral shoulder (Fig. 16-11).

Addition of retention and resistance features

After the tooth has been prepared according to the initial design, it should be evaluated for adequacy of retention and resistance. Conditions that require addition of supplemental retentive features are missing or weakened cusps, short preparations, excessive taper, and the use of the teeth as bridge abutments.

Retention and resistance are increased by adding surfaces aligned nearly perpendicular to the path of insertion and located so that they will oppose an intact wall, resisting tipping of the restoration. This can be accomplished by extending coverage onto axial surfaces that would otherwise be left intact, or by cutting grooves and pinholes into the remaining sound tooth structure to be occupied by ribs and pins of metal in the final cast restoration.

Grooves

Grooves placed in vertical walls of bulk tooth structure are, for all practical purposes, miniature boxes. To be effective, they must be well formed, at least 1.0 mm in diameter (depth as well as width), and as long as possible without encroaching on the finish line. Multiple grooves are as effective as box forms in providing resistance,[16] and they can be placed in axial walls without excessive destruction of tooth structure. They may also be added to the angles of over-

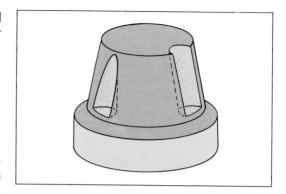

Fig. 16-12 The groove on the left has been cut parallel with the path of insertion. This is more effective for limiting the path of insertion and increasing resistance than is the groove on the right, which has been incorrectly cut to parallel the overtapered axial wall.

sized box forms to augment the resistance provided by the box walls. This is especially useful when the facial and lingual walls of a box are a considerable distance apart.

Grooves should be used judiciously in light of the finding of Tjan and associates that multiple grooves placed in full crown preparations adversely affect the seating of full veneer crowns.[17] However, a groove in the preparation that is not occupied by a corresponding rib of metal in the restoration serves very nicely as an internal escape channel for cement, improving casting seating by approximately 90 μm.[18]

Because the modulus of elasticity and ultimate yield strength of tooth structure is less than half that of cast gold,[19] the dentin separating multiple grooves should have twice the bulk that the metal ribs occupying the grooves do. For greatest resistance to tipping, a groove placed in an excessively tapered wall should be made nearly parallel with the path of insertion, rather than parallel with the outer surface into which it is cut (Fig. 16-12).

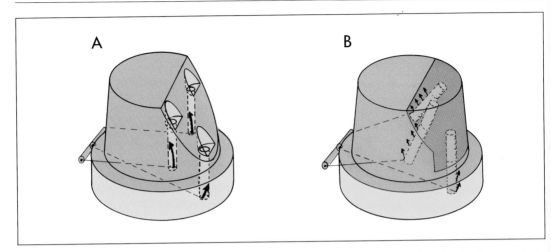

Fig. 16-13 Pinholes may be drilled parallel with the path of insertion to receive pins that are part of the casting *(A)*. The pinholes may be made nonparallel for individual pins to retain an amalgam core over which the cast restoration will be cemented *(B)*.

Fig. 16-14 *(A)* A pin at a relatively great distance from a tipping fulcrum provides effective resistance without being overstressed because the lever arm of the resisting force *(F₁)* is long in relation to that of the tipping forces *(F₂)*. *(B)* A pin near the fulcrum can easily be overstressed, resulting in distortion of the pin and/or fracture of the dentin around it. In both of these examples, a force from the direction opposite of that shown would be adequately resisted by the vertical wall of remaining tooth structure.

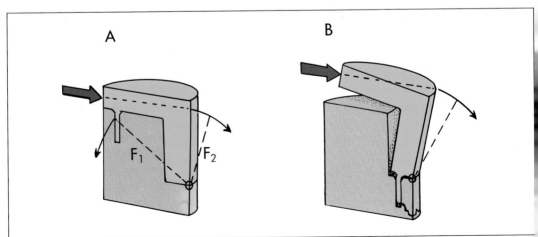

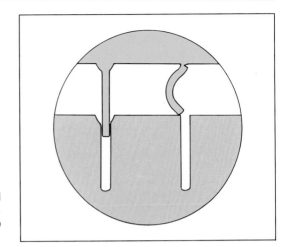

Fig. 16-15 The hole on the left has a small bevel at its mouth, which guides the pin to place. Without a beveled opening, the pin may fail to enter its hole, and be distorted *(right)*.

Pinholes

These are the only retention features that do not require existing vertical supragingival tooth structure for their placement. They can be used to generate additional length internally and apically rather than externally,[20] and are an effective means of increasing retention.[21,22] In addition to restoring damaged teeth, multiple parallel pins are very useful for augmenting partial veneer retainers.[23]

Pins can be used where there is insufficient axial wall length to place effective grooves, or where other retentive features would expose too much metal to view. They are commonly used in two ways. Pinholes parallel with the path of insertion can be made part of the final preparation to receive pins that are an integral part of the cast restoration (Fig. 16-13, *A*). The use of pins has been shown experimentally to be an effective way of enhancing the retention of seriously overtapered preparations.[24] Nonparallel pins can be cemented, threaded, or pressed into the tooth to retain an amalgam or composite resin core

in which a classic preparation for a cast restoration can be formed (Fig. 16-13, *B*).

Regardless of which type of pin is used, it should be surrounded by at least 0.5 mm of dentin.[25] Therefore, the use of pins is contraindicated on small, thin teeth.[26–28] Retention increases as the number, depth, and diameter of the holes increases.[29,30] As a rule, one pin should be used for each missing cusp,[31] line angle,[32] or axial wall.[33] Threaded pins are nearly five times as retentive as cemented pins. For this reason, threaded pins need only to be placed to a depth of 2.0 mm, but cemented pins, which are an integral part of the casting, should extend 4.0 mm into the tooth.[34]

For maximum resistance to tipping, the pinhole should be placed as far as possible from the fulcrum of the anticipated tipping motion (Fig. 16-14).

When the pin is to be part of the casting, the mouth of the hole should be countersunk slightly to form a funnel-shaped opening. This facilitates the impression and laboratory procedures, by strengthening the pin where it joins the

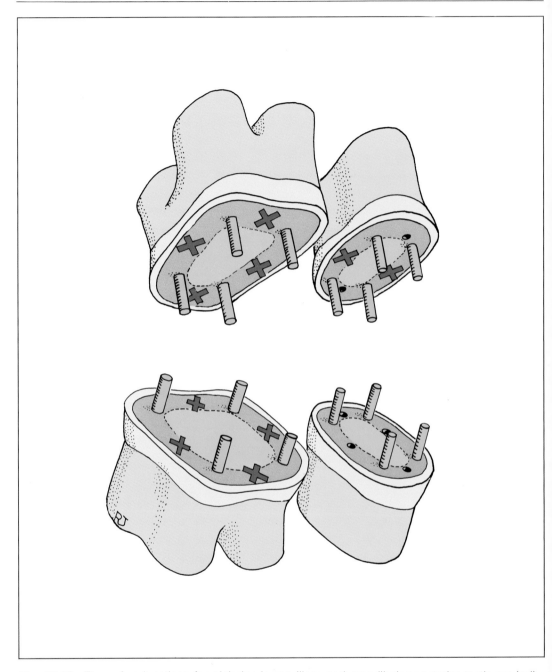

Fig. 16-16 The safest locations for pinholes in maxillary and mandibular posterior teeth are indicated by inserted pins. Secondary locations are indicated by unfilled pinholes. X's mark hazardous areas which must be avoided. The vital core *(broken line)* must not be impinged upon.

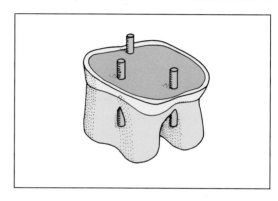

Fig. 16-17 Maxillary premolars usually have concavities on the mesial and distal aspects of the root, which make these areas unsuitable for pin placement.

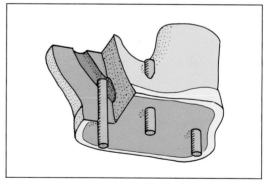

Fig. 16-18 The centers of the mesial, facial, and lingual surfaces of mandibular molars usually overlie root concavities, which precludes their use as pinhole locations.

Fig. 16-19 The trifurcations of maxillary molars are situated under the centers of the mesial, distal, and facial surfaces, making these areas unsuitable for pinhole placement. The midlingual surface must also be avoided because of the danger of encountering the lingual root canal.

body of the casting[35] and guiding the pin into the hole as the restoration is being seated (Fig. 16-15).

Pinholes must be placed carefully to avoid pulp exposures and perforations into the periodontal ligament. The safest locations for pinholes are the line angles or corners of the teeth (Fig. 16-16).[36] The least desirable areas for

placing pinholes lie in the middle of tooth surfaces,[36] especially overlying the furcations.[37] These and other areas which should be avoided to prevent penetrations into the pulp and the periodontal ligament are shown for maxillary premolars, mandibular molars, and maxillary molars in Figs. 16-17 to 16-19.

339

Table 16-1 Thickness of tooth structure in maxillary teeth (mm)[38]

	Thickness							
	CEJ				Root			
Tooth	M	F	D	L	M	F	D	L
Central incisor	2.2	2.5	2.3	3.1	2.3	2.5	2.2	2.8
Lateral incisor	1.8	2.2	1.7	2.4	1.7	2.5	1.6	2.6
Canine	2.0	2.7	2.2	2.9	2.0	2.7	1.9	3.0
First premolar	2.2	2.6	2.2	2.7	1.3	2.0	1.5	2.2
Second premolar	2.0	2.2	1.9	2.3	1.5	2.2	1.7	2.5
First molar	2.5	2.8	2.6	2.8	2.4	2.7	2.5	2.8
Second molar	2.6	2.9	2.6	3.0	2.4	2.7	2.5	2.8

Table 16-2 Thickness of tooth structure in mandibular teeth (mm)[38]

	Thickness							
	CEJ				Root			
Tooth.	M	F	D	L	M	F	D	L
Incisors	1.5	2.3	1.5	2.4	1.3	2.4	1.4	2.4
Canine	2.1	2.8	2.2	2.9	1.7	2.5	1.8	2.7
First premolar	2.1	2.5	2.1	2.8	1.9	2.3	1.6	2.7
Second premolar	2.2	2.6	2.2	2.5	2.1	2.7	1.9	2.9
First molar	2.5	2.8	2.7	2.6	2.3	2.7	2.5	2.6
Second molar	2.5	3.0	2.8	2.6	2.4	2.8	2.4	2.6

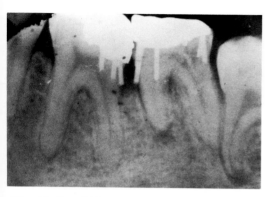

Fig. 16-20a This molar was lost because of injudicious placement of pins that perforated laterally into the periodontal membrane. Radiograph. (Courtesy of Dr. Dean L. Johnson, Oklahoma City.)

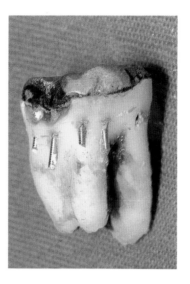

Fig. 16-20b Photograph of Fig. 16-20a. (Courtesy of Dr. Dean L. Johnson, Oklahoma City.)

To provide the reader with an idea of the bulk of tooth structure available for pinhole placement, the thickness of tooth structure measured from the pulp chamber to the outside of the tooth at the cemento-enamel junction (CEJ) and 3.0 mm down the root is shown for maxillary teeth in Table 16-1.[38] The same information for mandibular teeth can be seen in Table 16-2. These measurement levels were chosen because most pins are placed at or near the level of the cemento-enamel junction, and tooth structure is thinnest in that area. The values shown in these tables are, on the average, within 2 to 5% of the dimensions reported by Dilts and Mullaney[37] and by Stambaugh and Wittrock.[39] They differ more markedly from the dimensions reported by Gourley for molars.[36]

To avoid problems, the point of entry and direction of the drill must be carefully planned and controlled. The proper direction for the hole can be determined by studying the radiograph and by gently placing a probe,[36] or the drill itself,[40] into the gingival sulcus and holding it against the side of the tooth to get a clear picture of the direction of the outer tooth surface in the area of the pinhole. This limits the use of parallel pins that are an integral part of the casting, since the preparation path of insertion could dictate a pin direction that could lead to pulpal or periodontal complications.

Careless placement of pinholes can have disastrous results (Fig. 16-20). If blood is encountered during the drilling of a pinhole, it must be determined whether the pulp or the periodontal membrane is the victim. If it is the pulp, endodontic therapy must be performed before proceeding. If the hole exits the root surface, the pin should be carefully measured before insertion so that it neither overfills nor underfills the hole. Healing is then possible, although not guaranteed. A pin that extends into the periodontium coronal to the alveolar crest should be exposed with a surgical flap and trimmed flush with the root surface.

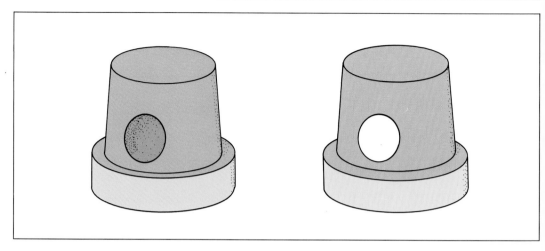

Fig. 16-21 A defect that has a bulk of sound dentin above it and lies at least 1.0 mm from the finish line should be filled with cement prior to making the impression. If additional retention were needed, the defect could have been converted into a box form as shown previously.

Cement bases and cores

Defects in tooth structure left by the removal of caries or old restorations can be filled in with a cement base if there is still adequate bulk of tooth structure to resist occlusal forces and enough axial wall surface area to provide retention for the restoration. Cement bases are used only to protect the pulp and to eliminate undercuts.

Polycarboxylate cement is an excellent material for this purpose, since it is nonirritating to the pulp and has some adhesive properties that make it less likely to become dislodged during subsequent preparation of the tooth. Cement bases do not have sufficient strength to effectively reinforce or replace weakened dentinal walls. For that purpose, amalgam or composite resin should be used. Placing retentive features such as grooves in cement is little more than an expression of good intentions.

An undercut created by caries removal can often be eliminated by forming a box. However, if the additional retention is not needed, and if excessive sound tooth structure would be sacrificed in creating the box, it is better to fill the defect with cement (Fig. 16-21). There should be 1.0 mm of sound tooth structure between a cement base and the finish line of the preparation to insure marginal integrity. If the defect is close to a finish line, amalgam should be used because of its strength and insolubility.

Pin-retained cores have been utilized for retaining cast restorations on broken down teeth for more than 30 years.[41-43] Both amalgam and composite resin can be used for replacing lost tooth structure. Composite resins are favored by some because they can be easily molded into large cavities and they set quickly, allowing the crown preparation to be made at the same appointment. Amalgam, however, has superior crush-

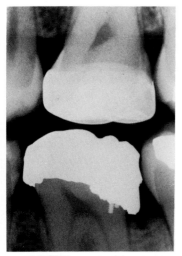

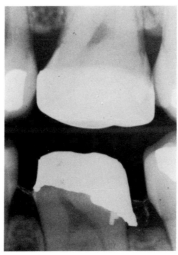

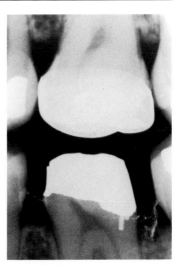

Fig. 16-22a An amalgam core may have overhangs because of subgingival extensions or other impediments to good matrix adaptation.

Fig. 16-22b If the crown finish line is placed on the amalgam core, the overhang will still be present.

Fig. 16-22c Only if the finish line is placed apical to the core is it possible to insure a smooth marginal area.

ing strength, and the new single-phase, copper-rich amalgams attain sufficient hardness to allow the crown preparation to be continued after only ten minutes.[44] Therefore, where maximum strength is needed, amalgam is still the preferred core material.

A pin-retained amalgam or composite resin core is indicated if less than half of the coronal structure of a vital tooth remains after removal of all caries and old restorations. All cusps thinner than half their height should be shortened or removed. Flatten cavity floors and walls for increased resistance, taking care not to traumatize the pulp or weaken the remaining walls. The core must be anchored firmly to the tooth and not just placed to fill the void. Otherwise it offers no advantage over allowing the bulk of the final casting to occupy the space.

Retention for an amalgam core can be achieved by using slots[45] as well as the nonparallel pins described previously. All retentive features for the core must be deep enough not to be eliminated by the axial reduction done in the subsequent crown preparation. The crown preparation may be completed as soon as the core material has hardened sufficiently. Or a properly contoured amalgam core may serve as a temporary restoration for several weeks, giving the tissue an opportunity to recover while more urgent treatment is being performed.

The preparation finish line for the cast restoration should extend beyond the core onto tooth structure.[46] The farther the core extends subgingivally, the more likely it is that it will have voids and overhangs, making it unsuitable to serve as the margin for the final restoration (Figs. 16-22a and b). If the core is amalgam, contacting dissimilar metals exposed to the oral environment are more prone to corrosion. If the exposed core is composite resin, it will be susceptible to leakage.

Solutions to common problems

Overtapered axial walls

The retention form of an overtapered preparation can be improved by plac-ing a beveled shoulder at the gingival finish line (Figs. 16-23a to c). Grooves have also been shown to be an effective way of augmenting resistance in preparations with tapered walls (Figs. 16-24a and b).[47]

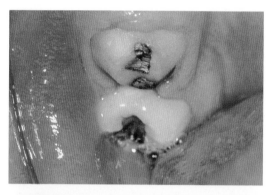

Fig. 16-23a The overtapered axial walls of a maxillary molar full crown preparation.

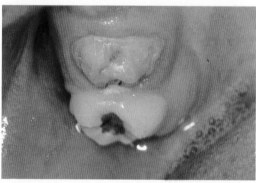

Fig. 16-23b Overtapering can be partially compensated for by uprighting the gingival segment of the axial walls.

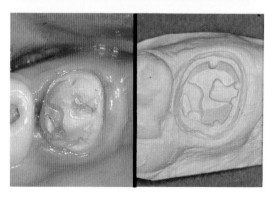

Fig. 16-23c Further compensation is gained by removing old amalgam restorations and incorporating their preparations into the crown preparation *(left)*. The various features are easily seen on a stone cast of the preparation *(right)*.

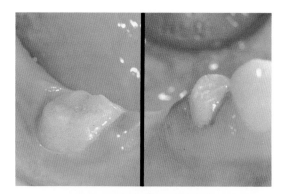

Fig. 16-24a Overtapered, overshortened preparations on two fixed bridge abutments.

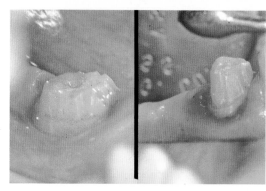

Fig. 16-24b The preparations are recouped by using shoulders and multiple grooves. The extent of tooth destruction did not permit the use of amalgam cores.

Short axial walls

A short preparation can be made more retentive by using multiple grooves in tooth structure (Fig. 16-25), or in a core (Fig. 16-26). Combinations of grooves in solid tooth structure and boxes incorporating caries can also be employed (Figs. 16-27a to d). Pinholes can be used in conjunction with limited internal wall retention or external sleeve retention (Figs. 16-28a to c).[48]

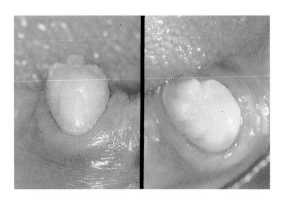

Fig. 16-25 The addition of multiple grooves can be used to enhance retention on a short preparation in natural tooth structure, as seen on this full veneer crown preparation on a mandibular premolar. *Left,* facial view. *Right,* occlusal view.

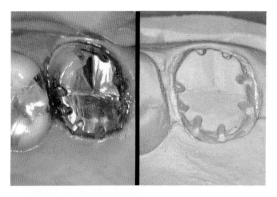

Fig. 16-26 Multiple grooves have been added to the amalgam core on a very short maxillary molar *(left)*. Detail of the grooves can be seen on a densite stone cast of the prepared tooth *(right)*.

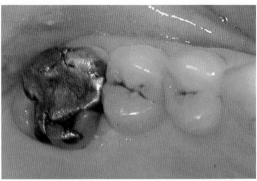

Fig. 16-27a An old extensive amalgam restoration must be replaced.

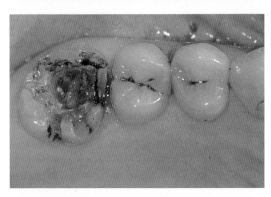

Fig. 16-27b Removal of the restoration reveals adequate bulk and length of tooth structure to restore the tooth without a core.

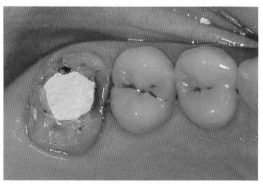

Fig. 16-27c The excavated area in the ''vital core'' is protected with a cement base.

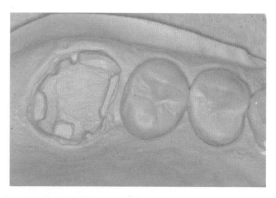

Fig. 16-27d A stone cast displays the various features of the preparation: the mesial box and the distolingual groove of the amalgam preparation have been converted to parts of the crown preparation. Caries on the distolingual aspect of the tooth has been incorporated into a box, and grooves have been placed in the solid tooth structure on the mesiolingual and distofacial aspects of the tooth.

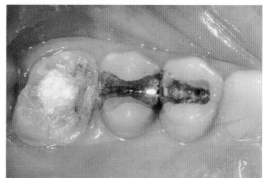

Fig. 16-28a Marginal axial wall length has been augmented in this porcelain-fused-to-metal crown preparation by placing a pinhole in each of the four corners of the tooth.

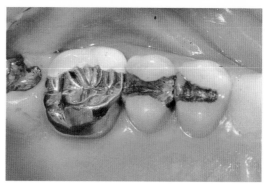

Fig. 16-28b The pins are visible inside the crown, where their length can be compared with that of the axial walls.

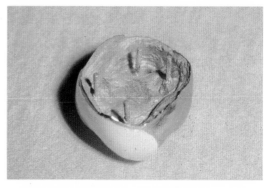

Fig. 16-28c The completed restoration is shown cemented in place.

Overextended box forms

If caries or trauma have caused the destruction of a wide expanse of tooth structure, producing an extremely wide box, grooves may be added to the corners to augment box resistance by forming small dovetails (Figs. 16-29a to c).[15]

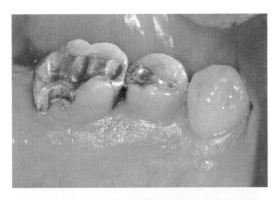

Fig. 16-29a A mandibular molar with an extensive amalgam has experienced a fractured distolingual cusp.

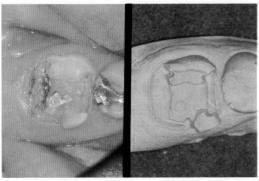

Fig. 16-29b The completed onlay preparation utilizes the distal and lingual axial walls in the box, as well as grooves in the angles of the routine mesial box and the extended "wraparound" distal box (*left,* intraoral view of preparation; *right,* stone cast).

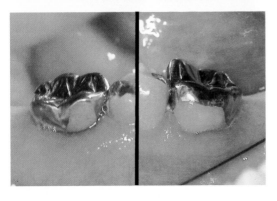

Fig. 16-29c The finished restoration is shown in lingual *(left)* and facial views *(right)*.

Undercuts in axial walls

Defects in long axial walls should be filled in with cement to eliminate undercuts before completion of the preparation (Figs. 16-30a and b). If such defects are left to be filled in on the die, the impression may be torn or distorted as it is withdrawn from the preparation. It also may be difficult for the inexperienced operator to visualize the proper configuration of the final preparation if large segments of it are missing.

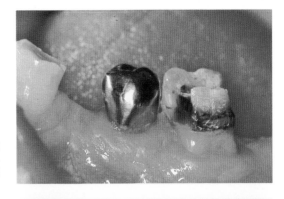

Fig. 16-30a Removal of a defective crown and associated caries leaves a molar with adequately sound tooth structure, but having axial undercuts and a large central defect.

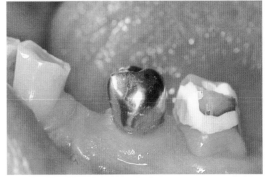

Fig. 16-30b After filling in the defects with a polycarboxylate cement base, a classic full veneer crown preparation can be done.

Fractured cusps

If a cusp fractures, producing a sloping surface, retention and resistance can be produced by cutting the inclined surface into steps that break the slope into horizontal and vertical components. The horizontal portions are perpendicular to the path of insertion, and the vertical ones are nearly parallel with the path of insertion (Figs. 16-31a to c).

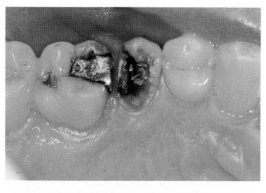

Fig. 16-31a A maxillary premolar with a sheared off lingual cusp is shown after removal of a disto-occlusal amalgam.

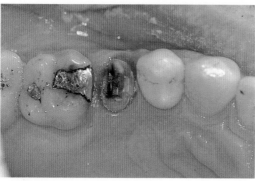

Fig. 16-31b Sufficient tooth structure remains for a satisfactory single tooth restoration if it is utilized properly. All sloping areas of the tooth are cut into vertical and horizontal components.

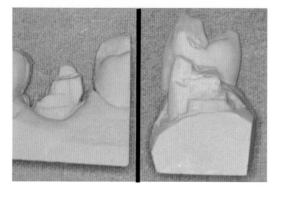

Fig. 16-31c A distal view of a stone cast shows the steps or terraces on the lingual and occlusal surfaces *(left)*. A lingual view of the cast shows them on the distal and occlusal surfaces *(right)*.

One missing cusp

When an entire cusp, including underlying dentin, is lost, existing amalgam preparation features, such as an isthmus or a box, can be incorporated into the crown preparation. This is usually accomplished by creating a box form in the tooth structure adjacent to the missing cusp. The restoration can be a partial veneer crown (Figs. 16-32a and b), or a full veneer crown (Figs. 16-33a and b), depending on caries rate, peripheral destruction, and the demands for retention placed on the tooth. Grooves can be placed in vertical surfaces of any length in the tooth structure surrounding the missing cusp (Figs. 16-34a to c). A pinhole can also be placed in the area of the missing cusp.

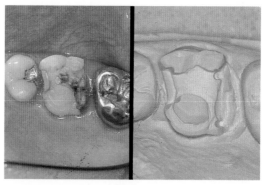

Fig. 16-32a A maxillary molar is shown with a fractured distolingual cusp after removal of an old amalgam restoration.

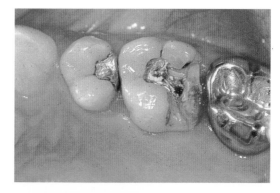

Fig. 16-32b The onlay preparation differs from the classic form by having a wide distal box, with grooves in the facial and lingual corners to augment retention (*left,* preparation; *right,* stone cast).

Figs. 16-33a and b The distolingual cusp has been lost from this mandibular molar. A full veneer crown has been selected because of decalcification and caries of the axial surfaces. A distinct extended box has been formed on the distal surface, with the isthmus extending through to the mesial surface.

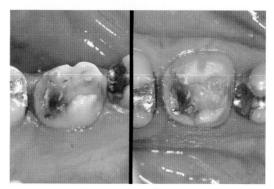

Fig. 16-33a Lingual *(left)* and occlusal intraoral views *(right)* of the preparation.

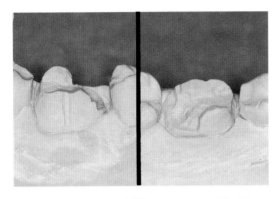

Fig. 16-33b Facial *(left)* and lingual views *(right)* of a stone cast of the preparation.

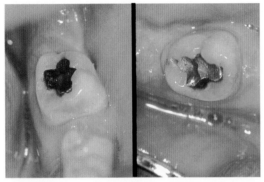

Fig. 16-34a The missing mesiolingual cusp on this mandibular molar *(left,* mesial; *right,* occlusal) will be incorporated into the planned full veneer crown bridge retainer that will restore the tooth.

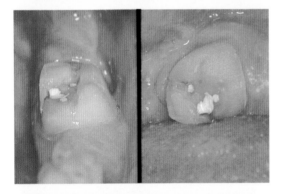

Fig. 16-34b Mesial *(left)* and occlusal views *(right)* show the converted amalgam isthmus and the four axial grooves that have been added to the preparation.

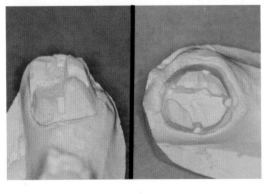

Fig. 16-34c Mesial *(left)* and occlusal views *(right)* show the detail of the preparation.

Two missing cusps

If two or more cusps are destroyed, a pin-retained core will be needed to provide retention and resistance (Figs. 16-35a to d).

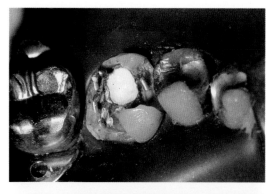

Fig. 16-35a Only a strong mesiofacial cusp and an undermined mesiolingual cusp remain on this mandibular molar. The number of pins used is probably greater than the situation called for.

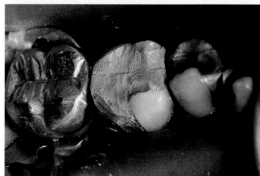

Fig. 16-35b Condensation of the amalgam core.

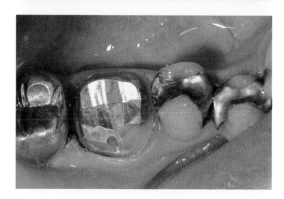

Fig. 16-35c Next, a full veneer crown preparation.

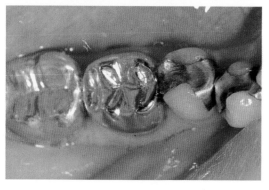

Fig. 16-35d The cast restoration can now be fabricated for the tooth.

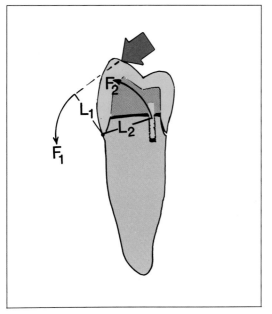

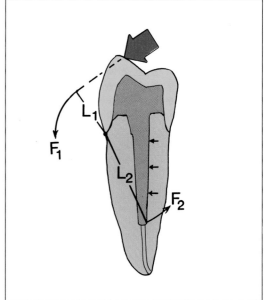

Fig. 16-36a A pin-retained amalgam core is inadequate for this narrow tooth. The dislodging force *(F₂)* at the pinhole is about as great as the applied force *(F₁)* because the lever arms *(L₁* and *L₂)* are nearly equal.

Fig. 16-36b Elective devitalization and placement of a dowel-core provides adequate resistance. *F₂* is now much smaller than *F₁* because it acts over a longer lever arm *(F₁ × L₁ = F₂ × L₂)*. In addition, the dislodging force is resisted by a more extensive area of tooth structure *(small arrows)*.

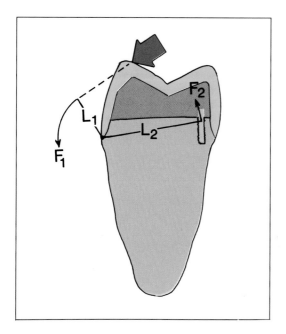

Fig. 16-36c A pin-retained amalgam core is usually adequate on a vital molar because the restored crown is wider than it is tall. Therefore, *F₂* is smaller than *F₁*.

Elective devitalization

There are situations in which intentional devitalization of a tooth to obtain retention is justified. These are instances where a crown is to be placed on a narrow single-rooted tooth that has an extremely short clinical crown remaining. A core on a badly broken down anterior tooth or premolar may not have sufficient resistance to dislodgment without a dowel extending into the root (Figs. 16-36a to c).

Endodontically treated teeth

Endodontic treatment of an anterior tooth does not of itself dictate placement of a crown.[49] If, however, a porcelain-fused-to-metal crown is needed because of coronal destruction, a dowel-core should be placed to support the final restoration. The axial reduction necessary for the crown preparation combined with the endodontic access preparation usually leaves insufficient sound dentin to support the restoration unaided.

The situation with posterior teeth is somewhat different. Because of their multicusp structure with a naturally divided occlusal surface, even caries-free teeth are in danger of fracturing vertically under heavy occlusal forces. No less should be done for an endodontically treated molar or premolar than the placement of a cast restoration with occlusal coverage, such as an MOD onlay.[50] Sorensen and Martinoff found that 94.2% of endodontically treated molars and premolars that were subsequently protected by coronal coverage were successful. On the other hand, the success rate for unprotected endodontical-

ly treated posterior teeth was only 56.3%.[51]

If a partial or full veneer crown is indicated because of moderate to severe loss of tooth structure, a core should be placed first. An amalgam or composite resin core is used for molars. If there is sound coronal tooth structure to provide resistance to laterally directed forces, pin retention alone can be used. If all coronal tooth structure is lost, two dowels are placed in the root canals for lateral resistance. Occasionally two-piece dowel-cores are used. Premolars, on the other hand, almost always require dowel-cores because of their narrow widths and lack of space for pin placement and core bulk.

At one time, it was common practice to make the dowel an integral part of the crown. This often resulted in a poor fit because the investment expansion necessary for a close-fitting crown is detrimental to the fit of the dowel, and vice-versa. A much better result is achieved by cementing a separate dowel-core before placing the crown. A further advantage of making a separate crown is the easier replacement of the crown if it should become necessary.

There are two general methods of forming a dowel-core. It may be cast of nickel-chrome from a custom acrylic or precision plastic pattern, or it can be made by combining a composite resin core with pins and a prefabricated stainless steel dowel. When a dowel-core fails, it is almost always because of loss of retention or fracture of the root into which it is cemented (Fig. 16-37). Both of these risks can be minimized by making the dowel space as long as possible without jeopardizing the apical seal. The margins of the final crown must be on sound tooth structure rather than on the core material. This encircling band of metal provides the "fer-

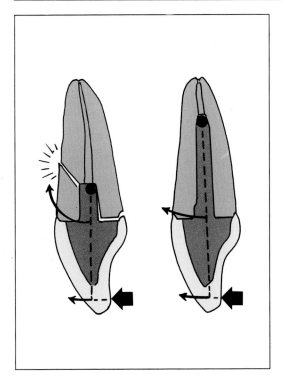

Fig. 16-37 The risk of root fracture is greater with a short dowel than with a long one. With a short dowel, the length of the lever arm through which the applied force acts is three times the length of the resisting arm (that part embedded in the root), making the stress three times as great as the applied force at the crown margin *(left)*. In a longer dowel, the lever arm is 1.8 times the length of the resisting arm. *(right)*. Therefore, the stress is only 1.8 times as great as the applied force at the margin. In addition, the longer dowel distributes the stress over a larger area of bone-supported root.

rule effect," which helps to protect the root from splitting by encircling it.[46] It also provides an optimal marginal seal. The strengthening effect of the cast crown whose margins extend beyond the core has been demonstrated by Hoag and Dwyer.[52]

References

1. Shillingburg, H. T., Jacobi, R., and Brackett, S. E. Preparation modifications for damaged vital posterior teeth. Dent. Clin. North Am. 29:305, 1985.
2. Shillingburg, H. T., Jacobi, R., and Dilts, W. E. Preparing severely damaged teeth. J. Calif. Dent. Assoc. 11:85, 1983.
3. Dilts, W. E. Pulpal considerations with fixed prosthodontic procedures. Quint. Int. 13:1287, 1982.
4. Ingber, J. S., Rose, L. F., and Coslet, J. G. The "biologic width"—A concept in periodontics and restorative dentistry. Alpha Omegan 10:62, 1977.
5. Murrin, J. R., and Barkmeier, W. W. Restoration of mutilated posterior teeth: Periodontal, restorative, and endodontic considerations. Oper. Dent. 6:90, 1981.
6. Ingraham, R. The application of sound biomechanical principles in the design of inlay, amalgam, and gold foil restorations. J. Am. Dent. Assoc. 40:402, 1950.
7. Holland, C. S. Cast gold restorations for teeth with large carious lesions. Br. Dent. J. 131:16, 1971.
8. Smith, G. E., and Grainger, D. A. Biomechanical design of extensive cavity preparations for cast gold. J. Am. Dent. Assoc. 89:1152, 1974.
9. Tinker, E. T. Fixed bridgework. J. Natl. Dent. Assoc. 7:579, 1920.
10. Dressel, R. P. The three-quarter crown as a bridge abutment for the posterior teeth. Dent. Cosmos 72:730, 1930.
11. Krause, O. G. Cast attachments for bridgework with special reference to vital teeth. J. Am. Dent. Assoc. 21:2104, 1934.
12. Silberhorn, O. W. Fixed bridge retainers—Design and retention features. Ill. Dent. J. 22:641, 1953.
13. Rhoads, J. E. Preparation of the Teeth for Cast Restorations. pp. 34–67 In G. M. Hollenback, Science and Technic of the Cast Restoration. St. Louis: The C. V. Mosby Co., 1964.
14. Ingraham, R., Bassett, R. W., and Koser, J. R. An Atlas of Cast Gold Procedures. 2nd ed. Buena Park, CA: Unitro College Press, 1969, 161–165.
15. Guyer, S. E. Multiple preparations for fixed prosthodontics. J. Prosthet. Dent. 23:529, 1970.
16. Kishimoto, M., Shillingburg, H. T., and Duncanson, M. G. Influence of preparation features on retention and resistance. II. Three-quarter crowns. J. Prosthet. Dent. 49:188, 1983.
17. Tjan, A. H. L., Sarkissian, R., and Miller, G. D. Effect of multiple axial grooves on the marginal adaptation of full cast gold crowns. J. Prosthet. Dent. 46:399, 1981.
18. Tjan, A. H. L., and Sarkissian, R. Internal escape channel: An alternative to venting complete crowns. J. Prosthet. Dent. 52:50, 1984.
19. Craig, R. G., Peyton, F. A., and Johnson, D. W. Compressive properties of enamel, dental cements, and gold. J. Dent. Res. 40:936, 1961.
20. Gilboe, D. B., and Teteruck, W. R. Fundamentals of extracoronal tooth preparation. I. Retention and resistance form. J. Prosthet. Dent. 32:651, 1974.
21. Lorey, R. E., and Myers, G. E. The retentive qualities of bridge retainers. J. Am. Dent. Assoc. 76:568, 1968.
22. Pruden, W. H. Full coverage, partial coverage, and the role of pins. J. Prosthet. Dent. 26:302, 1971.
23. Miller, L. L. Partial coverage in crown and bridge prosthesis with the use of elastic impression materials. J. Prosthet. Dent. 13:905, 1963.
24. Chan, K. C., Boyer, D. B., and Schulein, T. M. The effectiveness of pins with complete cast metal crowns. J. Prosthet. Dent. 51:765, 1984.
25. Clyde, J. S., and Sharkey, S. W. The pin ledge crown. A reappraisal. Br. Dent. J. 144:239, 1978.
26. Baum, L., and Contino, R. M. Ten years of experience with cast pin restorations. Dent. Clin. North Am. 14:81, 1970.
27. Hughes, H. J. Are there alternatives to the porcelain-fused-to-gold bridge? Aust. Dent. J. 15:281, 1970.
28. Crispin, B. J. Conservative alternatives to full crowns. J. Prosthet. Dent. 42:392, 1979.
29. Lorey, R. E., Embrell, K. A., and Myers, G. E. Retentive factors in pin-retained castings. J. Prosthet. Dent. 17:271, 1967.
30. Moffa, J. P., and Phillips, R. W. Retentive properties of parallel pin restorations. J. Prosthet. Dent. 17:387, 1967.
31. Courtade, G. L. Pin pointers. III. Self-threading pins. J. Prosthet. Dent. 20:335, 1968.
32. Roberts, E. W. Crown reconstruction with pin reinforced amalgam. Tex. Dent. J. 81:10, 1963.
33. Caputo, A. A., and Standlee, J. P. Pins and posts—Why, when, and how. Dent. Clin. North Am. 20:299, 1976.

34. Dilts, W. E., Welk, D. A., and Stovall, J. Retentive properties of pin materials in pin-retained silver amalgam restorations. J. Am. Dent. Assoc. 77:1085, 1968.

35. Racowsky, L. P., and Wolinsky, L. E. Restoring the badly broken-down tooth with esthetic partial coverage restorations. Comp. Cont. Educ. Dent. 2:322, 1981.

36. Gourley, J. V. Favorable locations for pins in molars. Oper. Dent. 5:2, 1980.

37. Dilts, W. E., and Mullaney, T. P. Relationship of pinhole location and tooth morphology in pin-retained silver amalgam restorations. J. Am. Dent. Assoc. 76:1011, 1968.

38. Shillingburg, H. T., and Grace, C. S. Thickness of enamel and dentin. J. South. Calif. Dent. Assoc. 41:33, 1973.

39. Stambaugh, R. V., and Wittrock, J. W. The relationship of the pulp chamber to the external surface of the tooth. J. Prosthet. Dent. 37:537, 1977.

40. Markley, M. R. Pin retained and reinforced restorations and foundations. Dent. Clin. North Am. 11:229, 1967.

41. Shooshan, E. D. The full veneer cast crown. J. South. Calif. Dent. Assoc. 23:27, 1955.

42. Markely, M. R. Pin reinforcement and retention of amalgam foundations and restorations. J. Am. Dent. Assoc. 56:675, 1958.

43. Kuratli, J. Restoration of broken down vital teeth for fixed partial denture abutments. J. Prosthet. Dent. 8:504, 1958

44. Nitkin, D. A., and Goldberg, A. J. Another look at placing and polishing amalgam in one visit. Quint. Int. 14:507, 1983.

45. Outhwaite, W. C., Twiggs, S. W., Fairhurst, C. W., and King, G. E. Slots vs. pins: A comparison of retention under simulated chewing stresses. J. Dent. Res. 61:400, 1982.

46. Eissmann, H. F., and Radke, R. A. Post-endodontic restoration. pp. 537–575 In S. Cohen and R. C. Burns (eds.) Pathways of the Pulp. St. Louis: The C. V. Mosby Co., 1976.

47. Woolsey, G. D., and Matich, J. A. The effect of axial grooves on the resistance form of cast restorations. J. Am. Dent. Assoc. 97:978, 1978.

48. Wagner, A. W. Pin retention for extensive posterior gold onlays. J. Prosthet. Dent. 15:719, 1965.

49. Shillingburg, H. T., and Kessler, J. C. After the root canal—Principles of restoring endodontically treated teeth. J. Okla. State Dent. Assoc. 74:19, 1984.

50. Frank, A. L.: Protective coronal coverage of the pulpless tooth. J. Am. Dent. Assoc. 59:895, 1959.

51. Sorensen, J. A., and Martinoff, J. T. Intracoronal reinforcement and coronal coverage: A study of endodontically treated teeth. J. Prosthet. Dent. 51:780, 1984.

52. Hoag, E. P., and Dwyer, T. G. A comparative evaluation of three post and core techniques. J. Prosthet. Dent. 47:177, 1982.

Chapter 17

Preparation Modifications for Special Situations

There are many circumstances in which the role to be played by the restored tooth will be significant in the selection of the preparation design. This role can also necessitate modification of a classic tooth preparation design on teeth that are relatively intact. Examples are: (1) the changes made in bridge abutment preparations because of increased mechanical load; (2) variations in preparations on removable partial denture abutment teeth because of the increased space requirements (occasioned by the placement of rest seats in the final crown); and (3) the special needs of the abutment preparation for an acid-etch resin-bonded bridge to enhance retention and resistance while keeping the preparation mostly or entirely in enamel.

Preparations for fixed bridge abutments

Modifications of the classic crown preparation designs are often required when the tooth is to be an abutment for a fixed bridge, in order to increase retention and resistance, to make provision for accessible margins adjacent to the pontic connectors, and to create space for precision attachments.

A bridge retainer is subjected to a greater range of forces from leverage and torque transmitted through the pontic. Therefore, more extensive coverage may be indicated for a tooth that is to serve as a bridge abutment than would be needed for a single restoration. Inlays and onlays are never indicated as bridge retainers. Three-quarter crowns on posterior teeth and pin-modified three-quarter crowns for anterior teeth are usually adequate for simple bridges replacing a single tooth or two single-rooted teeth, provided the abutment teeth are relatively intact and have adequate clinical crown lengths. For longer spans and for complex bridges with more than two abutments, seven-eighths or full-coverage crowns should be selected.

Additional grooves should be placed in bridge retainer preparations to help resist dislodgment. The most efficient location for a groove depends on the direction of anticipated torque. Each retainer of a long-span posterior bridge is subjected to torque around a faciolingual axis as the pontic span flexes under a load. Loosening of a crown by this type of torque can be prevented by addition of facial and lingual grooves (Fig. 17-1).

When a bridge curves around the arch so that the pontic lies facial to the interabutment axis, a load on the pontic will create torque around a more mesiodistal axis. Resistance to this type of torque can best be enhanced by ad-

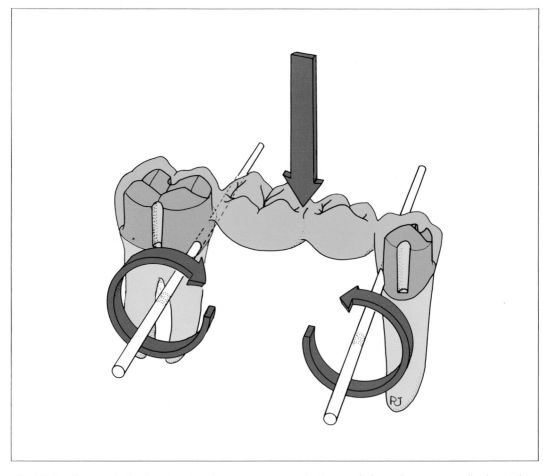

Fig. 17-1 The most effective location for a groove to resist torque is in a plane perpendicular to the axis of the torque. The load on a long-span bridge with straight pontics produces torque around faciolingual axes. Resistance can best be enhanced by the addition of facial and lingual grooves.

ding mesial and distal grooves (Fig. 17-2).

Consideration must be given to the location of the finish line in the area of a retainer adjacent to the pontic connector. The margin that will lie under the connector of a fixed bridge must extend far enough gingivally so that it will not be encroached upon by the connector (Fig. 17-3). On a short tooth this might require placement of the finish line at, or slightly below, the gingival crest.

Fig. 17-2 The load on a pontic that lies facial to the interabutment axis line produces torque primarily around that axis. The most effective location for supplemental grooves in this situation is on the mesial and distal surfaces.

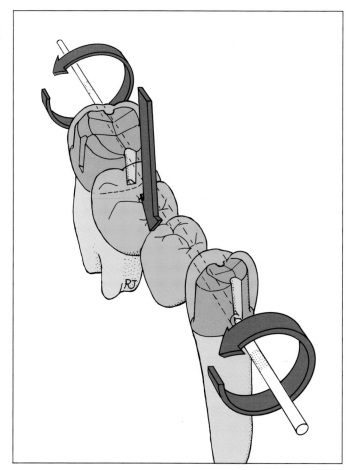

Fig. 17-3 The margin of this molar retainer lies too close to the pontic connector, making it difficult to finish, cleanse, and inspect. The finish line on the premolar has been carried farther facially and gingivally, placing it in a more accessible area.

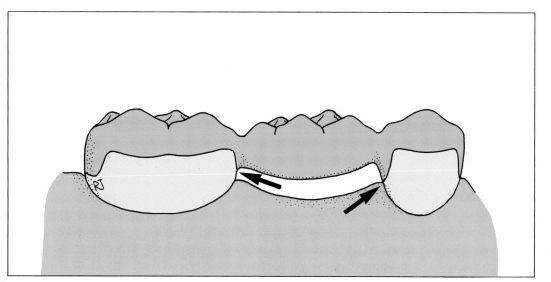

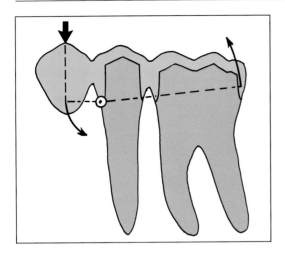

Fig. 17-4 An impact on a cantilevered pontic produces a strong lifting force on the distal retainer. Resistance can be increased by adding facial and lingual grooves, and by making the axial surface that is most distant from the pontic as nearly parallel with the wall nearest to the pontic as possible. The wall nearest the pontic must be as long as possible, thereby lowering the fulcrum and increasing the angle at which the arc of displacement strikes the distal wall.

A third type of modification sometimes required for a bridge abutment is the addition of a box to accomodate a nonrigid connector.[1] The box must be large enough for the bulk of the female portion of the connector to be contained within the normal contours of the completed crown. Otherwise the technician will have to grossly overcontour the crown, which will not only create a plaque-retentive area but also unfavorable tipping forces on the abutment tooth. The box must be aligned with the path of insertion of the other abutment preparation. If the abutments are not parallel, the box may have to be inclined several degrees in relation to the long axis of the tooth into which it is cut. In this case, its depth must be carefully gauged with the help of radiographs to avoid encroaching on the vital core of the tooth.

Cantilever bridges create a unique distribution of forces that their abut-ments must resist. Apical displacement of the pontic can often be resisted at the uncemented end by a rest that fits into a well-defined seat in a metal restoration. When a rest is not feasible, two adjacent teeth can be used as double abutments to reduce damaging stress concentrations in the periodontium. Under short-duration impact forces, teeth act as if they were immobile.[2] A torque created by an impact on the pontic of such a bridge is centered on the margin of the primary retainer nearest the pontic. The resultant lifting force on the secondary retainer is nearly parallel with its path of insertion because of the long radius of rotation (Fig. 17-4). Therefore, the preparation of the secondary abutment must be made as retentive as possible by adding grooves and forming the axial wall most distant from the pontic with a minimum of taper and a maximum of length.

Preparations for removable partial denture abutments

Rests are vital for the stabilization and proper function of removable partial dentures, and the seats for those rests frequently must be placed in cast restorations. Modification of the underlying tooth preparation by removing more than the normal amount of tooth structure is necessary to accommodate an adequate rest seat.[3–7] This must be done to meet the requirements of good partial denture design without compromising the integrity of the individual crown.

Cingulum rests

A properly formed cingulum rest on the lingual surface of an incisor or canine provides excellent resistance to apical or horizontal displacement of the partial denture. It also affords indirect retention by providing a positive vertical stop anterior to the fulcrum line on distal extension partial dentures. Although this type of rest can be used on an intact, unrestored tooth, it does require a tooth with considerable cingulum bulk. Therefore, the use of this type of rest, even when the tooth does not otherwise need restoration, may require the fabrication of a crown to allow placement of a rest seat of adequate depth and surrounding bulk.

The rest seat, in the form of a V with rounded internal angles,[8] is placed as far gingivally and as near the long axis of the tooth as possible (Figs. 17-5a to d). Perforation of the rest seat of the casting or overcontouring the wax pattern is likely to occur if no compensat-ing features are cut in the underlying tooth structure. This is accomplished by placing a groove on each side of the cingulum, joined by a flat, ledge-like offset in the sloped portion of the lingual surface (Fig. 17-6).

Occlusal rests

An occlusal rest, 1.4 mm thick[9] and occupying the middle third of a posterior tooth faciolingually, is needed to limit movement of a removable partial denture in an apical direction. It should be spoon-shaped, with rounded reduction of the marginal ridge and a floor sloping toward the center of the tooth (Figs. 17-7a and b).[10]

Unless the preparation is modified, the 1.4-mm-deep rest seat will perforate the occlusal surface of a crown made over 1.0 mm of occlusal reduction. While increasing the overall occlusal reduction would accomplish this end, it could easily overshorten the preparation and drastically reduce retention and resistance. Instead, a definite countersink, 0.5 to 1.0 mm deep, should be cut into the already prepared occlusal surface in the area of the proposed rest seat (Fig. 17-8).[11] Its outline should follow that of the rest, with approximately 0.5 mm of clearance between the countersink and the rest seat.

A countersink with definite vertical walls, rather than an amorphous dimple, is preferred. Its outline is easily seen, insures adequate extension, and can enhance both retention and resistance. A similar feature, the isthmus, adds significantly to the retention and resistance of the MOD onlay.[12]

Figs. 17-5a and b   Cingulum rest seat on a mandibular canine.

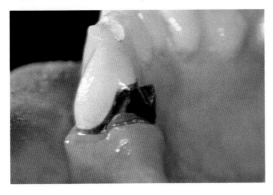

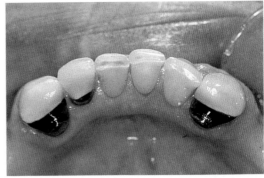

Fig. 17-5a   Distal view.

Fig. 17-5b   Incisal view.

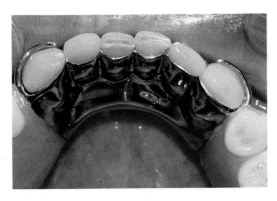

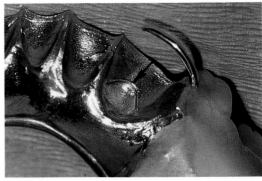

Fig. 17-5c   The partial denture is seen in place on the rest seat.

Fig. 17-5d   A view of the underside of the partial denture framework shows the rest *(arrow)*.

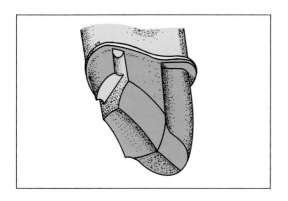

Fig. 17-6   The cingulum rest seat on an anterior crown is accommodated by grooves and an offset.

Figs. 17-7a and b   A properly done rest seat in a posterior crown.

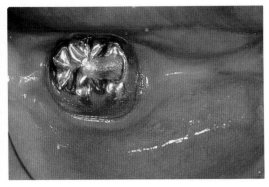

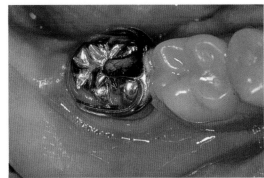

Fig. 17-7a   The occlusal rest is accommodated.

Fig. 17-7b   Stability is provided for the denture.

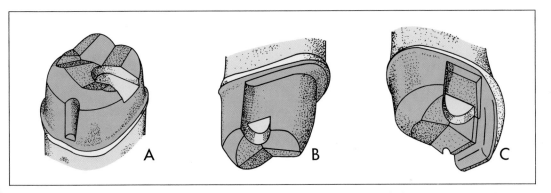

Figs. 17-8   The occlusal countersink for a rest seat. Shown alone for a full veneer crown preparation (A). Shown tied in with the wing for a porcelain-fused-to-metal crown preparation (B). Shown in conjunction with a proximal box on a three-quarter crown preparation (C).

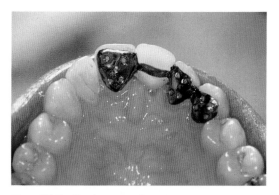

Fig. 17-9 Resin extruding through the small perforations in the metal framework were used by Rochette to retain resin-bonded bridges.[15]

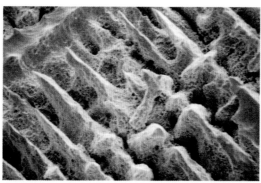

Fig. 17-10 A scanning electron micrograph of electrolytically etched metal reveals the extensive network of microscopic undercuts created by the etching process.

Preparations for resin-bonded bridges

Quality restorative dentistry has always had as one of its goals the conservation of tooth structure whenever possible. The development of the acid-etch bonding technique[13] has greatly enhanced our ability to maintain vital, structurally sound tooth structure. The technique for permanently bonding a cast metal bridge in place with resin was first described by Rochette,[14] who advocated the use of small perforations in the metal framework. Resin extruding through these holes locked onto the outer, or lingual, surface of the framework and retained the restoration (Fig. 17-9). Other clinicians and investigators began to explore the many avenues of treatment afforded by this technique.[15] They found the bond between the resin and the metal framework to be the weak link in the system.[16]

Livaditis and Thompson[17] adapted a technique introduced by Tanaka et al.[18] for selectively developing pitting corrosion on nickel-chromium alloys. This resulted in a system for bonding composite resins to metal and, in turn, to enamel, that is far stronger than previous techniques (Fig. 17-10). The bond between the resin and properly etched metal exhibits more than twice the tensile strength of the accepted value of resin to etched enamel.[17,19]

However, so much attention has been focused on the resin-to-metal bonding system that the necessity for proper preparation design has not been given proper notice.[20] In the rush to adapt this new treatment mode, some operators have paid scant attention to the need for adequate tooth preparation. If predictable long-term results are to be obtained, resistance form is just as critical in the preparation for this type of restoration as it is in standard crown preparations. The amount of tooth structure removed is minimal, but the preparation for the resin bonded bridge retainer and the overlying metal framework must be designed so that occlusal forces applied to the restoration will be

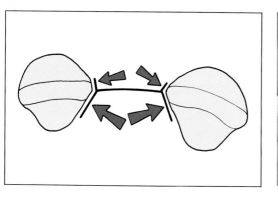

Fig. 17-11a The proximal reduction is done in two planes, which accommodate framework extension in facial and lingual directions, enhancing resistance.

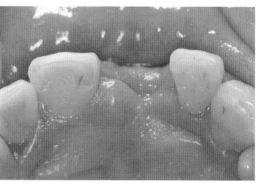

Fig. 17-11b When viewed from the incisal, the planes are obvious.

resisted by compression of the resin bond. The tensile strength of the resin should not be depended on as the sole source of retention.

Preparation design

This discussion of preparations for etched-metal resin-bonded bridges will be divided into anterior and posterior designs. While the majority of these restorations are placed in the anterior region, clinical experience indicates that this type of retainer can be used for replacing missing posterior teeth as well.[21]

Anterior preparation design

The preparation for anterior teeth can be broken into four separate and distinct segments:[21–26]

1. Proximal reduction
2. Vertical stops
3. Finish lines
4. Lingual reduction

The first, and possibly the most important, of these segments is the proximal reduction adjacent to the edentulous space (Figs. 17-11a and b). The prime function of the proximal preparation features is resistance form. Certainly any unsightly metal display should be avoided, so facial extension must be carefully planned. The classic design for proximal reduction consists of very subtle facial and lingual planes, and lowering the height of contour 2 to 3 mm (Fig. 17-12). The result appears as a curved or angled guide plane. When the metal framework is fabricated it is carried slightly onto the labial component of this guide plane and effectively resists lingual displacement (Fig. 17-13). This feature, at the same time, creates a definite line of draw for the preparation.

In many instances, because of the position or rotation of an abutment

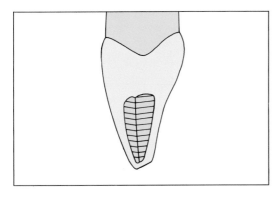

Fig. 17-12 Two-plane reduction, as viewed from the proximal surface, will result in the height of contour being lowered by 2.0 to 3.0 mm.

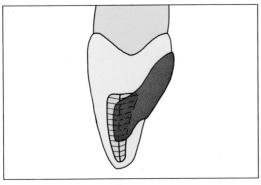

Fig. 17-13 A properly designed metal framework is extended onto the facial plane and resists lingual displacement.

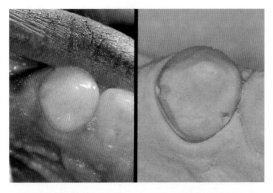

Fig. 17-14 Shallow, but definite, grooves can be used as proximal resistance features. They are shown on a canine in the mouth *(left)* and on a cast *(right)*.

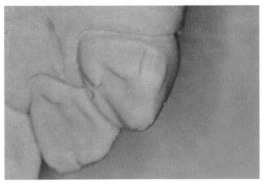

Fig. 17-15 The groove and the resulting path of insertion should parallel the incisal two-thirds of the facial surface.

tooth, creating a labial plane of reduction would result in an unacceptable show of metal. In these cases a shallow groove is placed in the proximal enamel (Fig. 17-14).[23] The groove is positioned far enough facially to have adequate length, but not far enough to allow metal to show through the more translucent proximal enamel. The line of draw is usually parallel with the incisal one-half to two-thirds of the tooth (Fig. 17-15). Again, having this groove recorded in the metal framework creates a definite path of insertion and provides resistance to lingual displacement.

The next features to consider in anterior preparation design are the vertical stops. These are necessary so that there is a definite and reproducible limit to gingival displacement during try-in and delivery of the restoration. Early resin-bonded bridges were designed with small hooks of metal extending over the incisal edges of the abutment teeth.[20] These hooks were not etched, allowing for their removal after the restoration was bonded in place. However, this was an inconvenience at delivery, and it left no resistance form to oppose functional forces from an incisal direction.

Small flat shelves can be placed on the lingual surface, usually in the marginal ridge areas where enamel thickness is greatest (Fig. 17-16). These form definite stops for the restoration. These stops are particularly important at delivery, when overseating the bridge could be disastrous. An even more definite feature can be placed on most canine teeth in the form of a cingulum rest (Fig. 17-17). This feature is designed so the depth of the preparation is gingival to the lingual lip of the rest. This configuration not only acts as a vertical stop, but also resists lingual displacement.

On most anterior teeth, the path of insertion is established with the proximal reduction, and the remainder of the preparation will draw freely with no undercuts. Therefore, the need for lingual reduction and finish lines is solely to allow for occlusal clearance. Approximately 0.5 mm of reduction is required for the typical lingual metal configuration.[20,21,26] This can usually be achieved on maxillary anterior teeth with slight lingual preparation (Fig. 17-18), sometimes accompanied by some reduction of the incisal edges of the mandibular teeth. Occlusions with a deep overbite in which the centric stops are in the gingival one-half of the maxillary teeth are considered contraindications to the resin-bonded retainer.

A very light chamfer may be prepared, always supragingivally (Fig. 17-19). This finish line can be carried to the opposite lingual interproximal embrasure, allowing for the maximum extension of the framework. This extension, across the marginal ridge opposite the edentulous space, is thought to be important because it will include enamel that, when etched and bonded to, will result in tags that are directed at different angles from those on the lingual and the opposite proximal surfaces. This circumferential design incorporates the maximum surface area and resin tags in as many different planes as possible, enhancing resistance to forces from varying directions.[21]

The addition of secondary abutments should be approached conservatively. All too often, it is felt that the increased surface area afforded by an additional retainer can only help. However, the tendency is for retainers on secondary abutments to debond.[27] In many cases, resistance and retention can be enhanced by auxiliary preparation features, such as grooves or boxes, elimi-

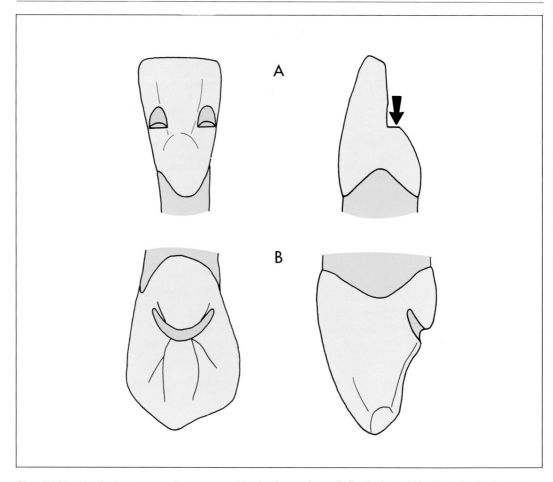

Fig. 17-16 Vertical stops can be prepared in the form of small, flat ledges *(A)*. When bulk of enamel permits, cingulum rests can act as vertical stops *(B)*.

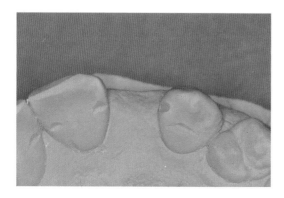

Fig. 17-17 The preparation on the central incisor incorporates two-plane proximal reduction and flat ledges for vertical stops, while the canine has grooves and a cingulum rest.

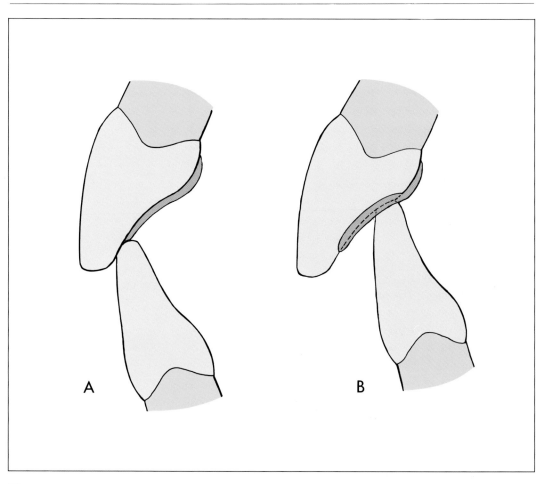

Fig. 17-18 Very slight reduction of 0.5 mm is adequate to allow an acceptable thickness of metal (A). An occlusion with a deep overbite in which the centric contacts occur in the gingival half of a maxillary tooth would require too much reduction of tooth structure to use a resin-bonded retainer (B).

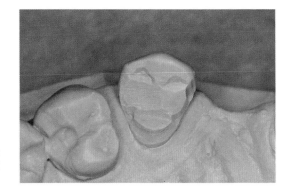

Fig. 17-19 The gingival finish line placed on an anterior tooth consists of a light supragingival chamfer.

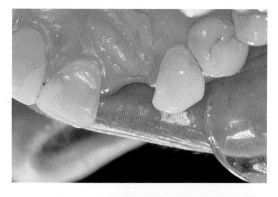

Fig. 17-20a Auxiliary preparation features enhance retention and resistance and may eliminate the need for secondary abutments. Both abutment preparations for a maxillary anterior bridge are shown in the mouth.

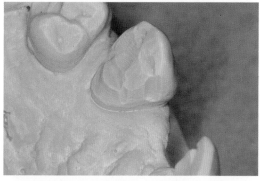

Fig. 17-20b The detail of the grooves and rests on the canine abutment are seen in this closeup of the stone cast.

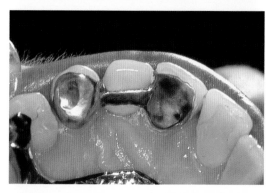

Fig. 17-21a A lingual view of the bridge whose abutments were shown in Figs. 17-19 and 17-20.

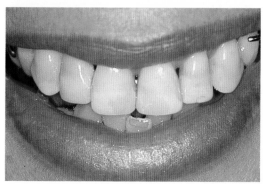

Fig. 17-21b A facial view of the bridge demonstrates the excellent esthetic results that are possible with this conservative design.

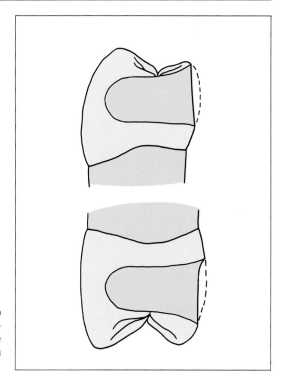

Fig. 17-22 The height of contour is lowered to within 1.0 mm of the gingiva on the lingual surface. The result is often a knife-edge finish line on a mandibular tooth and a light chamfer on a maxillary tooth.

nating the need for supplemental abutments (Figs. 17-20a and b and 17-21a and b). If the additional retainer is determined to be necessary, the tooth should be modified so that it will have definite features to resist lingual displacement of the framework resulting from facial movement of the tooth.

Posterior preparation design

The first step in preparing posterior teeth is to establish a path of insertion.[28–30] The height of contour should be lowered to within 1.0 mm of the gingiva whenever possible (Fig. 17-22). However, all of the preparation is carefully maintained in enamel. The interproximal height of contour is lowered a minimum of 2.0 mm, allowing for an adequate bulk of metal in the connector

area (Fig. 17-23). The lingual reduction is extended as far as possible to the embrasure opposite the edentulous space to insure maximum surface area is available for bonding.

As with the anterior preparation, creating resistance form is very important. The preparation and the framework must extend beyond the facial line angle of the abutment teeth. This extension of metal resists lingual displacement of the restoration. When properly extended, the framework for posterior retainers should extend at least 180 degrees around the circumference of each abutment tooth (Fig. 17-24).

An occlusal rest should be prepared with an outline form comparable to those used for removable partial dentures (Fig. 17-25). The facio-lingual dimension should be 1.5 to 2.0 mm; the mesial-distal, 1.5 to 2.0 mm; and the

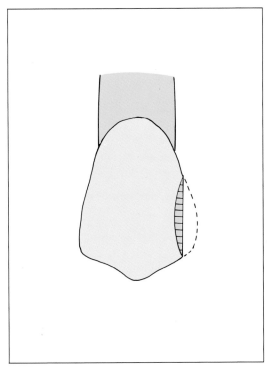

Fig. 17-23 The interproximal height of contour is lowered at least 2.0 mm to accommodate proper bulk in the connector.

Fig. 17-24 The metal framework should extend beyond the facial line angle and at least 180 degrees around the tooth to the lingual.

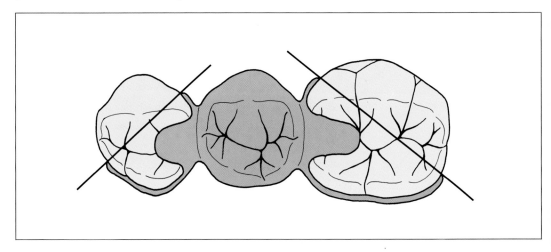

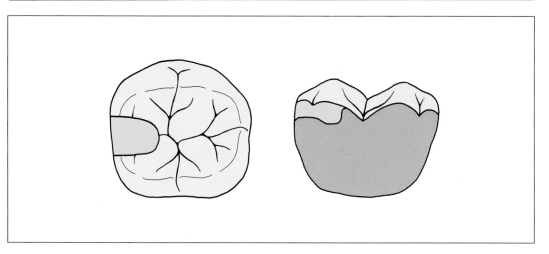

Fig. 17-25 The outline form for an occlusal rest seat for an acid-etch, resin-bonded bridge is comparable to that used for removable partial dentures.

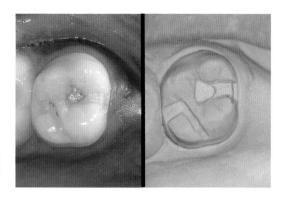

Fig. 17-26 Occlusal rests for resin-bonded bridges should be prepared with definite lingual walls that will resist lateral displacement.

depth, 1.0 to 1.5 mm. The difference in the design of this preparation is that the vertical walls are very distinct, minimizing the potential for lateral movement of the framework (Fig. 17-26). The preparation should be progressively deeper as it moves from the marginal ridge into the fossa.

Finally, the need for occlusal clearance is evaluated. In most cases, with careful preoperative treatment planning, the centric stops can be avoided by the framework. If some occlusal reduction is necessary, an occlusal clearance of 0.5 mm is required for the proper bulk of metal.

If there are any existing restorations, they should be conservative if the tooth is to be considered a good candidate for a resin-bonded retainer. A good rule of thumb when designing preparations on previously restored teeth is to either completely avoid or completely cover the existing restoration. This prevents the difficult situation that might result when a partially covered amalgam or composite resin restoration requires replacing for any reason. In cases where entire restorations cannot be avoided, access for their future replacement should certainly be a consideration during design of the metal framework.

References

1. Shillingburg, H. T., and Fisher, D. W. Nonrigid connectors for fixed partial dentures. J. Am. Dent. Assoc. 87:1195, 1973.
2. Muhlemann, H. R. Tooth mobility: A review of clinical aspects and research findings. J. Periodontol. 38(suppl.):686, 1967.
3. Dykema, R. W., Cunningham, D. M., and Johnston, J. F. Modern Practice in Removable Partial Prosthodontics. Philadelphia: W. B. Saunders Co., 1962, 167.
4. Zarb, G. A., Bergman, B., Clayton, J. A., and McKay, H. F. Prosthodontic Treatment for Partially Edentulous Patients. St. Louis: The C. V. Mosby Co., 1978, 484–485.
5. Boucher, L., and Renner, R. Treatment of Partially Edentulous Patients. St. Louis: The C. V. Mosby Co., 120.
6. Culpepper, W. D., and Moulton, P. S. Considerations in fixed prosthodontics. Dent. Clin. North Am. 23:21, 1979.
7. Gardner, F. M. Alterations in tooth preparations for surveyed crowns. Gen. Dent. 32:498, 1984.
8. Henderson, D., and Steffel, V. L. McCracken's Removable Partial Prosthodontics. 6th ed. St. Louis: The C. V. Mosby Co., 1981, 56.
9. Tsao, D. H. Designing occlusal rests using mathematical principles. J. Prosthet. Dent. 23:154, 1970.
10. Johnson, D. L., and Stratton, R. J. Fundamentals of Removable Prosthodontics. Chicago: Quintessence Publ. Co., 1980, 219.
11. Wiebelt, F. J., and Shillingburg, H. T. Abutment preparation modifications for removable partial denture rest seats. Quint. Dent. Technol. 9:449, 1985.
12. Kishimoto, M., Shillingburg, H. T., and Duncanson, M. G. Influence of preparation features on retention and resistance. I. MOD onlays. J. Prosthet. Dent. 49:35, 1983.
13. Buonocore, M. G. A simplified method of increasing the adhesion of acrylic filling materials to enamel surfaces. J. Dent. Res. 34:849, 1955.
14. Rochette, A. L. Attachment of a splint to enamel of lower anterior teeth. J. Prosthet. Dent. 30:418, 1973.
15. Howe, D. F., and Denehy, G. E. Anterior fixed partial dentures utilizing the acid-etch technique and a cast metal framework. J. Prosthet. Dent. 37:28, 1977.
16. Williams, V. D., Drennon, D. G., and Silverstone, L. M. The effect of retainer design on the retention of filled resin in acid-etched fixed partial dentures. J. Prosthet. Dent. 48:417, 1982.
17. Livaditis, G. J., and Thompson, V. P. Etched castings: An improved retentive mechanism for resin-bonded retainers. J. Prosthet. Dent. 47:52, 1982.
18. Tanaka, T., Atsuta, M., Uchiyama, Y., and Kawashima, I. Pitting corrosion for retaining acrylic resin facings. J. Prosthet. Dent. 42:282, 1979.
19. Thompson, V. P., Del Castillo, E., and Livaditis, G. J. Resin-bonded retainers. I. Resin bond to electrolytically etched non-precious alloys. J. Prosthet. Dent. 50:771, 1983.
20. Livaditis, G. J. Etched metal resin-bonded restorations: Principles in retainer design. Int. J. Periodont. Rest. Dent. 3(4):35, 1983.
21. Livaditis, G. J. Resin-bonded cast restorations: Clinical study. Int. J. Periodont. Rest. Dent. 1(4):71, 1981.
22. Simonsen, R., Thompson, V. P., and Barrack, G. General considerations in framework design and anterior tooth modification. Quint. Dent. Technol. 7:21, 1983.
23. McLaughlin, G. The etched-metal bridge: A new laboratory technique. Dent. Lab. Rev. 57:32, 1982.
24. Heymann, H. O. Resin-retained bridges: The porcelain-fused-to-metal "winged" pontic. Gen. Dent. 32:203, 1984.
25. Wood, M. Anterior etched cast-resin bonded bridges: An alternative for adolescent patients. Pediatr. Dent. 5:172, 1983.
26. Wood, M. Etched casting resin bonded retainers: An improved technique for periodontal splinting. Int. J. Periodont. Rest. Dent. 2(4):8, 1982.
27. Shaw, M. J., and Tay, W. M. Clinical performance of resin-bonded cast metal bridges (Rochette bridges). Br. Dent. J. 152:378, 1982.
28. Livaditis, G. J. Cast metal resin-bonded retainers for posterior teeth. J. Am. Dent. Assoc. 101:926, 1980.
29. Thompson, V. P., and Livaditis, G. J. Etched casting acid etch composite bonded posterior bridges. Pediatr. Dent. 4:38, 1982.
30. Thompson, V. P., Barrack, G., and Simonsen, R. Posterior design principles in etched cast restorations. Quint. Int. 3:311, 1983.

Author Index

The number in boldface indicates the page on which the full reference appears. The number following the colon is the number of the reference.

Subject Index